Neurology Case Studies

Second Edition

59 CASE HISTORIES
RELATED TO
NEUROLOGICAL DISᵣᴬᶜᵉˢ

by

D1521966

SHELDON M. WOLF, M.ᴅ.
Clinical Professor of Neurology
Los Angeles County —
University of Southern California Medical Center
Los Angeles, California

THEODORE L. MUNSAT, M.D.
Professor of Neurology
Los Angeles County —
University of Southern California Medical Center
Los Angeles, California

PETER B. DUNNE, M.D.
Associate Professor of Neurology
University of South Florida
Medical School
Chief of Neurology
Tampa Veterans Administration Hospital
Tampa, Florida

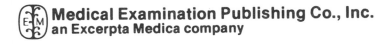
Medical Examination Publishing Co., Inc.
an Excerpta Medica company

Copyright © 1975 by
MEDICAL EXAMINATION PUBLISHING CO., INC.

Library of Congress Card Number
75-18354

ISBN 0-87488-006-8

October, 1975

PRINTED IN THE UNITED STATES OF AMERICA

FOREWORD

This book presents a series of actual case histories drawn from the practices of the authors and ranging over a wide spectrum of neurological disease, both common and esoteric.

In contrast to a CPC approach, in which historical, examination, and laboratory data are given, we have tried to place the reader in the position of the neurological clinician who is caring for the patient, and who must localize the probable site of the disease process, reach a diagnosis, consider differential possibilities, and then choose a treatment plan. The cases presented are interrupted by questions which give the reader the opportunity to make these decisions and then compare his choices and reasoning with those made by the neurologists who were actually managing the cases. In addition, we have asked the reader to consider problems of pathogenic and basic mechanisms underlying the patient's neurological symptoms and signs.

We recognize that experienced clinicians may differ in approaches to the same clinical problem, and the reader is encouraged to pursue his interest in the clinical and basic science questions raised by using the set of references given at the end of each case history. We believe that this "case study" method is both an instructive and enjoyable way to learn clinical neurology.

Sheldon M. Wolf, M.D.

Theodore L. Munsat, M.D.

Peter B. Dunne, M.D.

Dedicated to:

> *Barbara*
>
> *Carla*
>
> *Faith*
>
> *Madeline*

ABOUT THE AUTHORS

Sheldon M. Wolf, M.D. received his B.A. from Columbia College
and M.D. from the College of Physicians and Surgeons, Columbia University. He was an intern at Bellevue Hospital, New
York City, and then did his Neurology residency training at
the Neurological Institute of New York. This was followed by
a year as Visiting Fellow in Neurology and Physiology at the
Columbia Presbyterian Medical Center. He is currently Associate Clinical Professor of Neurology at the Los Angeles
County - University of Southern California Medical Center, and
a staff neurologist in the Southern California Permanente
Medical Group in Los Angeles.

Theodore L. Munsat, M.D. received his B.A. from the University
of Michigan and M.D. from the University of Vermont. He in-
terned at Mt. Sinai Hospital, New York and took his Neurology
Residency at the Neurological Institute of Columbia-Presbyte-
rian Medical Center. He is presently Professor of Neurology
at the Los Angeles County - University of Southern California
Medical Center, Director of its Muscular Dystrophy Clinic and
Chairman of the Medical Advisory Committee, Los Angeles
County, Chapter, Muscular Dystrophy Association. His area
of clinical and research interest is that of neuromuscular
diseases.

Peter B. Dunne, M.D., is a graduate of Harvard College and the
College of Physicians and Surgeons, Columbia University. He
was an intern and resident in medicine at Bellevue Hospital,
New York City, and then took his Neurology residency at the
Neurological Institute of New York. He then spent two years
in muscle research at the Columbia Presbyterian Medical
Center, as Instructor in Neurology. Clinical practice with the
Southern California Permanente Medical Group was interrupted
by service in the United States Army Medical Corps, including
one year as Neurologist in the Republic of Vietnam. He is
presently Associate Professor of Neurology at the University
of South Florida, and Chief of Neurology at the Tampa Veterans Administration Hospital.

ACKNOWLEDGMENTS

The authors would like to express their deep appreciation to Drs. I. Ackerman, E. Anderson, J. Braunwald, J. Donin, J. Feigenbaum, K. Fuchs, R. Hanson, R. Hubbard, W. Lusk, F. Pitts, J. Ratcliffe, J. Ruskin, R. Saul, and D. Sciarra for their review of these cases, and for their many helpful suggestions and corrections.

Drs. S. Davidson, A. Talalla and J. Wagner kindly allowed the use of their cases.

NEUROLOGY CASE STUDIES
SECOND EDITION

TABLE OF CONTENTS

CASE STUDY #1

Acute Onset of Double Vision in a Diabetic

HISTORY: A 57 year-old woman, an insulin-dependent diabetic, awoke one morning seeing double. The two images were side by side. The diplopia disappeared when either eye was covered. Visual acuity was 20/20 in each eye.

QUESTIONS:

1. THE SEPARATION OF IMAGES IN THE HORIZONTAL PLANE SUGGESTS THAT THE IMPAIRED EYE MUSCLE IS:
   A. Medial rectus or lateral rectus
   B. Superior rectus or inferior oblique
   C. Inferior rectus or superior oblique

2. IF THE DIPLOPIA PERSISTED AFTER SHE OCCLUDED EITHER EYE, (MONOCULAR DIPLOPIA) THIS WOULD LEAD YOU TO SUSPECT:
   A. Brain tumor
   B. Conversion reaction
   C. Transient ischemic attack
   D. Aneurysm of the posterior inferior cerebellar artery

She reported no headache, eye pain, hearing loss, tinnitus, dysphagia, dysarthria, numbness or weakness of her extremities. She had had a left Bell's palsy one year earlier. This cleared spontaneously three months after onset.

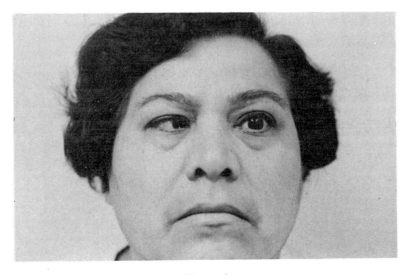

Figure 1

CASE STUDY #1

EXAMINATION: The neurological examination was normal except for decreased perception of vibration at both ankles, and the abnormality of eye movement noted in the photograph on attempted gaze to her left (Fig. 1).

QUESTIONS:

3. THE WEAK MUSCLE IS THE:
    A. Left lateral rectus
    B. Right superior oblique
    C. Left inferior oblique
    D. None of the above

4. THE WEAK MUSCLE IS INNERVATED BY THE:
    A. Oculomotor nerve
    B. Trochlear nerve
    C. Abducens nerve
    D. Optic nerve

5. THE NUCLEUS OF THIS NERVE IS LOCATED IN THE:
    A. Pons
    B. Medulla
    C. Mesencephalon
    D. Diencephalon

6. YOU WOULD EXPECT THE IMAGE SEPARATION TO BE MAXIMAL AS THIS PATIENT LOOKED:
    A. To her right
    B. To her left
    C. Up and to her right
    D. Down and to her right

7. THE MOST PROBABLE DIAGNOSIS IN THIS PATIENT IS:
    A. Brain stem infarct
    B. Acute diabetic cranial mononeuropathy
    C. Intracranial hemorrhage
    D. Aneurysm of the carotid artery

8. INITIAL TESTS SHOULD INCLUDE:
    A. Tensilon test
    B. 2 hour postprandial blood sugar
    C. Carotid angiogram
    D. Skull X-rays
    E. Pneumoencephalogram

LABORATORY DATA: Complete blood count, VDRL, sedimentation rate, X-rays of chest and skull were all normal. The 2 hour postprandial sugar was elevated. Intravenous injection of 10 mgms of tensilon did not alter the diplopia.

CASE STUDY #1

QUESTIONS:

9. IF THE MUSCLE RESPONSIBLE FOR THE DIPLOPIA IS ONLY SLIGHTLY PARETIC AND CANNOT BE READILY IDENTIFIED, THE RED GLASS TEST IS A USEFUL AID. FOR EXAMPLE, IF, IN THIS PATIENT WITH A WEAK LEFT LATERAL RECTUS, A RED GLASS WERE PLACED IN FRONT OF THE RIGHT EYE, THEN THE RED IMAGE BELONGS TO AND IDENTIFIES THE RIGHT EYE, THE WHITE IMAGE IDENTIFIES THE LEFT EYE. THE PATIENT IS ASKED TO LOOK AT A FLASHLIGHT IN DIFFERENT DIRECTIONS OF GAZE AND TO REPORT THE POSITION WHERE MAXIMUM IMAGE SEPARATION OCCURS. THE EYE THAT LAGS (IN THIS CASE THE LEFT EYE) PROJECTS THE IMAGE FARTHEST IN THE DIRECTION OF GAZE OR, STATED IN ANOTHER WAY, THE MORE PERIPHERAL OF THE DOUBLE IMAGES BELONGS TO THE PARETIC EYE. THUS:
    A. The red and white images would be maximally separated when looking to the left, with the red image then seen to the left of the white
    B. The red and white images would be maximally separated when looking to the right with the red to the left of the white
    C. The red and white images would be maximally separated when looking to the right with the white to the left of the red
    D. The red and white images would be maximally separated when looking to the left with the white to the left of the red

10. THERE ARE MANY NEUROLOGICAL COMPLICATIONS OF DIABETES MELLITUS. EXAMPLES ARE:
    A. Symmetrical motor and sensory polyneuropathy
    B. Polymyositis
    C. Coma
    D. Narcolepsy
    E. Cerebrovascular arteriosclerosis

11. THE MOST LIKELY PATHOGENETIC MECHANISM RESPONSIBLE FOR ACUTE DIABETIC MONONEUROPATHIES, BOTH CRANIAL AND PERIPHERAL, IS:
    A. Degenerative
    B. Ischemic
    C. Nutritional

12. THE MOST COMMON CRANIAL MONONEUROPATHIES OCCURRING IN DIABETICS INVOLVE CRANIAL NERVES:
    A. 1, 3, 5
    B. 2, 4, 7
    C. 3, 4, 10
    D. 3, 6, 12
    E. 3, 6, 7

ANSWERS AND DISCUSSION:

1. A   The medial rectus and lateral rectus muscles are horizontal rotators; the medial rectus is an adductor, the lateral rectus is an abductor. The superior rectus and inferior oblique are elevators, the inferior rectus and superior oblique are depressors. Paresis of any of the latter four muscles will result in vertical diplopia.

CASE STUDY #1

2. B Some complaints of monocular diplopia are accounted for by early cataracts, uncorrected irregular astigmatism or subluxated lenses. Rarely it may be cerebral in origin. Most commonly, the complaint indicates hysteria or malingering.

3. A Note that the photograph indicates a total inability of the patient to abduct her left eye.

4. C

5. A

6. B Separation of images is greatest on gaze to her left, in the field of action of the paretic left lateral rectus muscle.

7. B The brain stem is compact, with many important structures confined to a small area. When infarction occurs at this site, isolated injury to a single cranial nerve is not likely; rather, there may be various combinations of injury to cranial nerve nuclei, to long motor and sensory tracts and to cerebellar connections.

Intracranial hemorrhage is usually characterized by severe headache, which may be followed by convulsions, hemiparesis or a depressed level of consciousness. Blood in the subarachnoid space may produce signs of meningeal irritation: nuchal rigidity and a positive Kernig's sign.

An aneurysm of the internal carotid artery is a common cause of an isolated third nerve palsy. Rarely, an infraclinoid aneurysm may give rise to an isolated sixth nerve palsy.

8. ABD All patients with diplopia in whom the diagnosis is not readily apparent deserve a tensilon test to rule out myasthenia gravis. Skull films may reveal bony erosion, hyperostosis, abnormal calcification or pineal shift, thus providing important clues to diagnosis. Intracranial contrast studies are never indicated as initial studies.

9. D

10. ACE Acute cranial and peripheral mononeuropathies as well as symmetrical polyneuropathy occur in patients with diabetes mellitus. Coma can occur associated with acidosis and ketosis, or with marked hyperglycemia but without ketoacidosis (hyperosmolar nonketotic coma). Coma may result also in diabetics who have taken excessive medication and have developed hypoglycemia.

11. B Walsh and Hoyt have stated that ischemia from occlusive changes in small vessels is the essential cause of acute diabetic mononeuropathies. Raff[3] has suggested that diabetic asymmetric mononeuropathies may be vascular in origin whereas symmetrical polyneuropathies may be metabolic in origin. Dreyfus et al.[4] described a diabetic who developed a sudden third nerve palsy, and died five weeks later. Pathologic examination suggested an incomplete ischemic neuropathy. Weber et al.[6] suggested that in a typical diabetic third nerve palsy, "the complete or relative preservation of pupillary reaction, a valued sign in the recognition of this disorder, is apparently the result of sparing of the peripheral portion of the nerve, where pupillomotor fibers are said to traverse."

12. E

CASE STUDY #1

FOLLOW UP: This patient was reexamined two months later. She no longer complained of diplopia, and there was now a full range of ocular motion.

REFERENCES

1. Walsh, F. B., and W. F. Hoyt, Clinical Neuroopthalmology, 3rd Ed., Williams and Wilkins Co., Baltimore, 1969.

2. Haymaker, W., Bing's Local Diagnosis in Neurological Diseases, 15th Ed., C.V. Mosby, St. Louis, 1969.

3. Raff, M.C., V. Sangalang, and A.K. Asbury, Ischemic Mononeuropathy Multiplex Associated with Diabetes Mellitus, Arch Neurol 18:487, 1968.

4. Dreyfus, P.M., S. Hakim, and R.D. Adams, Diabetic Opthalmoplegia, Arch Neurol Psychiat 77:337, 1957.

5. Chopra, J.S., L.J. Hurwitz, and D. Montgomery, The Pathogenesis of Sural Nerve Changes in Diabetes Mellitus, Brain 92:391, 1969.

6. Weber, R.B., R.B. Daroff, and E.A. Mackey, Pathology of Oculomotor Nerve Palsy in Diabetics, Neurology 20:835, 1970.

7. Raff, M.C., and A.K. Asbury, Ischemic Mononeuropathy and Mononeuropathy Multiple· in Diabetes Mellitus, New Eng J Med 279:17, 1968.

8. Weingrad, A.I. Diabetic Neuropathy, New Eng J Med 286:1262, 1972.

CASE STUDY #2

Weakness in a Young Boy

HISTORY: The illustration is that of the patient at age seven (Figs. 2A and B). His prenatal history is unremarkable. He was a full-term, uncomplicated delivery with no evidence of neonatal distress. He sat at seven months of age and walked at eighteen months. In retrospect, his parents stated that he always seemed to have a peculiar gait but could be no more specific than this. At age four, his family became increasingly concerned when he began to fall easily, arose somewhat slowly, and was noted to have difficulty in climbing stairs. The family pediatrician, after checking the child over, was unable to find any definite abnormality and suggested a period of further observation.

QUESTION:

1. TRUE OR FALSE:
   A. Abnormality of gait is a common hysterical symptom in children
   B. In a myopathy, proximal weakness is more common than distal
   C. In a neuropathy, proximal weakness is more common than distal
   D. Pain is an uncommon feature of childhood neuromuscular disease
   E. In primary muscle disease the sensory pathways are usually spared

At age five, progressive gait difficulty was clearly present, he began to fall more frequently, and he was unable to hold heavy objects. His school playmates took advantage of his problem, frequently pushing him over and making fun of him during play. His mother noted that his back was "swayed" and his abdomen prominent.

-14-

CASE STUDY #2

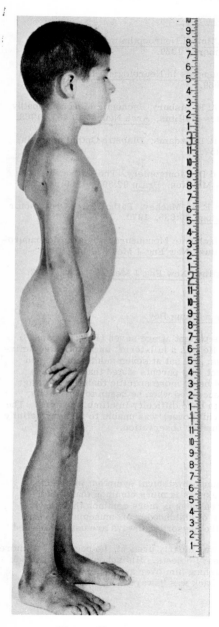 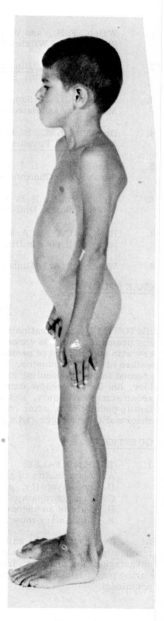

Figure 2A   Figure 2B

CASE STUDY #2

A maternal uncle had developed muscular weakness at age seven which was progressive in nature. This uncle became wheelchair-confined in his early teens and expired from respiratory insufficiency and progressive debilitation at age twenty. The patient has one sister, age nine, who is in good health. Otherwise there is no family history of neuromuscular disorder or other significant illnesses.

QUESTION:

2. THIS FAMILIAL PATTERN OF DISEASE IS MOST SUGGESTIVE OF A TYPE OF INHERITANCE TERMED:
   A. Autosomal dominant
   B. Sex-linked recessive
   C. Autosomal recessive
   D. Sporadic
   E. None of above

EXAMINATION: Blood pressure 105/65 right arm, sitting. Pulse 84 and regular. The heart was not enlarged. The lungs were clear and no organomegaly was present. Increased lumbar lordosis was noted as well as prominent scapular winging and protuberance of the abdomen. There was suggestive enlargement of the calves bilaterally. He was unable to walk on his heels because of tibialis anterior weakness and contracture of the heel cords. When arising from a supine position, the use of his upper extremities was required to elevate the trunk. There was questionable minimal facial weakness bilaterally. There was moderate weakness of the proximal extremity muscles of all four limbs in a symmetrical manner. The neck flexors were weak. All deep tendon reflexes were absent. There was no cerebellar deficit. The sensory examination was intact to all modalities. No fasciculations were noted and there was no myotonia.

QUESTIONS:

3. THE DESCRIPTION OF HIS LOWER EXTREMITIES SUGGESTS:
   A. Cerebellar deficit
   B. Spastic paraparesis
   C. Pseudohypertrophy
   D. Peripheral neuropathy
   E. Denervation

4. THE EPONYM APPLIED TO HIS DIFFICULTY IN RISING IS:
   A. Gower's sign
   B. Babinski's sign
   C. Brudzinski's sign
   D. Charcot's triad
   E. Myerson's sign

LABORATORY DATA: CBC, urinalyses and routine blood studies were all within normal limits. Serum SGOT 185, SGPT 160, Aldolase 102, CPK 500. Electrocardiogram was within normal limits as was an electroencephalogram. Electromyography showed polyphasic "miniature" motor units of markedly reduced voltage and duration. Rare fibrillatory activity was observed in the quadriceps on the right. These abnormal motor units were found mainly in the clinically affected muscles but in apparently normally strong muscles as well. Right median nerve conduction time was normal as was repetitive stimulation of the median nerve. A right quadriceps muscle biopsy was carried out. This revealed moderate variation of fiber size with scattered focal muscle necrosis and phagocytosis. There was a moderate increase of connective tissue and fat. The blood vessels and nerve terminals observed were normal.

QUESTIONS:

5. THE MOST LIKELY SITE OF THE DISEASE IS:
   A. Spinal cord
   B. Anterior horn cell
   C. Peripheral nerve
   D. Neuromuscular junction
   E. Muscle fiber

6. THE MOST LIKELY DIAGNOSIS IS:
   A. Duchenne muscular dystrophy
   B. Myasthenia gravis
   C. Guillain-Barré syndrome
   D. Polymyositis
   E. Friedrich's ataxia

CASE STUDY #2

7. INDICATE WHICH OF THE FOLLOWING ARE CONSIDERED AS TYPES OF MUSCULAR DYSTROPHY:
    A. Duchenne
    B. Polymyositis
    C. Limb-girdle
    D. Facioscapulohumeral
    E. Charcot-Marie-Tooth

8. THE MOST SENSITIVE INDICATOR OF A MYOPATHIC DISORDER IS:
    A. Urinary creatine
    B. Urinary creatinine
    C. Serum creatine phosphokinase (CPK)
    D. Serum creatinine
    E. Serum lactic acid

ANSWERS AND DISCUSSION:

1. A. False; B. True; C. False; D. True; E. True

    In almost all myopathies, with the exception of myotonic muscular dystrophy and a few very rare conditions, the preponderance of muscle wasting and weakness is proximal. This is in contradistinction to neuropathic disorders, such as diabetic neuropathy where the atrophy and weakness is more pronounced in the distal extremities. If weakness and wasting is present without sensory involvement, this suggests that the disease is located within the motor unit, i.e., from the anterior horn cell on out to the muscle fiber itself. Although purely motor neuropathies do occur, these are very rare.

2. B The hallmark of autosomal dominant inheritance is the occurrence of the disorder in both parent and child. In autosomal recessive inheritance, involvement of one generation only is the rule. The term sex-linked recessive refers to the fact that the abnormal gene or genetic defect is located on the sex, usually X, chromosome. In this situation, the female becomes the carrier while only males are affected.

3. C Pseudohypertrophy is a phenomenon limited almost entirely to muscular dystrophies. It refers to muscle tissue which becomes enlarged, but is in fact weak, which differentiates it from physiologic or work hypertrophy. This occurs as normal functioning muscle tissue is progressively replaced by fat and connective tissue. In Duchenne Muscular Dystrophy, which is the condition where pseudohypertrophy is most frequent, it is usually most prominent in the calves and thighs, but occasionally may be quite generalized, giving rise to an "infantile Hercules" appearance.

4. A Gower's sign refers to a phenomenon of the child "walking up" his lower extremities with his arms to achieve the upright position. This occurs when there is weakness of the pelvic musculature and low back muscles. It is not specific for muscular dystrophy, but can occur in any situation where weakness in these areas is present.

5. E

6. A

CASE STUDY #2

7. ACD The muscular dystrophies are a group of genetically determined, usual
ly progressive, primary degenerative diseases of the muscle fiber. The
Duchenne variety is most frequent, and is most aggressive in course,
beginning in the preschool years and usually leading to death by the early
20's. It is inherited in an x-linked recessive manner and the female carrier can be detected by a slight elevation in her serum creatine phosphokinase level which occurs in about 80% of known carriers of this disease.
The basic defect is unknown, but it is suspected that an absence or inadequate functioning of one or more enzymes is the underlying abnormality. Some have suggested that the abnormalities in muscle may be
secondary to disturbances of nerve or vascular supply. Therapy consists
of supportive care, physical therapy to prevent contractures, bracing,
occasionally surgical release of contracture, and proper genetic counselling which includes carrier detection.

The limb-girdle category appears to be a heterogenous group of muscle
disorders which begins in early adulthood, progresses slowly, and occurs equally in males and females. Usual mode of inheritance is autosomal recessive. These patients may simulate the chronic form of polymyositis.

Facioscapulohumeral dystrophy is an autosomal dominant disorder, very
slow in evolution, which primarily involves those muscles indicated by
its descriptive title. It appears that this group also may prove to be
heterogenous.

8. C Serum creatine phosphokinase (CPK) is one of many enzymes which appear in the serum in elevated concentrations when the muscle fiber is
destroyed. The CPK appears to be the most sensitive indicator of a
primary disease of muscle. Slight elevations may occur in denervating
diseases such as amyotrophic lateral sclerosis and chronic anterior
horn cell disease (Kugelberg-Welander syndrome). The evaluation of
serum enzymes has, for the most part, replaced the urinary creatine
and creatinine as biochemical indicators of muscle fiber disease. CPK
can also be elevated in myocardial disease and hypothyroidism, so that
these must be ruled out when appropriate.

REFERENCES

1. Bourne, G. H. and M. N. Golary, Muscular Dystrophy in Man and Animals,
Hafner Pub. Co., New York, 1963.

2. McComas, A., and R. Sica, Sick Motorneurons. A Unifying Concept of Muscle Disease, Lancet 1:321, 1971.

3. Takagi, A., D. Schotland, and L. Rowland, Sarcoplasmic Reticulum in
Duchenne Muscular Dystrophy, Arch Neurol 28:380, 1973.

4. Moosa, A., Muscular Dystrophy in Childhood, Develop Med Child Neur
16:97-111, 1974.

5. McComas, A., et al., Multiple Muscle Analysis of Motor Units in Muscular
Dystrophy, Arch Neurol 30:249, 1974.

6. Walton, J. N., Disorders of Voluntary Muscle, 3rd Ed., Churchill Living-
stone Publishing Co., 1974.

7. Appenzeller, O. and G. Ogin, Pathogenesis of Muscular Dystrophies,
Archives of Neurology 32:2, 1975.

8. Bradley, W., et al., Failure to Confirm a Vascular Cause of Muscular
Dystrophy, Arch Neurol 32:466, 1975.

CASE STUDY #3

A White Haired Man with an Unsteady Gait

HISTORY: A 58 year-old maintenance man noted progressive "numbness and stiffness in my arms" beginning about four months earlier. His gait gradually became more unsteady. He had no difficulty with bowel or bladder function. There was no history of alcoholism, diabetes, lues, exposure to toxins or familial neurological illness. He had noted no intellectual or emotional changes.

EXAMINATION: The patient appeared older than his stated age. There was slight limitation of movement of the head and neck to either side. There was no pain when the cervical spine was hyperextended. His hair was very white, his eyes blue and there was hyperemia of the tongue with depapillation. No cheilosis was observed.

QUESTIONS:

1.   IN THE CERVICAL REGION HYPEREXTENSION OF THE HEAD AND NECK:
     A.   Will put the cervical roots on the stretch
     B.   Will reduce tension on the cervical roots

2.   CHEILOSIS IS:
     A.   A red, sometimes oozing, lesion at the corners of the mouth
     B.   A sign of congenital syphilis
     C.   Seen in some vitamin deficiencies
     D.   A sign of lesions of the facial nerve

NEUROLOGICAL EXAMINATION: The gait was broad-based and hesitant. He was unable to walk a straight line, tending to fall to either side. He swayed but did not fall when he stood with his feet close together. When he then closed his eyes, the swaying increased and he tended to fall to either side or backwards. Coordination was normal in the arms but heel-to-shin test was ataxic and he was unable to hop on either foot rapidly or evenly. The deep tendon reflexes were 3+ in the arms, trace at the knees, and absent at the ankles. Both plantar responses were extensor. The jaw jerk was 2+ and there was a positive snout reflex. There was a stocking distribution hypesthesia to touch. He showed marked diminution of position sense in the toes and ankles and severe diminution of vibratory sense at the toes and malleoli. Cranial nerves were intact. He showed mild difficulty with memory and calculation.

QUESTIONS:

3.   DIFFICULTY WITH WALKING A STRAIGHT LINE (TANDEM WALKING) MAY BE SEEN WITH:
     A.   Cerebellar lesions
     B.   Posterior column disorders
     C.   Hysteria
     D.   Some lesions of the corticospinal tracts

4.   STANDING WITH THE FEET TOGETHER AND THEN CLOSING THE EYES IS KNOWN AS THE:
     A.   Romberg test
     B.   Lasegue test
     C.   Hoover's sign
     D.   Beevor's sign

CASE STUDY #3

5. IT MAY BE HELPFUL IN DIFFERENTIATING BETWEEN LESIONS OF:
   A. The cortico-spinal tracts and the spinothalamic tracts
   B. Muscle as opposed to peripheral nerve
   C. The cerebellum and the posterior columns
   D. None of the above

6. CHARACTERISTICALLY IN POSTERIOR COLUMN DISEASE WHEN STANDING WITH THE FEET CLOSE TOGETHER:
   A. The patient remains relatively stable if looking at his feet
   B. Falls even if looking at his feet
   C. Falls when he closes his eyes
   D. None of the above

7. THE NEUROLOGICAL DEFICITS DESCRIBED IN THIS PATIENT WOULD RESULT FROM LESIONS IN THE:
   A. Cerebrum
   B. Cerebellum
   C. Thalamus
   D. Basal ganglia
   E. Brainstem
   F. Spinal cord
   G. Nerve roots
   H. Peripheral nerves
   I. Neuromuscular junction
   J. Muscle

8. LOSS OF POSITION AND VIBRATION OCCUR IN SPINAL CORD LESIONS:
   A. In the posterior columns
   B. In the cortico-spinal tracts
   C. In the rubro-spinal tracts
   D. In the spino-cerebellar tracts
   E. In the spinothalamic tracts

9. THE BABINSKI RESPONSE INDICATES:
   A. Damage to the spinothalamic tracts or cells
   B. Damage to the cortico-spinal tracts or cells
   C. Damage to the posterior columns or cells
   D. That the lesion must be in the cerebral cortex
   E. That the lesion must be in the internal capsule
   F. That the lesion must be in the spinal cord

10. SENSORY SYMPTOMS DUE TO LESIONS IN THE CERVICAL SPINAL CORD MAY FIRST OCCUR IN THE LOWER EXTREMITIES:
    A. True
    B. False

11. LABORATORY TESTS THAT MIGHT BE OF HELP IN FURTHER EVALUATION:
    A. FTA absorption for lues
    B. Lumbosacral and cervical spine X-rays
    C. CBC
    D. ESR
    E. Two hour post-prandial sugar
    F. Diagnex blue for free HCl
    G. All of the above

CASE STUDY #3

LABORATORY DATA: Hemoglobin: 13.3; hematocrit: 39.2; RBC count: 3.79 x 10^6 (5.4 ± 0.8); mean corpuscular volume: 101 microns^3 (87 ± 5); mean corpuscular hemoglobin: 33 micra-micra grams (29 ± 2); mean corpuscular hemoglobin concentration 32% (34 ± 2). The smear was described as showing moderate to marked anisopoikilocytosis with ovalocytes. There was achlorhydria with the Diagnex blue test.

Normal or negative tests included FTA, X-rays of cervical and lumbo-sacral spines. ESR and blood sugar. Examination of the bone marrow and spinal fluid also were normal.

QUESTIONS:

12. OTHER USEFUL INFORMATION MIGHT NEXT BE OBTAINED FROM:
    A. Serum B_{12} level
    B. Reticulocyte count
    C. Barium enema
    D. Skull X-rays
    E. Schilling test
    F. All of the above
    G. None of the above

13. THE LACK OF ANEMIA, AND THE NORMAL BONE MARROW RULE OUT PERNICIOUS ANEMIA AS THE ETIOLOGY OF THE PATIENT'S PROBLEM:
    A. True
    B. False

A Schilling test was performed. The 24 hour urinary excretion of radioactive labelled vitamin B_{12} was less than 1%. The excretion rose to 10% after intrinsic factor was given. At this time, the patient recalled that he had taken oral supplementary vitamins. These were found to contain both folic acid and vitamin B_{12}.

QUESTIONS:

14. ORAL FOLIC ACID MAY REMEDY THE ANEMIA OF B_{12} DEFICIENCY:
    A. True
    B. False

15. BUT, IT DOES NOT PREVENT THE DEVELOPMENT OF NEUROLOGICAL DAMAGE:
    A. True
    B. False

The patient was immediately begun on a course of vitamin B_{12}, initially 1000 micrograms daily IM. Subjectively, he thought he "felt better". Objectively, the extensor plantar responses returned to flexor, his gait was slightly less ataxic, but there was no marked change in his posterior column sensibility loss. It was also thought that his mentation was improved, as judged by rapidity of calculations. The passage of further time, while continuing with parenteral B_{12} therapy at lower "maintenence dose levels", has resulted in additional objective and subjective improvement, and the patient has been able to return to work.

CASE STUDY #3

QUESTIONS:

16. VITAMIN DEFICIENCY STATES THAT COULD PRESENT WITH A PERI-
    PHERAL NEUROPATHY INCLUDE:
    A. Deficiency of nicotinic acid
    B. Deficiency of Thiamine
    C. Deficiency of Vitamin E
    D. Deficiency of Vitamin A

17. MATCH THE DEFICIENCY STATE TO ITS APPROPRIATE PRIMARY
    VITAMIN:
    A. Beriberi   1. Nicotinic acid
    B. Pellagra   2. Vitamin B_{12}
    C. Wernicke's syndrome   3. Thiamine
    D. Pernicious anemia   4. Vitamin E

ANSWERS AND DISCUSSION:

1. A   The use of this fact constitutes a useful test of cervical root
            lesions, often combined with valsalva maneuver. Conversely,
            maximal positional relief for the patient with cervical root dis-
            ease is usually obtained with the head and neck slightly flexed in
            the direction of the sternum.

2. AC   Vitamins implicated in the production of cheilosis include vitamin
            B_2 (riboflavin), niacin, and vitamin B_6 (pyridoxine).

3. ABCD   Cerebellar lesions may give unsteadiness due to tremor or poor
            coordination of one or both lower extremities, with lack of mid-
            line cerebellar integration of vestibular and proprioceptive input;
            the lack of position sense with posterior column disease will pre-
            vent smooth tandem gait, although being able to look at the feet
            helps; hysterical gaits are often bizarrely unsteady, the patient
            bouncing off walls if near, but rarely falling, or if falling, doing
            no harm to himself and usually with no distinct pattern discern-
            able; both spastic and flaccid limbs from corticospinal tract
            lesions may prevent walking of a straight line, with the most
            common gait the spastic "scissors" gait.

4. A

5. C

6. AC   Due to position sense input failure, he must use visual cues to
            remain upright. A patient with cerebellar ataxia will tend to
            sway and fall,even with his eyes open when he stands with feet
            together.

7. AFH   The positive snout reflex and memory loss are compatible with
            cerebral involvement. Peripheral nerve involvement is indicated
            by the stocking hypesthesia on examination. The correlation of
            the other abnormal findings with their location in the nervous
            system is discussed in questions eight and nine.

8. A   Vibration and position sense are generally considered to travel
            together in the posterior columns of the spinal cord.

9. B   Taken by itself there is no indication of the level of involvement
            of the neuraxis that is producing the Babinski sign.

CASE STUDY #3

10. A   This is because cervical lesions affecting the long ascending tracts of the spinal cord initially may affect predominantly fibers coming from the lower extremities. An example of this is compression of the lateral spinal cord causing a greater defect in pain and in temperature appreciation in the sacral dermatomes because of lamination of the spino-thalamic tract with the sacral fibers being pushed postero-laterally by fibers from higher regions as they ascend in the spinal cord.

11. G   All of these tests are important for evaluating this man for diseases that might affect the cerebral cortex, spinal cord, or peripheral nerves.

12. ABE

13. B   A patient's anemia may be obscured by folic acid but this does not alter the basic pathophysiological defect in the absorption across the gut wall of vitamin B_{12} due to lack of intrinsic factor that is by definition pernicious anemia.

14. A   To stress this again: an important fact is that the anemia of B_{12} deficiency may be corrected by oral folic acid.

15. A   To emphasize: the neurological abnormalities associated with B_{12} deficiency respond ONLY to B_{12} and will progress irrevocably if B_{12} is not administered parenterally.

16. AB   (see answer to 5 also) Although vitamin E deficiency has been linked in animal experiments to sterility and abortion, muscular dystrophy, cardiac muscle changes and other tissue dysfunction, clear correlation with disease in man thus far has been lacking. Vitamin A deficiency in man causes a gamut of symptoms and signs from nyctalopia (night blindness) to corneal and conjunctival dessication and ulceration, respiratory infections secondary to changes in bronchial epithelium, drying of skin, urinary calculi and diarrhea.

17.   A.   3
                                B.   1
                                C.   3
                                D.   2

Beriberi is a deficiency state primarily related to insufficient thiamine. There are two well recognized forms in the adult: wet beriberi, presenting acutely with edema and heart failure; and the dry form with chronic polyneuropathy, with the unpleasant quality of the dysesthesias that often occur, called the "burning foot syndrome." Pellagra is the deficiency state that results from lack of B vitamins, in particular nicotinic acid (niacin). Dementia, which may vary from mild signs of slowed mentation to states of hallucinosis and delirium, diarrhea, and dermatitis, primarily of areas of the body exposed to sun, are characteristic. It is presently thought that the neuropathy that may be seen in pellagrins is secondary to thiamine deficiency. Thiamine deficiency is associated with the Wernicke syndrome, a symptom complex with varying degrees of confusion, ophthalmoplegia, ataxia, and often peripheral neuropathy. It also is the major vitamin deficiency in Korsakoff's psychosis which presents with memory defects, confabulation, and peripheral neuropathy. Both of these conditions are now usually encountered in the alcoholic with poor nutrition. It remains unclear whether the peripheral neuropathy found in many alcoholics is entirely due to thiamine plus combinations of B_6, pantothenic acid and B_{12} deficiency, or whether a toxic effect of alcohol also plays a part. Pernicious anemia will be discussed further in the end of the section. Two indirect tests for thiamine deficiency are measurements of serum pyruvate and transketolase in the red cells.

DISCUSSION: This patient with pernicious anemia with neurologic manifestations illustrates several very important points. Although his corpuscular indices were suggestively abnormal, he was not anemic if judged only by hemoglobin and hematocrit determinations, done more than once. Despite repeated questions directed toward this point, it was not until late in the evaluation that the patient recalled that he had taken oral vitamins containing B_{12} and folic acid. If caught early enough, most of the neurological abnormalities in this problem are reversible when parenteral B_{12} is given consistently, while if untreated, or treated with folate, there is inexorable progression. The degeneration of white matter produces a spongiform state involving initially the spinal cord, particularly its posterior columns, and then ultimately affecting the cerebrum and other parts of the neuraxis. Pathological evidence for peripheral nerve involvement is debated, although clinically most feel it occurs.

Any patient presenting with paresthesias of the lower extremities, especially if accompanied by evidence of position and vibratory loss, must have pernicious anemia considered and ruled out. There may be other abnormal findings indicating involvement of other systems of the spinal cord, such as the corticospinal tracts, or pathology elsewhere in the central nervous system. A complete blood count and diagnex blue test for free HCl should be done. If these are abnormal, or there is any doubt, a bone marrow examination and Schilling test should be done. If the Schilling test has been performed, this is sufficient B_{12} (1000 microgm) to stimulate the marrow and may make the marrow not diagnostic. A serum B_{12} level may also be obtained before B_{12} is given.

Other diseases that can produce posterior column damage are multiple sclerosis, tabes dorsalis, cervical spondylosis, and cord tumors. Because B_{12} deficiency can affect multiple levels of the central nervous system, it may stimulate a variety of other diseases. (For example it rarely may present with dementia as the most notable feature.) It is vitally important that the diagnosis is considered and ruled in or out appropriately since it is a treatable condition.

This man will have to take parenteral vitamin B_{12} for the rest of his life. The vitamin B_{12} cannot be given orally because of the failure of absorption across the gut wall that is characteristic of the disease. The initial dose that he was given is higher than that suggested by some authorities, and was given for the first several weeks, in the hope that it would help the regression of his neurological deficits. He will be maintained with 100 micrograms of B_{12} every month.

CASE STUDY #3

REFERENCES

1. Carney, M.W.P., Serum Vitamin B_{12} Values in 374 Psychiatric Patients, Behav Neuropsychiat 1:19, 1969.

2. Foulds, W.S., I.A. Chisholm, J. Bronte-Stewart, and T.M. Wilson, Vitamin B_{12} Absorption in Tobacco Amblyopia, Brit J Ophthal 53:393, 1969.

3. Freeman, A.G., and J.M. Heaton, The Aetiology of Retrobulbar Neuritis in Addisonian Pernicious Anaemia, Lancet 280:908, 1961.

4. Halsted, J.A., P.M. Lewis, and M. Gasster, Absorption of Radioactive Vitamin B_{12} in the Syndrome of Megaloblastic Anemia Associated with Intestinal Stricture or Anastomosis, Amer J Med 20:42, 1956.

5. Herbert, V., Diagnostic and Prognostic Values of Measurement of Serum Vitamin B_{12}-Binding Proteins, Blood 32:305, 1968.

6. Holmes, J.M., Cerebral Manifestations of Vitamin B_{12} Deficiency, Brit Med J 2:1394, 1956.

7. Pollycove, M., and L. Apt, Absorption, Elimination and Excretion of Orally Administered Vitamin B_{12} in Normal Subjects and in Patients with Pernicious Anemia, New Eng J Med 255:207, 1956.

8. Pollycove, M., L. Apt, and M.J. Colbert, Pernicious Anemia Due to Dietary Deficiency of Vitamin B_{12}, New Eng J Med 255:164, 1956.

9. Richmond J., and S.P. Davidson, Subacute Combined Degeneration of the Spinal Cord in Non-Addisonian Megaloblastic Anemia, Quart J Med 27:517, 1958.

10. Silberstein, E.B., The Schilling Test, JAMA 208:2325, 1969.

11. Strachan, R.W., and J.G. Henderson, Psychiatric Syndromes Due to Avitaminosis B_{12} with Normal Blood and Marrow, Quart J Med 34:303, 1965.

12. Thompson, R.B., and C.C. Ungley, Megaloblastic Anemia Associated with Anatomic Lesions in Small Intestine, Blood 10:771, 1955.

13. Victor, M., and A.A. Lear, Subacute Combined Degeneration of the Spinal Cord, Amer J Med 20:896, 1956.

14. Herbert, V., Megaloblastic Anemias - Mechanisms and Management, Disease-a-month, August 1965.

15. Sullivan, L., Vitamin B_{12} Metabolism and Megaloblastic Anemia, Seminars Hematology 7:6, 1970.

16. Williams, W., et al., Hematology, McGraw-Hill Book Co., 1972.

CASE STUDY #4

A Housewife with Headaches

HISTORY: For many years this 37 year-old housewife had been bothered by headaches that occurred "off and on, " but for approximately the past eight months the headaches had become virtually constant. The pain invariably was bifrontal, but sometimes projected into the eyes, or at other times gradually moved backwards into the occiput   and the posterior cervical regions.

QUESTIONS:

1.   CERVICAL PAIN MAY BE NOTED BY THE PATIENT WITH:
       A. Muscle contraction headaches
       B. Meningeal irritation
       C. Cervical root disease
       D. Post traumatic musculo-ligamentous strain ("whiplash")

The quality of the pain was usually a constant, dull "steady ache." Occasionally, when most severe, she felt that her head throbbed. When the entire head was involved by pain, she described feeling that: "My brains are trying to push themselves out of my head sometimes; at other times it feels like someone put a band around my head and was tightening it."

QUESTION:

2.   THIS DRAMATIC DESCRIPTION IS MOST OFTEN FOUND WITH BRAIN TUMORS:
       A. True
       B. False

Associated with the headaches she intermittently felt nauseated. She noted no nasal occlusion or discharge, lacrimation, conjunctival suffusion, or change in facial color.

QUESTIONS:

3.   THE ABOVE SYMPTOMS PARTICULARLY MAY BE ASSOCIATED WITH HEADACHE IN:
       A. Trigeminal neuralgia
       B. Bell's palsy
       C. Migraine
       D. Cluster headaches (a migraine variety)

4.   MARKED PALLOR AND SWEATING WITH THE HEADACHE WOULD SUGGEST:
       A. Neuroblastoma
       B. Carcinoid
       C. Pheochromocytoma
       D. Hemangioma

She had no paresthesiae, diplopia or other visual symptoms, motor weakness or aphasia before, during or after her headaches.

QUESTION:

5.   ALL OF THE ABOVE SYMPTOMS MAY BE SEEN ASSOCIATED WITH HEADACHES IN:
       A. Migraine
       B. Arteriovenous malformations of the central nervous system
       C. Aneurysms of vessels of the circle of Willis
       D. Uncomplicated sinus disease

CASE STUDY #4

She denied ever losing consciousness, but frequently, sometimes "when a headache was building up" but at other times without headache, she noted episodes of dizziness. This was a lightheaded sensation accompanied by black spots in front of her eyes, and a lump in her throat.

QUESTION:

6. THIS IS A GOOD DESCRIPTION OF:
   A. A psychomotor epilepsy attack
   B. A bout of Meniere's syndrome
   C. Transient cerebral ischemia
   D. The hyperventilation syndrome
   E. Hypoxia secondary to tracheal obstruction

The patient was aware that "sometimes I pant when I get that feeling." She frequently found that she had a headache on awakening, but believed that the headache never awakened her.

QUESTION:

7. HEADACHES THAT AWAKEN THE PATIENT FROM SLEEP MOST OFTEN REPRESENT STRUCTURAL CONDITIONS OF THE CNS, SINUSES, ETC:
   A. True
   B. False

She did not note that her headaches occurred with consistency at any particular time of the day, and she was unaware of precipitating factors. The headaches did not change when she bent over, coughed, sneezed or strained.

QUESTIONS:

8. AN ALREADY PRESENT HEADACHE THAT INCREASES MARKEDLY WHEN BENDING OVER MAY BE SEEN WITH:
   A. Sinus disease
   B. Muscle contraction ("tension") headaches
   C. Some brain tumors
   D. All of the above
   E. None of the above

9. HEADACHES THAT BEGIN IMMEDIATELY UPON BENDING OVER ARE SUGGESTIVE OF INTRACRANIAL PATHOLOGY:
   A. True
   B. False

10. HEADACHES OCCURRING REPEATEDLY AT A CERTAIN TIME OF DAY OR NIGHT MAY BE ENCOUNTERED IN:
    A. Hypertensive headaches
    B. Cluster headaches
    C. Disease of the cervical spine
    D. Tension headaches

No other significant history was obtained referable to the headaches, but she did offer multiple other complaints including a constant sense that "I am very nervous and anxious," which she thought might be related to the headaches. She told of severe marital problems and also difficulties with her 16 year-old son who was taking narcotics and had been arrested several times for theft. Family history was negative for headaches or any other neurological disorders.

CASE STUDY #4

QUESTION:

11.   PATIENTS WITH "TENSION" HEADACHES:
       A.   Usually relate their occurrence to times of anxiety
       B.   May initially deny anxiety and stress
       C.   May have associated hyperventilation symptoms
       D.   May have co-existing migraine headaches

In the past, a number of medications gave her little relief. These included
chlordiazepoxid (Librium) in doses as high as 25 mg po tid, aspirin and many
other analgesics. He dizziness had not been helped by Meclyzine HCl and other
agents useful against vertigo.

QUESTION:

12.   MUSCLE CONTRACTION ("TENSION") HEADACHES OFTEN:

       A.   Do not respond consistently to a variety of analgesic agents
       B.   May respond to muscle relaxants, expecially prophylactically
       C.   May respond well to physical therapy such as massage, heat packs,
            and relaxing exercises
       D.   May respond to coolant sprays or ice packs over muscle in spasm

Normal laboratory examinations in the recent past included skull radiographs,
electroencephalogram, complete blood count, 2 hour post prandial sugar, and
normal thyroid studies. Cervical spine X-rays showed some straightening of
the normal cervical curve, felt to be compatible with cervical muscle spasm.

QUESTIONS:

13.   HELPFUL IN EVALUATING SKULL RADIOGRAPHS IN THE PATIENT
       WITH HEADACHE:
       A.   Is the presence of a calcified pineal gland
       B.   Frontal skull thickening (hyperostosis frontalis interna)
       C.   Is the status of the sella turcica
       D.   All of the above
       E.   None of the above
       F.   A and B
       G.   B and C
       H.   A and C

14.   ANOTHER USEFUL TEST IS THE ECHOENCEPHALOGRAPH BECAUSE
       IT:
       A.   Is without risk to the patient
       B.   Can be performed rapidly
       C.   Helps demonstrate presence or absence of intracranial midline
            shifts
       D.   All of the above
       E.   None of the above

15.   LOSS OF THE NORMAL CERVICAL CURVATURE:
       A.   Is a common sign of muscle spasm in the neck
       B.   May be seen after "whiplash" (musculoligamentous strain)
       C.   Is usually a benign sign
       D.   All of the above
       E.   None of the above

CASE STUDY #4

EXAMINATION: She was alert and cooperative, but very anxious, depressed, frowning and frequently sighing. Her palms were moist. General physical examination was unremarkable excepting marked, exquisitely tender occipital, posterior cervical and trapezius muscle spasm with several nodules tender to palpation by the examiner. There was full range of motion of the neck. Hyperventilation was moderately well performed; she was unable to continue beyond 45 seconds because: "I feel nauseated, weak in my legs and dizzy, just like when I have one of my attacks." Full neurological examination was within normal limits.

QUESTION:

16. THE ABOVE RESULTS OF THE PHYSICAL EXAMINATION ARE MOST
     COMPATIBLE WITH:
     A. Tension, muscle contraction, and hyperventilation sensitivity
     B. Meningitis
     C. Brain tumor
     D. Malingering

Treatment was begun with a daily program of massage, relaxing exercises, and hot packs primarily directed at the occipital, cervical and trapezius muscle spasm. She was instructed in bag rebreathing for use when symptoms of hyperventilation occurred. She was encouraged to try and avoid analgesics as much as possible. It was thought that in the future she might benefit from psychiatric counsel, and possibly also from an antidepressant. With further follow-up and supportive care, her headaches decreased in frequency, duration and severity. Although there was no particular change in the problems of her personal life, she appeared to be more aware of these problems and dealt with them more efficiently and realistically.

ANSWERS AND DISCUSSION:

1. ABCD   In differentiating between these problems: The patient with
                muscle contraction headaches usually has tender posterior
                cervical muscles, and may have some limited range of motion
                of the neck, but with the patient relaxed, the neck is usually
                supple in anterior-flexion onto the chest, while in meningeal
                irritation there will be pain and resistance and positive Kernig
                and Brudzinski signs. In cervical root compression, there is
                usually radiating pain, the location of which depends on the
                nerve root involved. The patient with "whiplash" may have
                generalized stiffness and guarding to cervical movement,
                rather than just in anterior flexion as seen in meningitis, and
                will have an appropriate history of trauma.

2. B   Although patients with tumors may give dramatic descriptions
                of their symptoms, this kind of statement is usually encountered
                with tension headaches.

3. CD   Bell's palsy is one cause of acute motor paralysis of the facial
                nerve. Migraine and cluster headaches frequently have the
                above associated symptoms. Except for the facial color change,
                sinus disease could also present with headaches and the other
                symptoms.

4. C   Carcinoid causes facial flushing, not pallor, and usually does
                not have headaches associated. The two other tumors should
                not have facial changes.

CASE STUDY #4

5. ABC   Although migraine may present with various neurological symptoms and signs, the physician must always be aware that a malformation or aneurysm may be underlying, especially if the symptoms or findings are stereotyped and always on one side. Sinus disease would give focal neurological symptoms and signs only if complicated by cerebral abscess, venous sinus thrombosis, or meningitis.

6. D   Maintained awareness, lack of automatisms would rule out psychomotor epilepsy. Although Meniere's syndrome may have headache, the lack of tinnitus, paroxysmal bouts of vertigo, (sensation of spinning of the environment around the patient, or of the patient herself), and no hearing loss make that diagnosis unlikely. Her age, absence of any focal neurological symptoms with the lightheadedness, rule against transient cerebral ischemia. The hyperventilation syndrome is very common, particularly as a symptom complex in tense and anxious persons. A part of the syndrome that may be described by the sufferer is globus hystericus - the sensation of a lump in the throat causing difficulty in swallowing. The intermittency, lack of progression, lack of stridor make tracheal obstruction very unlikely.

7. A   However, it should be noted that cluster vascular headaches quite frequently awaken the patient from sleep.

8. D   This maneuver may increase the severity of pain with virtually every type of headache.

9. A   This is not an absolute distinction but many observers note that this may be an ominous sign suggesting structural pathology intracranially.

10. ABCD   Hypertensive headaches are reported to occur at the same time each day, particularly in the morning. Patients suffering with cluster headaches with considerable frequency experience them at approximately the same time each day or night, especially when sleeping. Cervical spondylosis is liable to cause headache when the patient awakens. Tension headaches affect some people at approximately the same time each week, particularly at the end of the week when they have been under strain.

11. BCD   It is more common for the patient with tension headaches initially to be unaware of the relationship to anxiety and stress. The fact that migraine coexists with some frequency is not surprising, since emotional stress may precipitate migraine attacks in susceptible patients.

12. ABCD   The lack of consistent response to analgesics has been frequently noted, and makes therapy difficult for the ongoing muscle contraction headache. The other measures may be helpful in both therapy of the present headaches and in prophylaxis.

13. H   If the pineal gland is calcified sufficiently to be identified on skull films, it may be measured for shifts away from the midline on the anterior-posterior films, and for elevations, depressions, or anterior or posterior deviation on the lateral films. A mass lesion may shift the pineal to the opposite side.

CASE STUDY #4

Hyperostosis frontalis interna is thickening of the frontal calvarium, most often in middle-aged women, of no definite significance.

Atrophy or erosion of the sella turcica, particularly atrophy of the anterior portion of the dorsum sella, and of the posterior clinoid processes, is an early sign of increased intracranial pressure. Erosion of the floor of the sella may be seen with pituitary tumors and several other conditions.

14. D

15. D   There is normally a degree of lordosis in the cervical spine.

16. A   The lack of nuchal rigidity, fever, and other signs make men-
         ingitis very unlikely. Similarly, the normal exam, except for
         muscle spasm, along with the long history, make brain tumor
         a very distant possibility. Malingering is the conscious and
         deliberate assumption of signs and symptoms that are not
         present, which is not the case here.

COMMENTS: This case is an example of muscle contraction ("tension") headache. This is the most common type of headache encountered in medical practice.
The precipitants are emotional. The sequence of events usually is: emotional
conflicts - tension -- muscle spasm and contraction -- headache. The exact
pathophysiology is not entirely clear, but it has been suggested that sustained
contraction of the muscles of the neck and scalp leads to secondary effects on the
nerves and blood vessels in the area of the spasm, and causes the pain to spread
elsewhere in the calvarium. A frequent difficulty in helping the patient is that
he may not recognize, or may resist accepting, the underlying emotional factors.
The fact that the patient described a throbbing quality when the headaches were
the most severe suggests that she may have had an intermittent vascular component to her headaches. It is not uncommon to find "combination" headaches: the
patient who has muscle contraction and migraine, sometimes simultaneously, at
other times separately. Hyperventilation also is seen frequently in conjunction
with tension headaches.

Treatment is directed toward helping the patient understand his or her emotional
problems better, and relaxation techniques, all preferably used prophylactically.
Various analgesics may be used when the prophylactic measures do not prevent
the headache. Tranquilizers and "muscle relaxants" may help. Although heat is
most often suggested to help reduce muscle spasm, the work of Travell[2] and
others indicates that often topical coolants or ice packs also may be beneficial. A
major underlying concern facing the doctor is that muscle contraction is not the
entire story and that another process, such as a tumor, arteriovenous malformation or aneurysm might underly the headaches or coexist with it. It is for this
reason that the patient should be evaluated carefully with history and physical examination and then further tests ordered if there are any indications of underlying
pathology.

REFERENCES

1. Badran, R. H., et al., Hypertension and Headache, Scot Med J 15:48, 1970.

2. Travell, J., and S. H. Rinzler, The Myofascial Genesis of Pain, Postgrad
    Med J 11:425, 1952.

3. Kolb, L. C., Psychiatric and Psychogenic Factors in Headache, Headache,
    Diagnosis and Treatment, F. A. Davis, 1959.

4. Frazier, S. H., The Psychotherapy of Headache, Research and Clinical
    Studies in Headache, II, Williams and Wilkins, 1969.

CASE STUDY #4

5. Lance, J.W., The Mechanism and Management of Headache, Butterworths, 1970.

6. Vinhen, P.J., and G.W. Bruyn, Handbook of Clinical Neurology, V Ed., North-Holland Publishing Co., 1968.

7. Bastron, J.A., et al., Clinical Examinations in Neurology, W.B. Saunders, 1964.

8. Wilkinson, M., Cervical Spondylosis, W.B. Saunders, 1971.

9. Friedman, A., Reflections on the Treatment of Headache, Headache, 11:148, 1972.

10. Friedman, A., Current Concepts in the Diagnosis and Treatment of Chronic Recurring Headache, Medical Clin N America 56:1257, 1972.

11. Weber, R., O. Reinmuth, The Treatment of Migraine with Propanolol, Neurology 22:366, 1972.

12. Friedman, A., Treating Tension Headaches, Consultant, Feb. 1972, pp. 97-98.

13. Friedman, A., Headache, Postgraduate Medicine 53:172, 1973.

14. Dinsdale, H., Headache in Vascular Disease and Hypertension, Headache 13:85, 1973.

15. Hachinski, V., et al., Visual Symptoms in the Migraine Syndrome, Neurology 23:570, 1973.

16. Current Concepts of Headache, Postgraduate Medicine Vol.56, No. 3, Sept. 1974, pp.119-141.

CASE STUDY #5

Acute Hemiplegia in a Young Woman

HISTORY: A 32 year-old right-handed woman had been well until the morning of admission when she was found lying on the floor, attempting to reach the phone. For one year she had been taking an oral contraceptive. As a child she had rheumatic fever with no subsequent murmur or heart disease. Past medical history was otherwise unremarkable.

EXAMINATION: She was alert and normotensive. The neck was supple. The heart and carotid arteries were normal. There was a right hemiplegia, Babinski sign and homonymous hemianopsia. She was able to protrude her tongue and move her left extremities on command, and she could understand questions, responding by nodding her head yes or no. She was unable to speak.

QUESTIONS:

1. THE PATIENT'S COMMUNICATION PROBLEM IS CALLED:
   A. Receptive aphasia   C. Wernicke's aphasia
   B. Motor aphasia   D. Global aphasia

2. THIS TYPE OF DEFICIT IS ASSOCIATED WITH A LESION OF THE:
   A. Dominant posterior parietal lobe   E. Non-dominant parietal lobe
   B. Dominant frontal lobe   F. Brain stem
   C. Dominant occipital lobe   G. Any of the above
   D. Dominant posterior temporal lobe

CASE STUDY #5

3. THE DIFFERENTIAL DIAGNOSIS MIGHT INCLUDE ALL OF THE FOLLOW-
ING, EXCEPT:
   A. Brain tumor
   B. Arteriovenous malformation
   C. Barbiturate poisoning
   D. Intracranial hemorrhage
   E. Cerebral infarction

4. YOU MIGHT NOW ORDER:
   A. Skull films
   B. Spinal tap
   C. Pneumoencephalogram
   D. Myelogram
   E. Queckenstedt test
   F. Echoencephalogram

LABORATORY DATA: Normal studies included blood count, blood sugar, skull
and chest films, electrocardiogram and cerebrospinal fluid examination.

COURSE: A few hours after admission, a major motor seizure occurred, for which
anticonvulsant medications were given. Then she developed Cheyne-Stokes respiration, and a supraventricular tachycardia. The left pupil became fixed and dilated
and she died shortly afterwards.

QUESTIONS:

5. FROM THE HISTORY OF THE TERMINAL NEUROLOGICAL EVENTS, IT IS
MOST LIKELY THAT:
   A. She suffered a primary brain stem infarct
   B. Herniation of the cerebellum through the foramen magnum occurred
   C. Herniation of the temporal lobe through the tentorial incisura occurred
   D. None of the above

6. THE UNDERLYING PATHOLOGY IS PROBABLY:
   A. Cerebral infarction
   B. Cerebral hemorrhage
   C. Acute multiple sclerosis
   D. Brain abscess

At post mortem examination, a thrombosis of the left internal carotid artery was
seen, extending into the middle and anterior cerebral arteries. There was swelling and softening of the left cerebral hemisphere, with grooving of the uncus.
Microscopically no inflammatory or atheromatous changes were seen in the carotid arteries. No abnormalities were found outside the nervous system.

QUESTIONS:

7. WHEN CEREBRAL INFARCTION OCCURS IN A YOUNG PERSON, ONE
MUST CONSIDER THE POSSIBILITY OF:
   A. Embolism
   B. "Collagen" disease
   C. Lues
   D. Blood dyscrasias
   E. Atrial myxoma

8. ONE MUST ALSO CONSIDER SOME OF THE CAUSES OF ACCELERATED
ATHEROSCLEROSIS WHICH MAY BE CAUSED BY ALL, EXCEPT:
   A. Hypothyroidism
   B. Familial hyperlipidemia
   C. Occult carcinoma
   D. Hyperthyroidism
   E. Diabetes mellitus

CASE STUDY #5

9. BLOOD DYSCRASIAS ASSOCIATED WITH STROKES IN YOUNG PEOPLE
INCLUDE:
A. Sickle cell anemia
B. Polycythemia vera
C. Thrombotic thrombopenic purpura
D. All of the above

10. ORAL CONTRACEPTIVES HAVE BEEN ASSOCIATED WITH ALL OF THE
FOLLOWING, EXCEPT:
A. Thrombophlebitis
B. Pseudotumor cerebri
C. Meningiomas
D. Cerebral arterial occlusion
E. Pulmonary emboli

11. THE MOST COMMON NEUROLOGICAL COMPLICATION OF ORAL
CONTRACEPTIVE USE IS:
A. Bell's palsy
B. Strokes
C. Epilepsy
D. Migraine
E. Subarachnoid hemorrhage

12. BIRTH CONTROL PILLS HAVE ALSO BEEN THOUGHT TO CAUSE:
A. Orthostatic hypotension in some women
B. Hypertension in some women
C. No change in the blood pressure in the majority of women

13. THE BLOOD PRESSURE CHANGE WHICH OCCURS IN SOME WOMEN
TAKING ORAL CONTRACEPTIVES HAS BEEN PRIMARILY LINKED
WITH ALTERATIONS IN:
A. Norepinephrine   C. Dopamine
B. Epinephrine   D. Renin substrate

14. THE BEST TREATMENT FOR A WOMAN WHO DEVELOPS MIGRAINE
HEADACHES WHILE ON ORAL CONTRACEPTIVES IS:
A. Cafergot
B. Fiorinal
C. Stop the pill
D. A combination of analgesics and tranquilizers

TRUE OR FALSE:

15. Oral contraceptives always worsen epilepsy.
16. Oral contraceptives cause a decrease in the platelet count.
17. The incidence of thromboembolic disease and cortical venous thrombosis
is higher in pregnancy than in the postpartum period.

ANSWERS AND COMMENTS

1. B

CASE STUDY #5

2. B   Her ability to understand spoken questions and to respond by
         nodding her head appropriately rules out a Wernicke or recep-
         tive aphasia which is characterized by inability to comprehend
         spoken language. Motor or expressive aphasia is characterized
         by a great reduction in spontaneous verbal expression. Words
         are reduced to a minimum of sounds, or syllables, with pre-
         servation of auditory comprehension. The lesion in this type of
         aphasia has traditionally been localized to the base of the dom-
         inant third frontal convolution (Fig. 3).

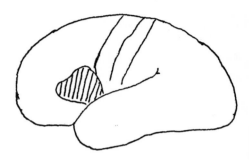

Figure 3

Global aphasia includes both expressive and receptive aphasia.

3. C   Barbiturate overdose produces the clinical picture of stupor or
         coma, depressed respiration and symmetrically hypoactive deep
         tendon reflexes and motor activity. All of the other choices can
         be present with acute hemiplegia.

4. ABF Skull films would provide useful information as to whether there
         were evidence of pineal shift, increased intracranial pressure, or
         pathological calcification. If the pineal were not calcified, an
         echoencephalogram should be obtained to see whether there were
         any shift of midline structures. A lumbar puncture would
         indicate whether there was evidence of intracranial bleeding.
         However, if the skull films or echoencephalogram showed a
         significant midline shift, a spinal tap should be deferred because
         of the increased risk of cerebral herniation. With a lateralized
         cerebral lesion, angiography is a much better choice than
         pneumoencephalography, since it can furnish not only information
         about the size of a cerebral lesion, but important evidence as to
         etiology - i.e. vascular disease, neoplasm, etc. Myelography
         is obviously inappropriate with a cerebral lesion. A Quecken-
         stedt test, in which bilateral compression of the jugular vein
         produces an increase of spinal fluid pressure as measured in the
         lumbar sac, is performed to identify a spinal block, where
         compression of the spinal cord is suspected. It is never a
         routine adjunct to a lumbar puncture, and in a patient with an
         intracranial mass lesion, may cause tentorial or tonsillar
         herniation and death.

CASE STUDY #5

5. C   The occurrence of a unilateral dilated pupil prior to death suggests transtentorial herniation of the medial portion of the temporal lobe with compression of the third nerve. This type of herniation, if not recognized and treated, is not infrequently followed by fatal hemorrhage within the brain stem.

6. A   The abrupt onset of neurological deficit, the pattern of abnormality are all consistent with cerebral infarction, although the age of the patient is quite unusual. The alertness and clear spinal fluid are against the diagnosis of cerebral hemorrhage. Brain abscess generally presents with a more gradual onset and evidence of a primary source of infection. Acute multiple sclerosis is an important possibility to consider with the abrupt onset of neurological abnormality in a young woman. It would be most unlikely that an episode of cerebral multiple sclerosis would lead to cerebral swelling to a degree which would cause transtentorial herniation.

7. ABCDE

8. CD

9. D

10. C

11. D   Many authors have noted the relationship between oral contraceptives and migraine headaches. Migraine can be either initiated or worsened by birth control pills, though paradoxically occasional migrainous women are improved after beginning the pill. The mechanisms which might explain this relationship between the pill and migraine are unknown.

12. BC

13. D

14. C

15. F   The literature is ambiguous about the relationship between oral contraceptives and seizures. The report of the World Health Organization Scientific Group on the Oral contraceptives states that "epilepsy may be made worse in some woman by the use of oral contraceptives. In other women, however, it may be improved." On one hand, several reports suggest that estrogens in animals and humans may have an epileptogenic effect.[5,6,10] On the other hand, other articles and reports[7,8] conclude that in some women birth control pills may decrease seizure frequency, or have no effect on epilepsy.[9,11]

16. F   The platelets of women on estrogen-containing pills have been reported to behave like those of patients with arterial disease.[12]

17. F

REFERENCES

1. Wolf, S.M., J.H. Wagner, and S. Davidson, Oral Contraceptives and Neurological Illness, Bull LA Neurological Soc 32:141, 1967.

2. Buchanan, D.S., and J.H. Brazinsky, Dural Sinus and Cerebral Venous Thrombosis, Incidence in Young Women Receiving Oral Contraceptives, Arch Neurology 22:440, 1970.

CASE STUDY #5

3. Heyman, A., M. Arons, M. Quinn, and L. Camplong, The Role of Oral Contraceptive Agents in Cerebral Arterial Occlusion, Neurology 19:519, 1969.

4. Contraceptives and Hypertension, Editorial, JAMA 214:136, 1970.

5. Logothetis, J., R. Harner, F. Morrell, and F. Torres, The Role of Estrogen in Catamenial Exacerbation of Epilepsy, Neurology 9:352, 1959.

6. Werboff, J., J. B. Corcoran, Effects of Sex Hormone Manipulations on Audiogenic Seizures, Am J Physiology 201:830, 1961.

7. Copeman, H., Letter to the Editor, Med J of Australia 2:969, 1963.

8. Sanchez-Longo, L., and L. Gonzales-Saldana, Hormones and their Influence in Epilepsy, Acta Neurol Latinoamer 12:29, 1966.

9. Toivakka, E., Oral Contraception in Epileptics, Arzneimittelforschung 17:1085 (Aug.) 1967.

10. Stitt, S. L., and W. J. Kinnard, The Effect of Certain Progestins and Estrogens on the Threshold of Electrically Induced Seizure Patterns, Neurology 18:213, 1968.

11. Espir, M., M. E. Walker, and J. P. Lawson, Epilepsy and Oral Contraception, Brit Med J 1:294, 1969.

12. Elgee, N. J., Medical Aspects of Oral Contraceptives, Ann Int Med 72:409, 1970.

13. Irey, N. S., W. C. Manion, and H. B. Taylor, Vascular Lesions in Women Taking Oral Contraceptives, Arch Pathology 89:1, 1970.

14. Carroll, J. D., Migraine and Oral Contraception, Hemicrania 1:4, 1969.

15. Bergeron, R. T., and E. H. Wood, Oral Contraceptives and Cerebrovascular Complications, Radiology 92:231, 1969.

16. Cole, M., Strokes in Young Women Using Oral Contraceptives, Arch Int Med 120:551, 1967.

17. Masi, M. T., and M. Dugdale, Cerebrovascular Disease Associated with the use of Oral Contraceptives, Ann Int Med 72:111, 1970.

18. Shafey, S., and P. Scheinberg, Neurological Syndromes Occurring in Patients Receiving Synthetic Steroids (Oral Contraceptives), Neurology 16:205, 1966.

19. Vessey, M. P., and R. Doll, Investigation of Relation Between Use of Oral Contraceptives and Thromboembolic Disease, Brit Med J 2:199, 1968.

20. McDowell, F., Strokes in Young Adults, Ann Int Med 66:932, 1967.

CASE STUDY #5

21. Mason, B., et al., Studies of Carbohydrate and Lipid Metabolism in Women Developing Hypertension on Oral Contraceptives, Brit Med J 3:317, 1973.

22. Vessey, M., Oral Contraceptives and Stroke, N Engl J Med 288:906, 1973.

23. Collaborative Group for the Study of Stroke in Young Women. Oral Contraception and Increased Risk of Cerebral Ischemia or Thrombosis. New Eng J Med 288:871, 1973.

24. Weir, J., et al., Blood Pressure in Women Taking Oral Contraceptives Brit Med J 1:533, 1974.

CASE STUDY #6

Vertigo and Diplopia in an Elderly Man

HISTORY: This 82 year-old right-handed male was driving his car when he suddenly became aware of a spinning sensation and feeling as though he were "drunk." He pulled the car over to the side of the road, and after a few minutes, he again was asymptomatic. A few hours later, he noted side by side double vision which cleared when either eye was closed. He began to experience a rotary or whirling sensation with rapid position change. Two days later he consulted you.

QUESTIONS:

1. THIS SYMPTOMATOLOGY SUGGESTS NEUROLOGIC DYSFUNCTION IN WHICH OF THE FOLLOWING AREAS?:
   A. Cerebral cortex
   B. Visual pathways
   C. Brain stem
   D. Cerebellar system

2. THE SUDDEN ONSET OF NEUROLOGIC DYSFUNCTION AT THIS AGE IS MOST SUGGESTIVE OF:
   A. Vascular disease
   B. Diabetes mellitus
   C. Central nervous system neoplasm
   D. A demyelinating disorder, such as late onset MS

Further history revealed that six months prior to the onset of these neurologic symptoms, he became aware of intermittent claudication. He has had no known cardiac disease, hypertension, or diabetes mellitus. About five years ago, he had two episodes of spontaneous epistaxis a few days apart, but otherwise, there has been no evidence of blood dyscrasia. Eight years ago, he had a subtotal gastrectomy for peptic ulcer disease, and since then has been asymptomatic.

The family history reveals that his mother died during the influenza epidemic in 1917. She had had diabetes late in life. One sister also possibly is a diabetic. His father died at age 42 from trauma. Two siblings have a history of heart disease.

CASE STUDY #6

Physical examination revealed an alert, well-nourished gentleman, who appeared considerably younger than his stated age. Blood pressure 195/80, both arms, sitting. The dorsalis pedis and posterior tibial pulses were absent bilaterally. The carotid pulsations were strong bilaterally. There was a Grade II systolic bruit in the left supraclavicular area. No intracranial bruit was present. There was no evidence of impairment of mentation. On gait testing there was unsteadiness and swaying with rapid turns and difficulty performing tandem walking. There was slight slowing of left foot tapping. The pupils were 2 mm bilaterally and reacted normally.

There were minimal atherosclerotic changes in the retinal vessels, and no papilledema was present. There was diplopia on left lateral gaze and to a greater extent on right lateral gaze. The images were horizontally displayed. With extreme right lateral gaze, there was unilateral nystagmus of the right eye with impairment of full medial gaze in the left eye. There was a suggestive, but not definite, left lateral rectus palsy. The rest of the cranial nerves were normal.

Sensory examination was intact to superficial, deep and discriminative modalities. Motor examination revealed no paresis or cerebellar deficit, and the reflexes were equal and active bilaterally with no abnormal reflexes present.

QUESTIONS:

3. THE ABNORMALITIES OF OCULAR MOTILITY CAN BEST BE ASCRIBED TO:
    A. A conversion reaction
    B. Drug effect
    C. Interruption of the median longitudinal fasciculus
    D. Involvement of the dentate nucleus of the cerebellum

4. WHICH OF THE FOLLOWING STATEMENTS ARE TRUE?:
    A. A bruit over an extracranial vessel in the neck always indicates stenosis of the artery being auscultated
    B. Because of flow patterns, a bruit may be present over the unobstructed side
    C. Significant stenosis may be present without a bruit
    D. All systolic bruits over the carotid arteries are pathological and require further investigation

COURSE: This patient was hospitalized, and was found to have normal skull films, an unremarkable electroencephalogram and brain scan and normal spinal fluid. He was mildly diabetic, and was placed on a diabetic diet. A surgical consultation was obtained. The vascular surgeon felt that consideration of surgical repair was not indicated because of the patient's age, and the fact that his disease most likely was in the basilar-vertebral distribution. Because of his history of peptic ulcer disease, epistaxis and absence of clinical evidence that his stroke was progressive or recurrent, it was elected not to give him anticoagulation. Over the next four months, his clinical signs gradually improved, although he continued to experience mild diplopia on extreme right lateral gaze.

QUESTIONS:

5. WHICH OF THE FOLLOWING SITUATIONS CALLS FOR ANTI-COAGULATION?:
    A. Transient insufficiency attacks
    B. Stroke-in-evolution
    C. Completed stroke
    D. Recurrent cerebral emboli

CASE STUDY #6

6. WHICH OF THE FOLLOWING SIGNS MAY BE SEEN IN VERTEBRAL-
BASILAR OCCLUSIVE DISEASE?:
   A. Nystagmus
   B. Horner's syndrome
   C. Bilateral Babinski's
   D. Hemiparesis
   E. All of the above

TRUE OR FALSE:

7. Chronic use of vasodilators is frequently indicated in atherosclerotic
cerebrovascular disease.

8. Vasodilators may be indicated in the initial management of the stroke
patient.

9. Seizures are common in basilar artery disease.

10. The basilar-vertebral distribution is a common site for cerebral emboli
from rheumatic heart disease.

11. Lumbar puncture is indicated in most patients with stroke.

12. WHICH OF THE FOLLOWING MAY PRECIPITATE A TRANSIENT INSUF-
FICIENCY ATTACK IN A PATIENT WITH UNDERLYING ARTERIAL
DISEASE?:
   A. Orthostatic hypotension
   B. Cardiac arrhythmia
   C. Embolic plaque from atherosclerotic lesion
   D. Hypercoagulable state
   E. All of the above

ANSWERS AND DISCUSSION:

1. C   The phenomenon of diplopia indicates a loss of normal conjugate
        eye movements. This is usually due to a lesion of the brain stem
        or one of the nerves innervating the eye muscles. In myasthenia
        gravis, diplopia can occur with the defect at the neuromuscular
        junction.

2. A   Neurologic deficit that begins suddenly, if it is not a seizure dis-
        order, is usually either vascular in origin or a manifestation of
        a demyelinating process such as multiple sclerosis. In demyelin-
        ating disease, the onset of neurologic deficit is rarely
        lightening-like, but rather evolves over a period of several hours
        at the least. Vascular disease, regardless of the kind of circula-
        tory disorder, characteristically begins abruptly. This is true
        regardless of whether the underlying mechanism is embolism,
        hemorrhage, or ischemic thrombosis. Since demyelinating dis-
        eases, especially those that are rapid on onset, involve primarily
        younger individuals, the sudden onset of neurologic deficit in an
        adult almost always indicates a disorder of blood supply of some
        variety.

3. C   Nystagmus of the abducting eye on attempted lateral gaze with
        limitation of movement of the adducting eye is termed internuclear
        ophthalmoplegia and is caused by a lesion of the median longitu-
        dinal fasciculus in the brain stem.

CASE STUDY #6

4. BC   Physiologic bruits are fairly common, especially in young males where they appear as rather localized systolic bruits at the base of the right carotid. This bruit increases with heart rate and can be altered with position. Pathologic bruit usually does not change significantly with alterations of heart rate or position. If a vessel is completely occluded, a bruit will not be present over that vessel, but may be heard over the contralateral vessel as flow in this channel shows a compensatory increase.

5. ABD   There is general agreement that 1) if the patient's clinical syndrome is one of transient insufficiency attacks, 2) if the diagnosis is reasonably certain, 3) if other correctable factors have been treated, and 4) if no contraindication is present, that anticoagulation will decrease the number of insufficiency attacks in most patients, and in some will stop them completely. It is not entirely clear, however, that anticoagulation in the patient with TIA's results in a decreased incidence of eventual cerebral infarction.

There is lesser agreement over the use of anticoagulation in the stroke-in-evolution syndrome and in recurrent cerebral emboli. Because of the not insignificant incidence of anticoagulation induced intracerebral hemorrhage, many have been reluctant to use anticoagulation in these two situations. Other evidence, however, indicates that on balance the patient will benefit from immediate anticoagulation. The evidence and clinical opinion is therefore divided in these two situations. Most authorities, however, tend to favor immediate anticoagulation in both situations. In the "completed stroke" syndrome there is general agreement that chronic anticoagulation does not prevent the recurrence of further cerebral infarctions and is therefore not indicated.

6. E   The major supply of the vertebral-basilar system is the brain stem and the occipital lobes. Thus, with either vertebral-basilar insufficiency or complete occlusion, one finds variable symptoms and signs referrable to brain stem dysfunction. Cerebellar signs may also occur. Nystagmus, hemiparesis and bilateral Babinski's are very common. Horner's syndrome may occur if the appropriate pathways in the brain stem are interrupted. Hypothalamic dysfunction as manifested by wide fluctuations in blood pressure and temperature may occur. "Crossed" motor and sensory syndromes may be found.

7. False

8. True

9. False

10. False

11. True   There is general agreement that chronic use of vasodilators is not of significant benefit in the patient with the usual variety of atherosclerotic cerebrovascular disease. In some patients, vasodilators may induce orthostatic hypotension which can be deleterious. In the initial phases of a vascular occlusion, however, several authors favor the use of vasodilators, especially papaverine hydrochloride. This has been debated in literature, however, since there is evidence that in certain situations vasodilation may shunt blood from an ischemic area. Seizures as a manifestation of cerebrovascular disease occur primarily with cerebral embolus and intracerebral hemorrhage. Although they do occur,

CASE STUDY #6

they are very infrequent in the acute stage of a cerebral thrombosis. They are extremely uncommon in any form of basilar-artery disease. The basilar-vertebral distribution is also a very uncommon site for a cerebral embolus regardless of its origin or etiology. In most patients who have sustained a stroke, a lumbar puncture is indicated. This is primarily to rule out subarachnoid or intracerebral hemorrhage.

12. E   The phenomenon of transient cerebral insufficiency attacks has received considerable interest and study over the past several years. At the present time, it would appear that many mechanisms are involved in precipitating such an event. In any one individual, these factors may be multiple and careful evaluation of each possibility is indicated. In some patients the episodes are clearly associated with mechanisms that cause orthostatic hypotension, such as urinating after arising from sleep. Occasionally, Stokes-Adams attacks and other cardiac dysrhythmias may present primarily as a TIA. It has been clearly documented that emboli may arise from an atherosclerotic lesion in the more proximal vascular bed. These emboli may consist of small thrombi or cholesterol crystals. TIA's also occur in the setting of hyperlipidemia, increased platelet adhesiveness, and other situations that result in a hypercoagulable state. The mechanism of vasospasm has been debated at great lengths and it is still unclear whether this is a significant factor in producing TIA's. Anemia and electrolyte disturbances may also be contributory.

REFERENCES

1.   Bradshaw, P., and P. McQuaid, The Syndrome of Vertebro-Basilar Insufficiency, Quart J Med 32:279, 1963.

2.   Williams, D., and T. G. Wilson, The Diagnosis of the Major and Minor Syndromes of Basilar Insufficiency, Brain 85:741, 1962.

3.   Gillilan, L. A., The Correlation of the Blood Supply to the Human Brain Stem with Clinical Brain Stem Lesions, J Neuropath Exp Neurol 32:279, 1963.

4.   Baker, R. N., W. S. Schwartz, and A. A. Rose, Transient Ischemic Strokes. A Report of a Study of Anticoagulant Therapy, Neurology 16:841, 1966.

5.   Leading Article: Anticoagulants and Cerebral Infarction, Lancet 1:245, 1966.

6.   Browne, T., Poskanzer, D., Treatment of Strokes, New Eng J Med 281:594, 1969.

7.   Hass, W., Occlusive Cerebrovascular Disease, Med Clin N Am 56:1281, 1972.

8.   Report of the Joint Committee for Stroke Facilities. Medical and Surgical Management of Stroke, Stroke 4:269, 1973.

9.   Heyman, A., et al., Transient Focal Cerebral Ischemia: Epidemiological and Clinical Aspects, Stroke 5:277, 1974.

10. Houser, O., et al., Atheromatous Disease of the Carotid Artery, J Neuro-surg 41:321, 1974.

CASE STUDY #7

Sudden Onset of Excruciating Headache

HISTORY: A 39-year-old woman was well until the night of admission when, while talking on the phone, she suddenly complained of an excruciating headache, dropped the phone and collapsed on the floor.

QUESTION:

1. THE HISTORY THUS FAR MIGHT SUGGEST:
    A. An acute migraine attack
    B. An intracranial hemorrhage
    C. An intracranial meningioma
    D. Sudden intraventricular obstruction of the cerebrospinal fluid pathway

She was brought to the hospital and noted to be disoriented and obtunded, with severe nuchal rigidity and a positive Kernig sign. The deep tendon reflexes were normal and there were no pathological reflexes. She was able to move all extremities, and examination of the cranial nerves was normal.

QUESTIONS:

2. PATHOLOGICAL REFLEXES INCLUDE:
    A. Snout   C. Unilateral Hoffman
    B. Babinski   D. All of these

3. THE MOST IMPORTANT PROCEDURE TO DO AT THIS POINT IS A:
    A. Blood count   D. Blood glucose
    B. Skull X-ray   E. Spinal tap
    C. Electroencephalogram

A lumbar puncture was performed, which showed grossly bloody fluid under increased pressure. The supernatant was xanthochromic.

QUESTIONS:

4. XANTHOCHROMIA OF THE SPINAL FLUID USUALLY RESULTS FROM THE PRESENCE OF:
    A. Oxyhemoglobin   C. Carotene
    B. Bilirubin   D. All of these

5. THE DIFFERENTIATION BETWEEN A TRAUMATIC SPINAL TAP PRODUCING BLOODY FLUID, AND A TRUE SUBARACHNOID HEMORRHAGE, IS A COMMON PROBLEM. IMPORTANT LABORATORY INDICES OF A TRUE SUBARACHNOID BLEED ARE:
    A. The amount of blood in the spinal fluid
    B. Xanthochromia in the supernatant portion of the centrifuged spinal fluid
    C. Crenation of the red cells
    D. No clearing of successive tubes as cerebrospinal fluid is collected

6. NONHEMORRHAGIC SPINAL FLUID CAN BE XANTHOCHROMIC IF:
    A. The patient is deeply jaundiced
    B. The spinal fluid protein is greater than 150 mgm%
    C. Either of the above
    D. Neither of the above

CASE STUDY #7

7. THE MOST COMMON CAUSE OF SUBARACHNOID HEMORRHAGE IS:
    A. ·Trauma   C. Encephalitis
    B. Hemorrhage into a brain tumor   D. None of these

8. THE MOST COMMON NON-TRAUMATIC CAUSE OF SUBARACHNOID
    HEMORRHAGE IN A NORMOTENSIVE PATIENT IS:
    A. An arteriovenous malformation   C. Anticoagulant therapy
    B. Blood dyscrasias   D. None of these

9. IN THIS PATIENT, THE MOST VALUABLE DIAGNOSTIC STUDY AT
    THIS POINT WOULD BE:
    A. Pneumoencephalography   D. Brain scan
    B. An electroencephalogram   E. Isotope cisternography
    C. Carotid angiography

COURSE: A right carotid arteriogram was performed.

An aneurysm is seen, arising at the origin of the posterior communicating
artery from the internal carotid artery (Fig. 4). There is no evidence of arterial
spasm or intracerebral hematoma.

QUESTIONS:

10. THE MORTALITY FROM THE INITIAL BLEED OF A RUPTURED
    ANEURYSM IS ABOUT:
    A. 3-5%   C. 20-35%
    B. 5-10%   D. 70-90%

11. THE CHANCES OF RE-BLEEDING WITHIN THE FIRST MONTH, IN A
    PATIENT WITH A RUPTURED ANEURYSM, WHO HAS SURVIVED THE
    INITIAL BLEED, AND WHO HAS BEEN TREATED ONLY WITH BED
    REST, ARE ABOUT:
    A. 3%   C. 35%
    B. 5%   D. 70%

12. THE MORTALITY RATE OF A SECOND BLEED IS ABOUT:
    A. 3%   C. 20%
    B. 10%   D. 40%

COURSE: A craniotomy was performed. The frontal and temporal lobes were
edematous and blood stained. The aneurysm was seen to arise from the posteri-
or aspect of the carotid artery and a clip was placed across its neck. Postoperatively the patient has done well.

13. IF THIS PATIENT WERE TO DEVELOP, IN SUBSEQUENT MONTHS, THE
    INSIDIOUS ONSET OF DEMENTIA AND GAIT DISTURBANCE, YOU
    MIGHT SUSPECT:
    A. Cerebral atrophy   C. Another aneurysm
    B. Hydrocephalus   D. Brain tumor

14. DIFFERENT TYPES OF ANEURYSMS INCLUDE:
    A. "Congenital"   D. Arteriosclerotic
    B. Mycotic   E. Traumatic
    C. Luetic   F. All of these

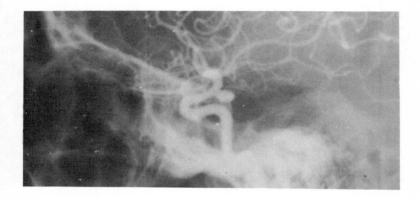

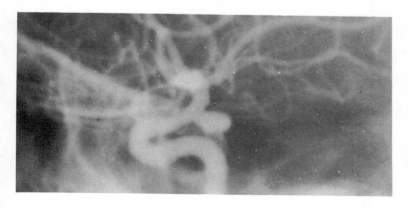

Figure 4

CASE STUDY #7

QUESTIONS:

15. ALTHOUGH THE WALLS OF SO-CALLED "CONGENITAL" ANEURYSMS OFTEN SHOW DEFECTS IN THE MEDIA, THESE ANEURYSMS ARE PROBABLY NOT SIMPLY CONGENITAL MALFORMATIONS SINCE:
   A. Aneurysms are very rare in infancy and childhood
   B. There is some correlation between increasing age and size of aneurysms
   C. Medial defects are found at sites of blood vessel walls where aneurysms do not develop
   D. All of the above

16. THE MOST IMPORTANT GUIDE TO PROGNOSIS FOLLOWING RUPTURE OF AN ANEURYSM IS:
   A. The size of the aneurysm
   B. The presence of multiple aneurysms
   C. The patient's level of consciousness
   D. Presence or absence of hemiplegia
   E. Level of blood pressure

17. ALTHOUGH NECESSARY TO DIAGNOSE THE ETIOLOGY OF A SUB-ARACHNOID HEMORRHAGE, ANGIOGRAPHY IS NOT WITHOUT RISKS, WHICH INCLUDE:
   A. Cerebral infarction   D. Cervical hematoma
   B. Seizures   E. All of the above
   C. Hypotension

ANSWERS AND DISCUSSION:

1. BD   The onset of a migraine headache is gradual, not abrupt and cataclysmic. Meningioma is a slow growing tumor and one would also not expect an apoplectic onset of headache.

2. D

3. E   The evidence of meningeal irritation makes it mandatory to examine the cerebrospinal fluid to determine whether there is meningitis or subarachnoid hemorrhage present.

4. AB   Oxyhemoglobin is released with lysis of red cells and may be detected in the supernatant within about two hours after the release of blood in the subarachnoid space. It reaches a maximum in the first 36 hours and gradually disappears over the next 7-10 days. Bilirubin is an iron free derivative of hemoglobin, produced in vivo following hemolysis of red cells. It is first detected about 10 hours after subarachnoid bleeding, reaches a maximum at 48 hours and may persist for 2-3 weeks.

5. BD   Cell counts or hematocrits should be made on the first and last tubes of fluid. In a traumatic tap, the fluid in the last tube will be clearer and the red cell count lower. After obtaining bloody fluid, the supernatant of a centrifuged specimen should be quickly examined. It should be clear if the red cells have been present for less than two hours. However, if a traumatic tap contains more than 12,000 red cells, oxyhemoglobin may stain the fluid within a half hour after the puncture, and if the red cell count exceeds 150,000, enough serum chromogens will be present to tinge the supernatant yellow. The presence or absence of crenation of red cells is of no importance in distinguishing a traumatic tap from subarachnoid hemorrhage. The exact pigment present in the supernatant fluid can be determined by spectrophotometric analysis.

CASE STUDY #7

6. C

7. A

8. D   The correct answer would be a ruptured aneurysm.

9. C   This is the procedure of choice where a cerebral vascular lesion
              is suspected.

10. C

11. C

12. D

13. B   One would suspect the development of a communicating hydro-
               cephalus due to obliteration of the subarachnoid space beneath
               and over the cerebral hemispheres by fibrous adhesions secondary
               to the subarachnoid hemorrhage.

14. F

15. D

16. C

17. E

REFERENCES

1.   Intracranial Aneurysms and Subarachnoid Hemorrhage, A Cooperative
      Study, Sahs, A.L., G.E. Perrett, H.B. Locksley, and H. Nishioka, Ed.,
      J.B. Lippincott Co., 1969.

2.   McKissock, W., A. Richardson, L. Walsh, and E. Owen, Multiple
      Intracranial Aneurysms, Lancet 1:623, 1964.

3.   McKissock, W., et al., Posterior Communicating Aneurysms, Lancet
      1:1203, 1960.

4.   McKissock, W., et al., Middle Cerebral Aneurysms, Lancet 2:417, 1962.

5.   McKissock, W., et al., Anterior Communicating Aneurysms, Lancet
      1:1391, 1965.

6.   Fishman, R.A., Cerebrospinal Fluid, Clinical Neurology, A.B. Baker,
      and L.H. Baker, Ed., Harper and Row, 1971.

7.   Browne, T.R., and D.C. Poskanzer, Treatment of Strokes, Part 2,
      New Eng J Med 281:650, 1969.

8.   Tourtellotte, W.W., et al., A Study on Traumatic Lumbar Punctures,
      Neurology 8:129, 1958.

9.   Wolfson, L., Katzman, R., Infusion Manometric Test in Experimental
      Subarachnoid Hemorrhage in Cats, Neurology 22:856, 1972.

10.   Alvord, E., et al., Subarachnoid Hemorrhage due to Ruptured Aneurysms,
      Arch Neurol 27:273, 1972.

11.   Zervas, N., et al., Cerebral Arterial Spasm, Arch Neurol 28:400, 1973.

12.   Petito, F., Plum, F., The Lumbar Puncture, New Eng J Med 290:225, 1974.

13.   Hunt, W.E., Kosnik, E., Timing and Perioperative Care in Intracranial
      Aneurysm Surgery, pp. 79-89, in Clinical Neurosurgery, Wilkins, R.H.
      editor, Williams and Wilkins Co., 1974.

14.   Slosberg, P., Nonoperative Management of Ruptured Intracranial
      Aneurysms, pp. 90-99, in Clinical Neurosurgery, Wilkins, R.H., editor,
      Williams and Wilkins Co., 1974.

15.   Cooperative Study of Intracranial Aneurysms and Subarachnoid Hemorrhage,
      Stroke 5:557, 1974.

CASE STUDY #7

16. Millikan, C., Cerebral Vasospasm and Ruptured Intracranial Aneurysm, Arch Neurol 32:433, 1975.

CASE STUDY #8

Confusion in a Patient with a Hilar Lung Mass

HISTORY: A 66 year-old man was admitted to the hospital because of fever, anorexia, cough, and weight loss, of two months duration. He was a heavy smoker. On admission his temperature was 100.5°F. He was confused and had a moderately enlarged liver. Examination was otherwise normal.

QUESTIONS:

1. CONFUSION IN A PATIENT WITH CANCER OF THE LUNG MIGHT BE DUE TO:
   A. Metastases
   B. Hyponatremia
   C. Hypercalcemia
   D. Multifocal leukoencephalopathy
   E. Any of the above

2. AS THE NEUROLOGICAL CONSULTANT YOU MIGHT REQUEST:
   A. Electroencephalogram
   B. Myelogram
   C. Skull films
   D. Brain scan
   E. All of the above

3. THE MOST COMMON PRIMARY SITE OF METASTATIC BRAIN TUMOR IS THE:
   A. Lung
   B. Breast
   C. GI tract
   D. Kidney

LABORATORY DATA: Hemoglobin was 8.3 gm%. The white blood cell count was 12,600. Urine contained a few white cells per high power field. There was 1+ proteinuria. The spinal fluid was clear, under normal pressure, with a protein of 43mgm%, no cells, normal sugar and negative serology. The electroencephalogram showed a left temporal slow wave focus. Skull films were normal, but the pineal was not calcified. Intravenous pyelogram, histoplasmin, coccidioidin, and ppd skin tests, serum electrolytes, multiple blood cultures, bronchoscopy, examination of the bone marrow, brain scan, scalene node biopsy were all negative or normal. X-ray of the chest revealed a left hilar mass (Fig. 5).

A hematology consultant felt that the anemia was of the type seen with chronic neoplasia or infections.

COURSE: He continued to run a low grade temperature, and he was begun on cephalothin and given transfusions for his anemia. He did well for a few days, but then one morning was noted to be obtunded with nuchal rigidity. A right Babinski sign was found.

QUESTIONS:

4. THE MOST IMPORTANT TEST TO DO AT THIS TIME WOULD BE:
   A. A repeat brain scan
   B. An arteriogram
   C. A repeat spinal tap
   D. A pneumoencephalogram

CASE STUDY #8

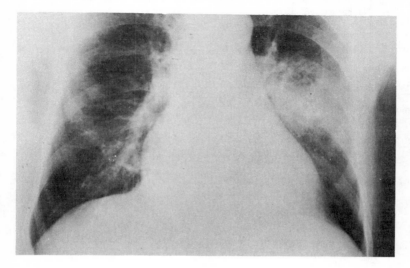

Figure 5

5.   MOST LIKELY THIS PATIENT HAS DEVELOPED:
       A. Subarachnoid hemorrhage
       B. Meningitis
       C. Transtentorial herniation
       D. Hemorrhage into a malignant tumor

6.   IN VIEW OF THIS COMPLICATION, THE BRAIN LESION IS MOST
       LIKELY:
       A. Glioblastoma
       B. Metastasis
       C. Abscess
       D. Medulloblastoma

A spinal tap was performed.   The fluid was cloudy and under increased pressure.
There were 890 white cells/cu mm, 95% of which were polymorphonuclears.
Protein was 78 mgm%, sugar 37 mgm%.   Gram stain, pyogen culture, india ink
and acid fast stains were negative.   He was placed on high doses of ampicillin
intravenously and given isoniazid and streptomycin also, because of the possibility of tuberculous infection.   An echoencephalogram revealed a left to right shift
of 5 mm.

QUESTION:

7.   THE MIDLINE ECHO WHICH IS CONVENTIONALLY MEASURED COR-
       RELATES BEST WITH THE POSITION OF THE:
       A. Anterior cerebral artery
       B. Middle cerebral artery
       C. Pineal gland
       D. Lateral ventricle

CASE STUDY #8

Neurological examination now showed weakness of the right arm and leg, with slight internal rotation of both eyes. Neither eye was able to abduct fully. The left pupil was two mm larger than the right and slightly more sluggish in its reaction to light. The patient was lethargic.

QUESTIONS:

8. THE BILATERAL INTERNAL DEVIATION OF THE EYES SUGGESTS INVOLVEMENT OF THE:
   A. Median longitudinal fasciculus
   B. Corticobulbar tracts
   C. Mesencephalon
   D. Sixth cranial nerves

9. ABNORMALITIES OF FUNCTION OF THIS STRUCTURE ARE FREQUENTLY SEEN WITH:
   A. A lesion within the medulla
   B. Increased intracranial pressure
   C. Spread of the pathological process to the diencephalon
   D. None of the above

10. THE PUPILLARY ABNORMALITY SUGGESTS:
    A. A left sixth cranial nerve palsy
    B. A right Horner's syndrome due to a brainstem lesion
    C. A left third cranial nerve lesion
    D. Possible transtentorial herniation of the left cerebral hemisphere

11. AN IMPORTANT DRUG TO GIVE QUICKLY WOULD BE:
    A. Neostigmine
    B. Mannitol
    C. Neomycin
    D. Pilocarpine

12. THE MOST APPROPRIATE DIAGNOSTIC PROCEDURE NOW WOULD BE:
    A. Ventriculogram
    B. Pneumoencephalogram
    C. Left vertebral angiogram
    D. Left carotid angiogram

A left carotid angiogram suggested a deep frontal mass with a 1.5 cm shift of the anterior cerebral artery from left to right (Fig. 6).

At craniotomy, an abscess cavity, containing yellow-green pus was encountered below the cortex. Culture of the abscess revealed Nocardia Asteroides, (an aerobic, gram positive acid-fast fungus) and he was treated with sulfadiazine and ampicillin. Postoperatively he improved, becoming much more alert for about a week, but then again became lethargic and obtunded. He was clinically well hydrated and there was no cardiomegaly or peripheral edema. The neurological examination was unchanged. A repeat carotid angiogram showed no evidence of a mass lesion. The blood urea nitrogen was 6, serum sodium 114 meq/l, chloride 80, and potassium 3.5 meq/l.

QUESTIONS:

13. THE PATIENT MOST LIKELY SUFFERS FROM:
    A. Adrenal insufficiency
    B. Insufficient intravenous fluid and salt replacement
    C. Inappropriate antidiuretic hormone secretion
    D. Congestive heart failure

CASE STUDY #8

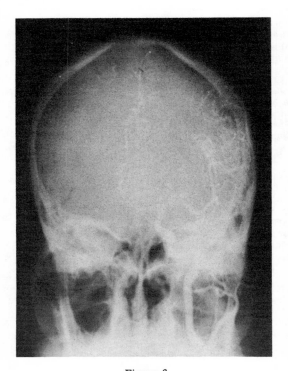

Figure 6

14. THE DIAGNOSIS WOULD BE STRONGLY SUPPORTED BY FINDING:
   A. Pulmonary rales
   B. Decreased urinary delta amino levulinic acid
   C. Decreased serum and increased urine osmolality
   D. Increased serum and decreased urine osmolality

15. THE TREATMENT FOR THIS PROBLEM IS:
   A. Sodium lactate
   B. Isotonic sodium chloride
   C. Fluid restriction
   D. Dextrose and water
   E. None of the above

CASE STUDY #8

COURSE: Serum osmolality was 235 mo.m, urine 335 mosm, confirming the clinical impression of inappropriate antidiuretic hormone secretion. Fluid restriction was begun. Electrolytes gradually became normal. The patient became much more alert, but remained confused. Over the next three months, his mental status greatly improved, and the ampicillin and sulfadiazine were then discontinued. Since then he has done well, but still has the neurologic residua of a slight organic mental syndrome.

QUESTIONS:

16. NOCARDIA IS CAPABLE OF INITIATING DISEASE IN THE ABSENCE OF ANY KNOWN PREDISPOSING FACTORS. AS WITH OTHER CENTRAL NERVOUS SYSTEM FUNGAL INFECTIONS, THE RISK AND FREQUENCY INCREASE IN PATIENTS RECEIVING:
   A. Dilantin
   B. Corticosteroids
   C. Cytotoxic agents
   D. All of the above

17. THE MOST FREQUENT PORTAL OF ENTRY, IN MOST CASES OF CENTRAL NERVOUS SYSTEM NOCARDIOSIS, IS THE:
   A. Lung
   B. Ear
   C. GI tract
   D. GU tract

ANSWERS AND DISCUSSION:

1. E   Hyponatremia might occur as a result of antidiuretic hormone secretion either from the neoplasm itself, or in association with cerebral metastases. Hypercalcemia could result from secretion of parathormone by the cancer or secondary to bony metastases. Multifocal leukoencephalopathy is a rare demyelinating disease which occurs, in most instances, as a complication of lymphoma or leukemia.[10] Electron microscopic studies suggest that the etiologic agent may be a virus belonging to the popova group.

2. ACD   All of the tests mentioned would be appropriate and indicated, except for the meylogram, since there is at this point no indication of disease of the spinal portion of the nervous system.

3. A

4. C   Fever, obtundation, and a stiff neck require a lumbar puncture to determine whether meningitis is present.

5. B   One might also consider the possibility of a subarachnoid hemorrhage from an aneurysm, either congenital or perhaps mycotic, associated with an endocarditis. However, there were no heart murmurs, and multiple blood cultures were negative in this patient.

6. C

7. C

8. D   Bilateral internal ocular deviation indicates weakness of the lateral recti, innervated by the sixth cranial nerves. The sixth cranial nuclei are located in the pons; the third in the mesencephalon. The ocular syndrome seen with lesions of the median

CASE STUDY #8

longitudinal fasciculus is ipsilateral limitation of adduction and nystagmus of the abducting eye.

9. B   The abducens nucleus is in the pons, and so neither a diencephalic or a medullary lesion would involve it. However weakness of sixth nerve function is not infrequently seen in various conditions causing increased intracranial pressure. Such palsies, according to Walsh and Hoyt, are related to the long course of the nerve and the resultant liability to compression, stretching, pressure at the petrous ridge and impairment of blood supply.

10. CD   A right Horner's syndrome would produce pupillary irregularity with the right pupil smaller, as in this case, but one would expect that the right pupil would be miotic, that there would be an associated ptosis of the right upper lid and that there would be no impairment of the pupillary light reflex as was present in this patient. The dilated sluggishly reactive pupil suggests the ominous possibility of third nerve compression by transtentorial herniation of the left temporal lobe secondary to a left cerebral mass lesion. If the significance of these early findings of transtentorial herniation of the uncus of the temporal lobe are not appreciated and the situation treated, fatal hemorrhages into the brainstem may follow.

11. B   Mannitol renders the blood more osmotically concentrated than the brain cells, causing a shift of water out of the brain, with a resultant shrinkage in brain size, and a transient improvement in the symptoms and signs of increased intracranial pressure.

12. D   A lateralized cerebral mass lesion is best studied with carotid arteriography which gives information about the size of the mass, the shift of adjacent structures, and may also furnish clues as to the histological diagnosis, depending on the degree and pattern of vascularity, the rapidity of blood flow through the mass, etc.

13. C   Fichman and Bethune[6] divide hyponatremia into three catagories: 1) Hypoosmolar states with dehydration secondary to primary salt depletion 2) hyponatremia with overhydration and edema due to an increase in total body water in excess of sodium and 3) a group of hypoosmolar states associated with normal hydration and frequently a relatively high urine sodium in the absence of any apparent abnormality of cardiac, hepatic, renal or adrenal function. An example of this latter is the syndrome of inappropriate secretion of antidiuretic hormone, which has been described in association with varied chest lesions, as well as with different types of central nervous system disease, including subdural hematomas, meningitis, acute intermittent porphyria, etc.

In this patient the lack of evidence of congestive failure, or dehydration, the very low blood urea nitrogen, and the presence of central nervous system disease should lead to the suspicion of the inappropriate antidiuretic hormone syndrome as the cause of the hyponatremia. The patient did not show the pigmentation, hypotension, or hyperkalemia of Addison's disease. However, since Addison's disease can simulate the inappropriate ADH syndrome, Bartter[7] suggests that urine or plasma corticoid levels should be determined on every patient suspected of having uncomplicated inappropriate ADH release.

CASE STUDY #8

14. C

15. C

16. BC   Recent reviews have emphasized the role of Nocardia Asteroides
as an opportunistic pathogen in patients with severe underlying illness who are receiving intensive medical therapy. The great majority of cases have been associated with such underlying conditions
as cancer, systemic lupus, immunosuppression after organ trans-
plantation, sarcoidosis, etc.

17. A

REFERENCES

1. Fetter, B.F., G.K. Klintworth, and W.S. Hendry, Mycoses of the Central
Nervous System, Williams and Wilkins, 1967.

2. Richter, R., M. Silva, H. Neu, and P. Silverstein, The Neurological Aspects
of Nocardia Asteroides Infection, Assoc for Res in Nervous and Mental Dis
44:424, 1968.

3. Clinico-Pathologic Conference, Mayo Clinic Proc 42:565, 1967.

4. Young, L., D. Armstrong, A. Blevins, and P. Lieberman, Nocardia
Asteroides Infection Complicating Neoplastic Disease, Am J Med 50:356, 1971.

5. Fichman, M., and J. Bethune, The Role of Adrenocorticoids in the Inappropriate Secretion of Antidiuretic Hormone Syndrome, Ann Int Med 68:807, 1968.

6. Bartter, F., and W. Schwartz, The Syndrome of Inappropriate Secretion of
Antidiuretic Hormone, Am J Med 42:790, 1967.

7. Fichman M., C. Kleeman, and J. Bethune, Inhibition of Antidiuretic Hormone
Secretion by Diphenylhydantoin, Arch Neur 22:45, 1970.

8. Bolton, C., and B. Rozdilsky, Primary Progressive Multifocal Leukoencephalopathy, Neurology 21:72, 1971.

9. Adams, A., J. Jackson, J. Scopa, G. Lane, and R. Wilson, Nocardiosis,
Diagnosis and Management, Med J Australia (March 27) 1971.

10. Turner, E., J. Whitby, Nocardia Cerebral Abscess with Systemic Involvement Successfully Treated by Aspiration and Sulphonamides, J Neurosurg
31:227, 1969.

11. Mendoza, S., Keller, M., Inappropriate Secretion of Antidiuretic Hormone,
Western J Med 121:45-49, 1974.

12. Schrier, R., Inappropriate vs Appropriate Antidiuretic Hormone Secretion,
Western J Med 121:62, 1974.

13. Maderazo, E., Quintiliani, R., Treatment of Nocardial Infection with Tri-
methoprim and Sulfamethoxazole, Am J Med 57:671, 1974.

CASE STUDY # 9

Hypotension and Impotence in a Middle-Aged Male

HISTORY: A 59-year-old right-handed male was admitted with a chief complaint of "low blood pressure." Fifteen years before admission, he noted the onset of impotence. Four years before he began to have progressive generalized weakness. About this time, he experienced episodes of lightheadedness and occasional syncope upon standing. No convulsive movements ever occurred. He consulted a physician who recorded a standing blood pressure of 60/20 and placed him on ephedrine, which gave moderate relief of his symptoms. Three years before admission, he began to have alternating diarrhea and constipation without abdominal pain. He denied nausea or vomiting.

During the year prior to admission, he noted progressive distal weakness and paresthesia in the upper and lower extremities. On several occasions, he burned his hands without experiencing pain. His ambulation was limited by symptoms of orthostatic hypotension. In the year prior to admission, he also noted delayed healing of skin abrasions, and several ulcerated lesions of the hands and feet appeared. He remarked that he no longer sweated in warm weather. Hoarseness without dyarthria or dysphagia had been present for eighteen months. Three years before admission, he was placed on 5 mg of Prednisone daily without therapeutic effect.

QUESTIONS:

1. ORTHOSTATIC HYPOTENSION, IMPOTENCE AND GI DYSFUNCTION ARE MOST SUGGESTIVE OF:
   A. Cerebrovascular disease
   B. Autonomic nervous system abnormality
   C. Brain stem disorder
   D. Myasthenia gravis
   E. Parietal lobe disorder

2. THE HISTORY IS MOST SUGGESTIVE OF:
   A. Multiple sclerosis
   B. Frontal lobe mass
   C. Peripheral neuropathy
   D. Transverse myelopathy

3. AUTONOMIC NEUROPATHY IS PROMINENT IN:
   A. Chronic lead intoxication
   B. Amyloidosis
   C. Diabetes
   D. Alcoholism
   E. Charcot-Marie-Tooth Disease

The patient was born in Valencia, Spain, and moved to the United States at age 18. He did not smoke and rarely drank alcohol. After coming to this country, he worked as a handyman at various odd jobs. Fifteen years before admission, he worked for a short time in a plant which manufactured paints. Otherwise, there was no history of exposure to neurotoxins.

The family history revealed no evidence of significant systemic or neurologic disease nor was he aware of any endemic syndrome of a nature similar to his in his birthplace.

EXAMINATION: A cachectic, chronically ill male who was in no acute distress while in the supine position. He was unable to maintain a sitting position because of symptoms of hypotension. Supine blood pressure was 130/70. On standing, the pressure varied from 120/60 to 55/20. The tongue was normal. There was no evidence of vitreous opacities on funduscopic examination. Examination of the

CASE STUDY #9

heart and lungs revealed no abnormalities. The spleen and liver were not palpable. The skin had poor turgor, and several small trophic ulcerations were present on the feet.

Gait could not be tested because of orthostatic hypotension. The cranial nerves were unremarkable except for mild hoarseness with normal oropharyngeal sensation and motor function. There was atrophy and weakness of the interosseous muscles and distal forearms. Moderate dysmetria was present in all extremities. There was generalized areflexia with a flexor response to plantar stimulation bilaterally. Sensory examination revealed decreased pin, touch, and temperature perception in the distal extremities to the level of the wrist and knees, being most marked distally. Position and vibration sense were absent in the toes and impaired in the ankles and fingers.

LABORATORY DATA: Urinalysis was unremarkable. There was no Bence Jones protein in the urine. Hemoglobin was 14 gm percent, hematocrit was 41.5%, and white count was 4,950 with a normal differential count. The following studies were within normal limits: serum calcium, phosphorus and alkaline phosphatase, serum glutamic oxalacetic transaminase, fasting blood sugar, Bromsulphalein excretion, protein bound iodine, VDRL, serum carotene, cholesterol, creatine, and electrolytes. Serum protein electrophoresis revealed a normal pattern. Twenty-four hour urine collection for arsenic, lead, uroporphyrins, coproporphyrins, porphobilinogen, creatine, and creatinine revealed no abnormalities. Stools for ova and parasites on 3 occasions were negative. Lumbar puncture revealed an opening pressure of 80 mm with clear and colorless spinal fluid. No cells were present. The cerebrospinal fluid protein was 74.4 mg percent, sugar 94 mg percent and chloride 125.8 meq per liter.

Chest films were normal. The electrocardiogram was interpreted as showing sinus tachycardia, marked left-axis deviation, and old anteroseptal myocardial infarction. Electromyography revealed diffuse fibrillation potentials in all extremities, somewhat more marked distally. Schilling test was normal. Direct visualization of the vocal cords revealed no abnormalities. Skin, muscle and rectal biopsies were done soon after admission. The tissues were fixed in formalin and Zenker's solutions and stained with Congo red and crystal violet. In the skin biopy, the panniculus and lower dermis contained amorphous pools of hyaline material, which stained metachromatically with crystal violet and gave a positive Congo red reaction. Several of the smaller arterioles contained Congo red positive material in their walls. Muscle biopsy showed degenerative changes with moderate sarcolemmal nuclei proliferation and muscle fibers which varied considerably in size and in degree of eosinophilic staining. There was no inflammatory reaction and no amyloid material could definitely be identified, although several vessels showed medial thickening of their walls.

The most impressive findings, however, were those revealed by rectal biopsy. The mucosa and submucosal connective tissue were unremarkable. Most of the arterioles showed marked thickening and hyalinization of their walls with frequent encroachment on the lumen, although no thromboses or completely occluded vessels could be found (Fig. 7).

This hyaline material reacted in a strikingly positive manner with Congo red. The sections fixed in formalin demonstrated these changes much better than the material fixed in Zenker's solution.

CASE STUDY #9

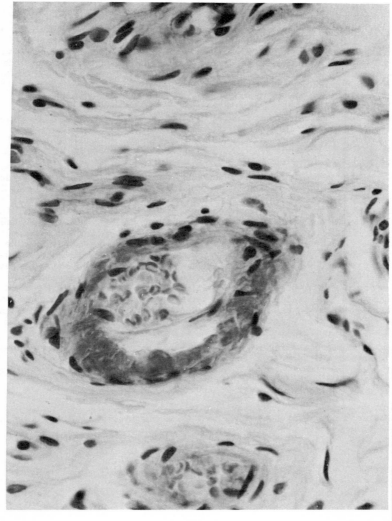

Figure 7

CASE STUDY #9

QUESTIONS:

TRUE OR FALSE

4. Primary and secondary amyloidosis overlap in their clinical and bio-chemical attributes and cannot be clearly differentiated

5. Nerve conduction times constitute one of the most sensitive lab tests for peripheral nerve disorder

6. In most peripheral neuropathies, vibration sense is lost before touch perception

7. In peripheral nerve disease, the sensory loss is more marked proximally than distally

8. Intracranial deposits of amyloid are a frequent cause of seizures in primary amyloidosis

9. INDICATE OTHER CAUSES OF PERIPHERAL NEUROPATHY:
   A. Guillain-Barre Syndrome
   B. Charcot-Marie-Tooth Disease
   C. Multiple sclerosis
   D. Alcoholism
   E. Wilson's Disease

ANSWERS AND DISCUSSION:

1. B

2. C

3. BC   This patient presents with rather prominent findings of inadequacy of the autonomic nervous system. He has difficulty controlling blood pressure with episodes of orthostatic hypotension, he has become impotent, and his sweat production has become impaired. All of these suggest that at some level the autonomic nervous system is impaired. This could occur anywhere from a hypo-thalamic level to the neuroeffector mechanism, but is most frequent when the peripheral nervous system is involved. Later in his course, he developed clinical evidence that the peripheral nervous system was, indeed, affected with weakness, most marked distally, and paresthesiae in all four extremities. Thus the history is extemely suggestive of peripheral neuropathy with a prominent component of autonomic neuropathy. This aspect is most suggestive of amyloidosis or diabetes. Although autonomic dysfunction can occur in any peripheral neuropathy, it is much more frequent in those two disorders.

4. True

5. True

6. True

7. False

8. False

9. ABD   A symmetrical peripheral neuropathy produces a somewhat similar clinical syndrome regardless of the etiology in most cases.

CASE STUDY #9

Characteristically, the involvement begins distally and progresses in a distal to a proximal manner. This is true for both sensory and motor involvement. Eventually all four extremities are affected, although initially in most neuropathies, the legs show the greatest degree of involvement. Some neuropathies begin asymmetrically or may affect individual large nerve trunks, so-called "mononeuritis multiplex." When this occurs, one should consider an underlying vasculopathy such as occurs in the neuropathy of diabetes and the collagen-vascular disorders. In certain disorders, such as the Guillain-Barré syndrome, the motor involvement may be more marked proximally. Multiple sclerosis and Wilson's disease primarily affect the central nervous system and do not produce clinical neuropathy. Spinal fluid protein may be elevated in any neuropathic disorder, but may be especially high in the Guillain-Barré syndrome and in certain patients with diabetic neuropathy. The cell count is usually normal, although a modest elevation can occasionally occur. Peripheral nerve conduction times are very helpful in determining the presence, distribution, and severity of the peripheral neuropathy. Initially, since the peripheral portions of the nerve are usually involved first, only the terminal conduction (terminal latency time) may be affected. The electromyogram is somewhat less helpful in peripheral neuropathy, but can demonstrate fibrillatory activity as the muscle fibers become denervated. Sensory nerve conduction times are somewhat more sensitive but are subject to more errors of interpretation.

The neuropathy of amyloidosis, as is demonstrated in this patient, is a somewhat unusual and relatively rare cause of peripheral neuropathy. Nonetheless, most patients with this disorder usually remain undiagnosed for many months, or even many years. An accurate diagnosis can only be made by obtaining tissue which shows the characteristic staining for amyloid deposition. The autonomic manifestions in amyloid neuropathy frequently antedate the more typical sensory-motor phenomena. Amyloid polyneuropathy may occur in a familial setting or sporadically. If obviously pathologic tissue isn't available for biopsy, a rectal biopsy seems to offer the highest yield in undiagnosed patients.

REFERENCES

1. Brandt, K., E.S. Cathcart, and A.S. Cohen, A Clinical Analysis of the Course and Prognosis of 42 Patients with Amyloidosis, Am J Med 44:955, 1968.

2. Munsat, T.L., and A.F. Poussaint, Clinical Manifestations and Diagnosis of Amyloid Polyneuropathy. Report of Three Cases, Neurology 12:413, 1962.

3. Gafni, M., and E. Sohar, Rectal Biopsy for the Diagnosis of Amyloidosis, Am J of Med Sci 240:332, 1960.

4. Primary Amyloidosis: Clinical Staff Conference at the National Institutes of Health, Ann Int Med 69:787, 1968.

5. Henson, R., Urich, H., Metabolic Neuropathies, Chapter 1, Diseases of Nerves, Part II, in Handbook of Clinical Neurology, Vinken, P.J., and Bruyn, G.W., ed., North-Holland Publishing Co., Amsterdam, 1970.

6. Kaeser, H., Nerve Conduction Velocity Measurements, Chapter 5, p. 116, Diseases of Nerves, Part I, in Handbook of Clinical Neurology, Vinken, P.J., and Bruyn, G.W., ed., North-Holland Publishing Co., Amsterdam, 1970.

7. Dyck, P.J., Mulder, D. Differential Diagnosis of Neuropathy, Chapter 21, Diseases of Nerves, Part II, p. 357, in Handbook of Clinical Neurology, Vinken, P.J., and Bruyn, G.W., ed., North-Holland Publishing Co., Amsterdam, 1970.

CASE STUDY #9

8. Cohen, M., Differential Diagnosis of Toxic Neuropathy, Chapter 22, p. 552, in Handbook of Clinical Neurology, Vinken, P.J., and Bruyn, G.W., ed., North-Holland Publishing Co., Amsterdam, 1970.

9. Case Records of the Massachusetts General Hospital, New Eng J Med 286:534, 1972.

10. Novak, D., Victor, M., The Vagus and Sympathetic Nerves in Alcoholic Polyneuropathy, Arch Neurol 30:273, 1974.

11. Thomas, P., King, R., Peripheral Nerve Changes in Amyloid Neuropathy, Brain 97:395, 1974.

12. Diabetic Autonomic Neuropathy, Editorial, British Medical Journal 6 July 1974.

CASE STUDY #10

Sudden Facial Paralysis

HISTORY: This 24-year-old man was in good health until he awoke one morning with an aching pain behind the right ear, followed a day later by twisting of his face to the left, and diminished taste on the right side of his tongue. He found loud noises unusually disagreeable. He complained of a constant feeling of irritation in his right eye. There was no diplopia, dizziness, dysarthria, weakness, hearing loss or tinnitus.

EXAMINATION: Was negative except for weakness of the upper and lower portions of the right side of the face. (Fig. 8, taken as the patient attempts to grimace).

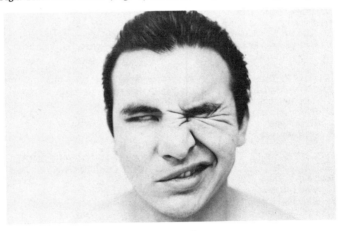

Figure 8

The weakness was present both when the patient voluntarily grimaced and when he spontaneously laughed. Taste was decreased over the anterior right portion of the tongue.

QUESTIONS:

1. THE LESION IS IN THE:
    A. Corticobulbar tract
    B. Facial motor nucleus
    C. Facial nerve
    D. Trigeminal nerve
    E. Neuromuscular junction

CASE STUDY #10

2.   IF THE FACIAL WEAKNESS WERE MUCH MORE MARKED ON VOLUN-
      TARY THAN EMOTIONAL EXPRESSION, THIS WOULD SUGGEST THAT
      THE LESION IS:
      A. Central
      B. Peripheral
      C. Muscular

3.   THE BEST DIAGNOSIS IN THIS PATIENT IS:
      A. Pontine infarct
      B. Cerebellopontine angle tumor
      C. Multiple sclerosis
      D. Bell's palsy
      E. Pontine glioma

4.   IF VESICLES WERE FOUND OVER THE RIGHT EAR, HERPES ZOSTER
      WOULD BE SUSPECTED AS THE ETIOLOGIC AGENT, AND THE SYN-
      DROME WOULD BE GIVEN THE EPONYM OF:
      A. Dejerine-Sottas
      B. Refsum
      C. Ramsey-Hunt
      D. Von Recklinghausen

5.   IN THE DIFFERENTIAL DIAGNOSIS OF IDIOPATHIC BELLS PALSY,
      ONE SHOULD RULE OUT:
      A. Diabetes mellitus
      B. Sarcoid
      C. Middle ear infection
      D. Cerebellopontine angle tumor
      E. All of above

6.   TOUCHING THE RIGHT CORNEA OF THIS PATIENT WITH A WISP OF
      COTTON SHOULD PRODUCE BLINKING OF:
      A. The left eye
      B. The right eye
      C. Both eyes
      D. Neither eye

7.   IN CONTRAST, A PATIENT WITH A NEUROMA OF THE RIGHT FIFTH
      NERVE MIGHT SHOW, WHEN THE RIGHT CORNEA WAS STIMULATED,
      BLINKING OF:
      A. The left eye
      B. The right eye
      C. Both eyes
      D. Neither eye

8.   A "CENTRAL" FACIAL WEAKNESS, AS MIGHT BE SEEN WITH A LESION
      OF THE OPPOSITE CEREBRAL HEMISPHERE, DIFFERS FROM A
      PERIPHERAL TYPE OF WEAKNESS IN THAT IN THE FORMER:
      A. Taste is not impaired
      B. Weakness of the lower face is much greater than in the forehead
          muscles
      C. Lacrimation is often impaired
      D. All of the above

CASE STUDY #10

9. ONE PATIENT WITH BELL'S PALSY FINDS, AFTER SEVERAL MONTHS, THAT HIS EYE INVOLUNTARILY CLOSES WHEN HE GRIMACES; ANOTHER THAT HIS EYE TEARS WHEN HE EATS. THESE PHENOMENA ARE BEST EXPLAINED BY:
   A. Failure of the nerve to reinnervate denervated structures
   B. Nerve degeneration
   C. Conditioned reflexes
   D. Regeneration of nerve fibers along the wrong pathway

10. DEFINITIVE TREATMENT FOR IDIOPATHIC BELL'S PALSY IS CONTROVERSIAL. STEROIDS AND SURGICAL DECOMPRESSION OF THE FACIAL NERVE BOTH HAVE THEIR ADVOCATES. EVALUATION IS DIFFICULT SINCE IN THE NATURAL COURSE OF THE DISEASE, WITHOUT TREATMENT, FULL RECOVERY OCCURS IN:
   A. 15%
   B. 35%
   C. 65%
   D. 85%

11. THIS PATIENT'S INTOLERANCE TO LOUD NOISE SUGGESTS THAT:
   A. The 8th nerve or nucleus is involved and the pathology may extend to the brain stem
   B. The cochlea may be damaged
   C. The lesion is in the facial nerve at or above the emergence of the branch which innervates the stapedius muscle

ANSWERS AND DISCUSSION:

1. C   A lesion of the corticobulbar tract would produce an upper motor neuron type of facial paresis, with the upper portion of the face less affected than the lower because of the bilateral upper motor neuron innervation of the facial motor nuclei supplying the upper portion of the face in contrast to the contralateral upper motor neuron innervation of the portion of the nucleus innervating the lower half of the face. Also, with a lesion of the corticobulbar tract one usually sees associated corticospinal tract damage, with weakness, hyperreflexia, etc.

   The lesion is not in the facial motor nucleus, since the sensation of taste is impaired, which is represented in the brain stem by the nucleus and tractus solitarius. The trigeminal nerve is the sensory nerve to the face and the motor nerve to the muscles of mastication, not facial expression.

   Myasthenia gravis often produces facial weakness, but bilaterally and with intact sensation.

   The lesion is in the facial nerve, impairing motor fibers which innervate the facial muscles causing paralysis and twisting of the mouth to the opposite side (because of the unopposed pull of the intact muscles). In addition sensory fibers carrying taste from the anterior 2/3 of the tongue are affected.

2. A   A lesion of the facial muscles or nerve would produce the same impairment with either volitional or emotional expression. With central lesions one may see a difference in facial strength between emotional and volitional expression, suggesting that there are divergent and separate central neuroanatomical pathways.

CASE STUDY #10

3. D   Bell's palsy is an acute lesion of the facial nerve which may involve motor, sensory and autonomic fibers in varying severity. With lesions of the facial nucleus in the pons as due to vascular, demyelinating or neoplastic disease, one would expect involvement of contiguous cranial nuclei as well as the long sensory and motor tracts, rather than the isolated 7th nerve paresis typical of Bell's palsy. In a cerebellopontine angle tumor, the onset of illness is gradual, the course progressive, and other structures besides the 7th cranial nerve are compromised, such as cranial nerves 5 and 8, cerebellar pathways and the pyrimidal tract.

4. C   There are several Ramsay-Hunt syndromes. One is herpes zoster affecting the 7th cranial nerve. The 7th cranial nerve supplies sensory fibers to the tympanic membrane and external auditory canal.

The Dejerine-Sottas syndrome is one of hypertrophic peripheral neuropathy. Refsum's syndrome is hereditary ataxic polyneuropathy with accumulation of phytanic acid. The Von Recklinghausen syndrome includes neurofibromatosis and café-au-lait skin pigmentation.

5. E   Diabetes mellitus exists in a high percentage of patients with Bell's palsy[6]. The other conditions listed can all cause impairment of facial nerve function.

6. A   Because the afferent arc of the corneal reflex is intact, but the efferent arc on the right is damaged.

7. D   Because the afferent arc (5th cranial nerve) is damaged, the impulses could not reach the pontine reflex center or the efferent arcs.

8. AB   The pre-ganglionic parasympathetic fibers to the lacrimal glands originate in the superior salivatory nucleus in the pons, and so tearing would not be impaired with a lesion of the corticobulbar tract above that level producing a "central" facial palsy. Other differences between central and peripheral facial weakness are discussed in the answer to Question 1 above.

9. D   In the first example, regenerating nerve fibers which should have gone to the obicularis oris find their way to the obicularis oculi. In the second example, fibers are misdirected to the lacrimal glands which should have gone to the salivary glands.

10. D   Various techniques including electrogustometry, nerve conduction latency, nerve excitability testing and electromyography have been used to pick those patients with Bell's palsy who have an increased risk of poor prognosis, including incomplete return of facial strength and abnormal associated movements. However, it remains to be definitively proven whether surgery, steroids or other treatment significantly changes the prognosis.

11. C   This patient's Bell's palsy involved motor fibers going to innervate the stapedius muscle. This tiny muscle inserts on the stapes of the middle ear. Its contraction restricts the motion of the middle ear ossicular chain, damping sound transmission and protecting the hearing mechanism against intense and possibly damaging sounds. Stapedius weakness due to a 7th nerve lesion may produce, as in this case, hyperacusis, especially for low tones.

CASE STUDY #10

REFERENCES

1. May, M., Facial Paralysis, Peripheral Type, Laryngoscope 80:331, 1970.

2. Marinacci, A., and K.O. Von Hagen, The Prognosis in Bell's Palsy, Bull Los Angeles Neuro Soc 36:83, 1971.

3. Korczyn, A., Bell's Palsy and Diabetes Mellitus, Lancet 1:108, 1971.

4. Giancarlo, H., and K. Mattucci, Facial Palsy (Facial Nerve Decompression), Arch Otolaryng 91:30, 1970.

5. Kendall, D., Facial Paralysis, Practitioner 204:523, 1970.

6. Mechelse, K., E. Huizing, A.N. Van Bolhuis, G. Goor, E. Hammelburg, A. Staal, and A. Uerjaal, Bell's Palsy, Prognostic Criteria and Evaluation of Surgical Decompression, Lancet 2:57, 1971.

7. Adour, K., et al., Prednisone Treatment for Idiopathic Facial Paralysis, New Eng J Med 287:1268, 1972.

8. Rowland, L.P., Treatment of Bell's Palsy, New Eng J Med 287:25, 1972.

9. Jongkees, L.B.W., Practical Application of Clinical Tests for Facial Paralysis, Arch Otolaryngol 97:220, 1973.

10. Alford, B., et al., Neurophysiology of Facial Nerve Testing, Arch Otolaryngol 97:214, 1973.

11. Groves, J., Facial Palsies, Proc Roy Soc Med 66:545, 1973.

12. Adour, K., J. Wingerd, Idiopathic Facial Paralysis: Factors Affecting Severity and Outcome in 446 Patients, Neurology 24:1112, 1974.

13. Adour, K., J. Wingerd, Nonepidemic Incidence of Idiopathic Facial Paralysis, JAMA 227:653, 1974.

14. Symposium, Bell's Palsy: Drugs or Decompression, Modern Medicine, August 19, 1974, pp. 30-39.

CASE STUDY #11

Amnesia In An Elderly Woman

HISTORY: A 69-year-old woman was referred because of an episode of amnesia. Three days previously, she had driven to her niece's house, bringing several gifts for different members of her family. She appeared normal on arrival. After about an hour, though, her family noted that she seemed confused. She recognized her relatives, knew who and where she was, but had no recollection of how she had arrived there. She kept repeatedly and nervously asking how she had gotten to her niece's house. She had no remembrance of her activities earlier that day, but could recall events of days, weeks, months or years ago with complete clarity. She was fully alert and oriented, but very anxious that something was wrong with her mind. Her speech was normal, and there was no evidence of motor or visual abnormality. Eight hours later, she was completely well, but has remained amnesic for the events of that entire day.

QUESTION:

1. IN THE HISTORY, YOU MIGHT WISH TO INQUIRE ABOUT:
   A. A history of convulsions   D. Emotional conflict
   B. A family history of convulsions   E. All of the above
   C. Olfactory or gustatory hallucinations

CASE STUDY #11

There was no history of seizures, trauma, abnormal olfactory or taste phenomena, diabetes, drug use, emotional illness, hypertension, heart disease or
other serious illnesses.

The general physical and neurological examinations were entirely normal.
Orientation, calculating ability and other tests of mental function were all normal.

QUESTIONS:

2.   THE DIFFERENTIAL DIAGNOSIS MIGHT INCLUDE ALL OF THESE,
      EXCEPT:
      A. Korsakoff's syndrome
      B. Wernicke's syndrome
      C. Psychomotor seizures
      D. Stroke
      E. Lesch-Nyhan syndrome

3.   HELPFUL, IN EXCLUDING A PSYCHOMOTOR SEIZURE, WOULD BE:
      A. Absence of prior seizures of any type
      B. Normal wake and sleep electroencephalogram
      C. No aura
      D. No motor automatisms during the episode
      E. All of the above

4.   AGAINST THE DIAGNOSIS OF HYSTERIA IS THE:
      A. Preservation of personal identity during the attack
      B. Patient's anxious concern about her condition
      C. Lack of history of prior psychiatric disease
      D. Lack of history of prior emotional conflict
      E. B, C, D

5.   AGAINST THE DIAGNOSIS OF A TRANSIENT ISCHEMIC EPISODE IS
      THE LACK OF:
      A. Motor symptoms
      B. Sensory symptoms
      C. Visual symptoms
      D. Speech abnormality
      E. All of the above

6.   THE MOST PROBABLE DIAGNOSIS IS:
      A. Cerebrovascular accident
      B. Transient global amnesia
      C. Petit mal
      D. Stokes-Adams syndrome

7.   YOU MIGHT NOW REQUEST:
      A. Psychiatric consultation
      B. Wake and sleep EEG
      C. Bilateral carotid angiograms to exclude a brain tumor
      D. Pneumoencephalogram

LABORATORY DATA: Blood count, urinalysis, glucose tolerance test, skull and
chest films, serology, wake and sleep electroencephalograms, brain scan,
lumbar puncture, echoencephalogram, calcium, protein bound iodide, serum
electrolytes, sedimentation rate, and electrocardiogram were all normal.

CASE STUDY #11

QUESTIONS:

8. THE MAJOR DEFICIT IN THIS PATIENT WAS ONE OF:
   A. Immediate recall   C. Language function
   B. Recent memory   D. Remote memory

9. SELECTIVE IMPAIRMENT OF MEMORY, WITH RELATIVE PRESERVATION
   OF OTHER COGNITIVE FUNCTIONS, HAS BEEN ASSOCIATED WITH LESIONS
   INVOLVING:
   A. The anterior portions of the frontal lobes
   B. The occipital lobes
   C. The parietal lobes
   D. The Hippocampal portions of the temporal lobes

10. RECENT MEMORIES ARE:
    A. Vulnerable to a variety of injurious agents
    B. Typically impaired in Korsakoff's syndrome
    C. Often impaired following severe head trauma
    D. None of the above

11. STIMULATION OF THE TEMPORAL LOBES IN EPILEPTIC PATIENTS:
    A. Has evoked distant memories if done on the dominant side
    B. Has evoked recent memories if done on the nondominant side only
    C. Has evoked memories if done on either side

12. REMOVAL OF BOTH TEMPORAL LOBES RESULTS IN:
    A. Gilles de la Tourette syndrome   C. Eaton-Lambert syndrome
    B. Kluver-Bucy syndrome   D. Decerebrate rigidity

13. THIS SYNDROME IS CHARACTERIZED BY:
    A. Opisthotonus   D. Placidity
    B. Increased sexual activity   E. Profound impairment of mem-
    C. Coprolalia   ory learning ability

14. THE PROGNOSIS FOR THE PATIENT DESCRIBED IN THIS CASE REPORT IS:
    A. Very grave   C. Unpredictable
    B. Guarded   D. Good

15. MEDICAL MANAGEMENT WOULD INCLUDE:
    A. Dilantin   E. Zarontin
    B. Phenobarbital   F. Papaverine
    C. Primidone   G. Vasodilan
    D. Mesantoin   H. None of the above

ANSWERS AND DISCUSSION:

1. E   The differential diagnosis of an episode of memory loss includes both
        temporal lobe seizures and psychogenic illness.

2. ABE Korsakoff's psychosis is a chronic illness with a disproportionate loss
        of memory in an otherwise clear sensorium. There is retrograde am-
        nesia for a period of months or years, and impaired ability to acquire
        new information. Confabulation may be present, but is not essential
        for the diagnosis. Wernicke's syndrome includes ophthalmoplegia,
        ataxia, and mental confusion. Peripheral neuropathy is usually pre-
        sent. The illness results from thiamine deficiency, and most often
        is seen in alcoholics. The Lesch-Nyhan syndrome is a rare pediat-
        ric condition and includes self mutilation and hyperuricemia.

CASE STUDY #11

3. E

4. ÁBCD   The hysterical amnesic episode is often characterized by "loss" of personal identity. This contrasts sharply with memory loss of "organic" cause in which personal identification is maintained in spite of severe impairment of memory, temporal and spatial orientation, attention span and other cognitive functions. Typical also in hysterical amnesia is the patient's seeming unconcern about it, "la belle indifférénce." The explanation for this is the role of the symptom in resolving emotional conflict and alleviating anxiety.

5. E

6. B   This patient's episode of amnesia is a good example of the transient global amnesia syndrome. This syndrome generally occurs in persons over 50. Most recent evidence suggests that it is caused by ischemia in the distribution of the vertebro-basilar-posterior cerebral arteries, affecting the medial portions of the temporal lobe bilaterally. The onset during the 6th to 8th decades; the occurrence of the syndrome, following presumed arterial embolism during cardiac angiography; the regional reduction of cerebral blood flow in the temporal areas; and angiographic evidence of stenotic or occlusive arteriosclerotic lesions in the vertebro-basilar posterior cerebral arteries, in some patients, support a vascular explanation. The absence of a prior history of seizures, loss of consciousness, automatic motor movements, purposeless behavior, prodromal aura, illusions, hallucinations, delusions, deja or jamais vu phenomena in these patients are against an epileptic etiology. Where amnestic seizures do occur, they are usually at an earlier age and are not characterized by repetitive questioning and a pure recent memory defect. The neurological examination in these patients is generally normal except for the memory deficit. The results of usual laboratory tests including cerebrospinal fluid examinations are normal. The electroencephalogram is usually normal, but temporal slowing or spike discharges have been reported in some cases.

7. AB   If the clinical and laboratory criteria of this syndrome are present, contrast studies would represent an unwarranted risk to the patient.

8. B

9. D

10. ABC

11. C

12. B   Eaton and Lambert described a myasthenic syndrome in association with carcinoma of the lung. Giles de la Tourette's syndrome includes multiple tics, stereotyped movements, use of obscene words and evidence of regressive behavior.

13. BDE

14. D   The prognosis is generally excellent. A minority may have repeated attacks. Permanent memory deficit or dementia have been reported in occasional patients.

15. H   Medical management should be directed toward the reduction of predispositions to occlusive cerebrovascular disease, including control of hypertension, diabetes, hyperlipidemia and cardiac dysrhythmia. Mathew and Meyer suggest that in cases where embolism is suspected from atherosclerotic plaques, agents which prevent platelet aggregation should be considered.

CASE STUDY #11

REFERENCES

1. Patten, B.M., Transient Global Amnesia Syndrome, JAMA 217:690, 1971.

2. Victor, M., R.D. Adams, and G.H. Collins, The Wernicke-Korsakoff Syndrome, Contemporary Neurology Series, F.A. Davis, Co., 1971.

3. Penfield, W., and B. Milner, Memory Deficit Produced by Bilateral Lesions in the Hippocampal Zone, Arch Neurology and Psychiatry 79:475, 1958.

4. Victor, M., J. Angevine, E. Mancall, and C.M. Fisher, Memory Loss with Lesions of Hippocampal Formation, Arch Neurology 5:244, 1961.

5. Fisher, C.M., and R.D. Adams, Transient Global Amnesia, Acta Neur Scand 40 (suppl 9):7-83, 1964.

6. Steinmetz, E., F. Vroom, Transient Global Amnesia, Neurology 22:1193, 1972.

7. Heathfield, K., et al., The Syndrome of Transient Global Amnesia, Brain 96:729, 1973.

8. Shuttleworth, E., G. Wise, Transient Global Amnesia Due to Arterial Embolism, Arch Neurol 29:340, 1973.

9. Mathew, N., J.S. Meyer, Pathogenesis and Natural History of Transient Global Amnesia, Stroke 5:303, 1974.

10. Jaffe, R., M. Bender, Further Studies in the Pathophysiology of Transient Global Amnesia, (Abstract), Neurology 24:395, 1974.

11. Rowan, A.J., L. Protass, Transient Global Amnesia: Clinical and EEG Findings in Eight Cases, Neurology 24:350, 1974 (Abstract).

12. Greene, H., Transient Global Amnesia with a Previously Unreported EEG Abnormality, Electroenceph and Clin Neurophys 36:409, 1974.

CASE STUDY #12

Paraparesis in a Middle-Aged Man

HISTORY: This patient was a 54 year-old salesman who was in good health until five months previously, when he began to note aching behind the left calf followed by a sense of numbness in and about the left knee. In the ensuing weeks, he noted progressive weakness of the left leg, and progressive numbness which extended both distally and proximally to the level of the lower rib cage. During the few weeks prior to evaluation, a similar process had begun in the right lower extremity. He began using crutches, and eventually became wheelchair-confined. During recent weeks he had become aware of urinary hesitancy and frequency as well as of increasing constipation. He denied any recent back pain or injury. He was not aware of any difficulty with cranial nerve or upper extremity function.

QUESTIONS:

1. THE MOST LIKELY CAUSE FOR THIS PATIENT'S URINARY COMPLAINTS IS:
A. Benign prostatic hypertrophy   C. Neurogenic bladder
B. Metastatic disease to the bladder D. Conversion reaction

CASE STUDY #12

2. THE FOLLOWING FEATURES ARE CHARACTERISTIC OF A SPASTIC OR "UPPER MOTOR NEURON" BLADDER:
    A. Urinary incontinence
    B. Pain in and about the rectum
    C. Frequency
    D. Urgency
    E. Large bladder capacity

3. THE FOLLOWING ARE CHARACTERISTIC OF A DENERVATED OR "LOWER MOTOR NEURON BLADDER":
    A. Frequent irregular, low density, involuntary bladder contractions
    B. Large bladder capacity
    C. Incontinence
    D. Urgency
    E. Pain in and about the rectum
    F. Frequency

Past medical history included hypercholesterolemia, spontaneous pneumothorax in 1949, renal calculus in 1964, and pleurisy in 1943. There was no family history of neurological disorder.

PHYSICAL EXAMINATION: Vital signs were normal. There was minimal bilateral pretibial ankle edema. There was an irregularly shaped midline cherry red nevus on the forehead. No vertebral spine tenderness was present. He was alert and intellectually normal. No abnormalities of cranial nerve function could be detected. Deep tendon reflexes were normal in the upper extremities, but symmetrically hyperactive in the legs. Bilateral Babinski reflexes were present. There was a moderately severe paraparesis. No fasciculations were seen. At the T7-8 level, there was a well-demarcated sensory level below which touch and pin sensation were markedly reduced.

QUESTION:

4. THIS MAN'S CLINICAL NEUROLOGIC SYNDROME IS THAT OF A TRANSVERSE MYELOPATHY. IN THIS AGE GROUP, THE FOLLOWING WOULD HAVE TO BE CONSIDERED IN THE DIFFERENTIAL DIAGNOSIS:
    A. Demyelinating disease, such as multiple sclerosis
    B. Primary intramedullary or extramedullary spinal neoplasm
    C. Wilson's disease
    D. Renal insufficiency
    E. Metastatic disease of the spinal cord
    F. Heavy metal toxicity

LABORATORY DATA: Plain films of the thoracic spine were normal. Lumbar puncture revealed clear and colorless spinal fluid. The opening pressure was normal and manometrics revealed no evidence of a block in dynamics. There were four lymphocytes per cu. mm. Spinal fluid protein was 187 mgm%.

QUESTION:

5. A LOGICAL, AND PERHAPS DEFINITIVE,NEXT PROCEDURE MIGHT BE:
    A. Nerve conduction velocity
    B. Myelography
    C. Electromyography
    D. Electroencephalography

A pantopaque myelogram was carried out. This revealed what appeared to be an extramedullary mass lesion, primarily on the left, at the T-6 spinal cord level. An aortogram (Fig. 9) was carried out in an attempt to visualize a suspected arteriovenous malformation of the cord. Laminectomy was performed, at which time a large arteriovenous malformation of the spinal cord was uncovered.

CASE STUDY #12

Using microneurosurgical techniques, the major feeding vessels were ligated and the major part of the lesion was successfully removed. Postoperatively the patient's condition remained essentially unchanged, with neither worsening nor significant improvement over the subsequent months.

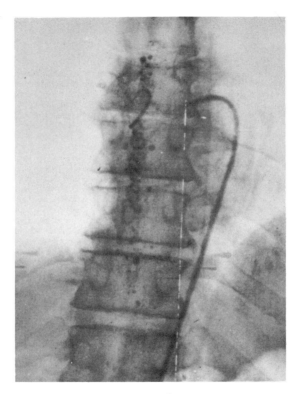

Figure 9

QUESTIONS:

6.   COMMON COMPLICATIONS OF MYELOGRAPHY ARE:
      A. Post LP headache
      B. Disc herniation
      C. Chronic adhesive arachnoiditis
      D. Acute bacterial meningitis
      E. Low pressure hydrocephalus

      TRUE OR FALSE:

7.   Lhermitte's sign refers to acute pain in the low back when the patient coughs.

CASE STUDY #12

8. Spinal fluid protein greater than 100 is frequently observed in disc disease.

9. Pain is a frequent concomitant of extramedullary spinal cord compression.

10. Disc disease frequently results in lower motor neuron signs.

11. In contrast to intracranial arteriovenous malformations, those of the spinal cord do not bleed and cause subarachnoid hemorrhage.

ANSWERS AND DISCUSSION:

1. C

2. ACD

3. BCF Micturition is basically a spinal cord reflex function which is modulated by cortical influences. Thus, there are both voluntary and involuntary control aspects. When the bladder is denervated (lower motor neuron lesion) it becomes flaccid, enlarged, and loses its capacity to empty reflexly. This type of bladder demonstrates overflow incontinence with almost constant leaking of small amounts of urine. Frequently in this situation, sensory pathways are also interrupted and the patient is unaware of his bladder distention. This type of bladder disorder occurs frequently in cauda equina lesions. When there is bilateral upper motor neuron involvement, as occurs in any form of transverse myelopathy, the bladder becomes spastic with frequent, low intensity, uncontrolled bladder contractions. The bladder capacity is small and sensation usually is intact. This combination of abnormality leads to urgency, frequency and incontinence which is more episodic. Patients with bilateral cortical disease, especially in the frontal lobe, may demonstrate a type of urinary incontinence analogous to the situation in the child before bladder control is developed. These individuals may show a lack of concern about the incontinence. Usually the history and physical examination are sufficient to allow the clinician to decide what kind of bladder dysfunction is operative. Cystometrograms can provide useful additional information when necessary.

4. ABE This patient presents the historical aspects and physical findings of a transverse lesion of the spinal cord, i.e., transverse myelopathy. Wilson's disease, renal insufficiency, and heavy metal intoxication are not processes which damage the spinal cord in this manner. When beginning later in life, multiple sclerosis may present as a slowly progressive transverse myelopathy. This is quite different from the usual course of M.S. in the younger patient where exacerbations and remissions are to be expected and multiple lesions are found within the central nervous system. The main extramedullary lesion of middle age, more frequent in females than in males, is the meningioma which usually occurs at a midthoracic level. This is histopathologically benign and a total cure is possible. Intramedullary neoplasms are less common in later life and consist primarily of gliomas. Metastatic disease to the spinal cord usually presents as a rapidly progressive mass producing a transverse myelopathy. The most common sources in a male this age would be lung, GI tract and kidney.

5. B

6. A Positive contrast myelography is a relatively safe procedure. Infection occurs rarely and is usually caused by inadequate sterilization of equipment. Cases of chronic adhesive arachnoiditis have been reported, but also are infrequent. By far the most common compli-

CASE STUDY #12

cation is a headache syndrome which characteristically is initiated or intensified by assuming the upright position and rapidly relieved by lying down. The exact mechanism of this headache is unclear. It may be related to the amount of fluid removed, the size of the needle used, the number of dural punctures and the amount of leaking after the needle is withdrawn. In most patients undergoing myelography, clinically inapparent "aseptic" meningitis occurs. Air myelography is a technique whereby air is injected into the subarachnoid space. It is somewhat more effective in outlining the cervicomedullary junction. At times, both procedures are necessary for definition of the problem. Recently, angiographic visualization of the spinal cord has been used with increasing success. This is the most effective way of defining an arteriovenous malformation of the cord, although on occasions, even with proper technique the malformation is not seen. Occasionally, positive contrast myelography can visualize such lesions, although less effectively.

7. False   Lhermitte's sign is a sudden electric-like sensation spreading down the body or into the limbs on flexion of the neck and is present with lesions of the cervical spinal cord, of diverse etiology.

8. False

9. True

10. True

11. False

REFERENCES

1. Gregorius, F., and S. Weingarten, The Natural History of Vascular Malformation of the Spinal Cord, Bull LA Neuro Soc 35:25, 1970.

2. Ommaya, A., G. DiChiro, and J. Doppman, Ligation of Arterial Supply in the Treatment of Spinal Cord Arteriovenous Malformations, J Neurosurg 30:679, 1969.

3. Krayenbuhl, H., M. Yasargil, and H. McClintock, Treatment of Spinal Cord Vascular Malformations by Surgical Excision, J Neurosurg 30:427, 1969.

4. Doppman, J., F. Wirth, G. DiChiro, and A. Ommaya, Value of Cutaneous Angiomas in the Arteriographic Localization of Spinal Cord Arteriovenous Malformation, New Eng J Med 281:1440, 1969.

5. Wyburn-Mason, R., The Vascular Abnormalities and Tumors of the Spinal Cord and Its Membranes, Henry Kimpton, London, 1943.

6. Aminoff, M., V. Logue, Clinical Features of Spinal Vascular Malformations, Brain 97:197, 1974.

7. Aminoff, M., V. Logue, The Prognosis of Patients with Spinal Vascular Malformations, Brain 97:211, 1974.

8. Logue, V., et al., Results of Surgical Treatment for Patients with a Spinal Angioma, J Neurology Neurosurgery and Psychiatry 37:1074, 1974.

CASE STUDY #13

A Paralyzed Man From Mexico

HISTORY: This 29 year-old Mexican male was admitted to the hospital in February 1965 because of paralysis of his legs and difficulty in breathing for several hours. He had been well until six months previously when he developed diarrhea, nervousness, excessive perspiration, and tremor of his hands. In spite of a hearty appetite and normal food intake, he lost 20 lbs in two months.

Five weeks before, he began to suffer from episodes of weakness of his legs and arms lasting several hours, usually following heavy meals. The night before admission he developed weakness of all extremities followed the next day by difficulty in breathing. There was no family history of weakness or neurological disease. There was no history of diabetes, alcoholism, recent immunization or exposure to toxins.

EXAMINATION: Revealed a dyspneic, tachypneic male in respiratory distress. He was afebrile. The neck was supple. The general physical examination was otherwise normal, except for a soft apical systolic cardiac murmur.

NEUROLOGICAL EXAMINATION: Deep tendon reflexes were absent in all extremities. Plantar responses were flexor. The legs were totally paralyzed. There was severe weakness of the arms both distally and proximally so that he could barely lift them against gravity. The neck and intercostal muscles were also very weak. Muscle tone was diminished in the extremities. No fasciculation were seen. All sensory functions were normal as was the remainder of the neurological examination.

QUESTIONS:

VARIOUS DISEASES MUST BE CONSIDERED IN THE DIFFERENTIAL DIAGNOSIS OF THIS CASE. INDICATE WHETHER THE FOLLOWING ARE TRUE OR FALSE:

1. The normal sensation with severe paralysis makes an acute cervical cord lesion unlikely.

2. Polio is improbable because of the lack of fever, signs of meningeal irritation and the symmetry of the paralysis.

3. In the Landry-Guillain-Barré syndrome one sees a flaccid acute areflexic paralysis, but the history of episodic weakness in this case would be against that diagnosis.

4. This is not likely to be myasthenia gravis, since in that disease the patient, although weak, has normal deep tendon reflexes, and the extra-ocular muscles are often affected.

5. Muscular dystrophy is a chronic, slowly progressive disease.

6. The periodic paralyses typically produce attacks of flaccid paralysis with loss of the deep tendon reflexes.

LABORATORY DATA AND COURSE: Serum potassium was 2.9 meq/1. Other electrolytes were normal. An infusion of 40 meq of potassium was given intravenously and within two hours he was able to move his arms and legs. By the next morning strength and the deep tendon reflexes were normal. When re-examined after the disappearance of the paralysis, the thyroid was found to be diffusely enlarged, and there was a tremor of the outstretched hands. I-131 uptake was 76%, PBI 15. Normal or negative studies included complete blood

CASE STUDY #13

count, urinalysis, lumbar puncture, sedimentation rate, tensilon test, serology, calcium and blood sugar.

QUESTIONS:

7. THE MOST LIKELY DIAGNOSIS IS:
    A. Polymyositis
    B. Hyperaldosteronism
    C. Hypokalemic periodic paralysis associated with thyrotoxicosis
    D. None of the above

A week later, the patient was given 125 grams of glucose orally with 20 units of regular insulin subcutaneously. Baseline strength was entirely normal. In three hours he complained of weakness in arms and legs. Examination again showed distal and proximal weakness in all extremities. He was given oral potassium, and in an hour strength was again normal. During this provocative test, the baseline potassium was 4.5 meq/l. At the time of weakness it dropped only to 4.1 meq/l. Other electrolytes remained unchanged.

The thyrotoxicosis was treated with radioiodine. When seen in the clinic one month later, his strength was excellent, but he still complained of experiencing mild episodes of weakness after eating large meals. Several months later he was euthyroid and asymptomatic. He has since been followed for four years without recurrence of any weakness.

TRUE OR FALSE:

8. In hypokalemic periodic paralysis,the potassium during paralysis may be normal or only minimally decreased, but an attack can often be induced by glucose and insulin.

9. In other conditions of potassium depletion, weakness does not occur until serum potassium falls to 2.5 meq/l or less.

10. The electrocardiogram is always normal during an attack of hypokalemic paralysis.

11. In the thyrotoxic form of periodic paralysis, restoration of the euthyroid state abolishes the attacks of weakness.

12. THE MORTALITY OF AN ATTACK OF PERIODIC PARALYSIS IS:
    A. None
    B. 10%
    C. 50%
    D. 80%

ANSWERS AND DISCUSSION:

1. True

2. True

3. True

4. True

5. True

CASE STUDY #13

6. True

7. C

8. True

9. True

10. False

11. True

12. B   Periodic paralysis is rarely associated with hyperthyroidism except in Japan, where between 2% and 8% of hyperthyroid patients suffer from periodic paralysis. In thyrotoxic adult Japanese males the incidence may be as high as 33%.

Thyrotoxic periodic paralysis resembles familial hypokalemic periodic paralysis in clinical features (flaccid, areflexic paralysis), and the triggering of attacks by exercise, ingestion of large amounts of carbohydrate, salt, or alcohol, and the administration of glucose and insulin or corticosteroids. In both, a shift of potassium from extracellular fluid into muscle occurs during an attack and administration of potassium generally shortens the duration and lessens the severity of the weakness. Intramuscular vacuoles, which seem to be due to dilation of the sarcotubular system, have been found in both familial and thyrotoxic periodic paralysis during paralytic episodes.

Differences between familial and thyrotoxic periodic paralysis include the predilection of the latter for Japanese males, the thyrotoxic state, and, most importantly, the elimination of paralytic attacks when the patient becomes euthyroid.

REFERENCES

1. Pearson, C.M., The Periodic Paralyses, Differential Features and Pathological Observations in Permanent Myopathic Weakness, Brain 87:341, 1964.

2. Satoyoshi, E., K. Murakami, H. Kowa, M. Kinoshita, and Y. Nishiyama, Periodic Paralysis in Hyperthyroidism, Neurology 13:746, 1963.

3. Engel, A.G., Electron Microscopic Observations in Primary Hypokalemic and Thyrotoxic Periodic Paralyses, Mayo Clin Proc 41:797, 1966.

4. Okihiro, M., and R. Nordyke, Hypokalemic Periodic Paralysis, Experimental Precipitation with Sodium Liothyronine, JAMA 198:949, 1966.

5. Shy, G.M., Periodic Paralyses, Textbook of Medicine, P. Beeson, and W. McDermott, Ed., 12th Ed., W.B. Saunders Co., 1968.

6. Brody, I., and A. Dudley, Thyrotoxic Hypokalemic Periodic Paralysis, Arch Neurology 21:1, 1969.

7. Macdonald, R.D., N.B. Rewcastle, and J.G. Humphrey, Myopathy of Periodic Paralysis, Arch Neurology 20:565, 1969.

8. Norris, F., B. Panner, and J. Stormont, Thyrotoxic Periodic Paralysis, Arch Neurology 19:88, 1968.

9. Engel, A., and E. Lambert, Calcium Activation of Electrically Inexcitable Muscle Fibers in Primary Hypokalemic Periodic Paralysis, Neurology 19:851, 1969.

CASE STUDY #13

10. Dyken, M. , W. Zeman, and T. Rusche, Hypokalemic Periodic Paralysis, Children with Permanent Myopathic Weakness, Neurology 19:691, 1969.

11. Bergman, R. A. , A. K. Afifi, L. M. Dunkle, and R. J. Johns, Muscle Pathology in Hypokalemic Periodic Paralysis with Hyperthyroidism, John Hopkins Med J 126:88, 1970.

12. Bernard, J. , M. Larson, and F. Norris, Thyrotoxic Periodic Paralysis in Californians of Mexican and Filipino Ancestry, Calif Med 116:70, 1972.

13. Takagi, et al. , Thyrotoxic Periodic Paralysis, Neurology 23:1008, 1973.

14. Conway, M. , et al. , Thyrotoxicosis and Periodic Paralysis: Improvement with Beta Blockade, Ann Int Med 81:332, 1974.

15. Yeung, R. , T. Tse, Thyrotoxic Periodic Paralysis, Effect of Propanolol, Am J Med 57:584, 1974.

16. Layzer, R. , E. Goldfield, Periodic Paralysis Caused by Abuse of Thyroid Hormone, Neurology 24:949, 1974.

CASE STUDY #14

Weakness, Diplopia and an Abnormal Chest Film

HISTORY: A 42 year-old woman was told of an abnormal chest X-ray in 1944. She was, however, asymptomatic until 1965 when she began to note difficulty in elevating her arms above her head. Her eyelids began to droop in the late afternoon, and she complained of double vision.

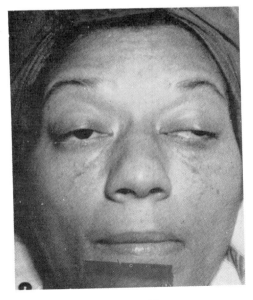

Figure 10

CASE STUDY #14

EXAMINATION: There was ptosis of the eyelids which worsened on repeated blinking, and all the extraocular muscles were weak. She was able to elevate her arms above her head for only thirty seconds and there was proximal weakness of the legs. She showed facial weakness, but had no dysphagia or dysarthria. Reflexes and sensation were normal, and there was no muscle atrophy or fasciculation.

QUESTIONS:

1. ON THE BASIS OF THE INFORMATION THUS FAR, THE MOST LIKELY DIAGNOSIS IS:
    A. Guillain-Barré syndrome
    B. Muscular Dystrophy
    C. Myasthenia Gravis
    D. Polymyositis
    E. Amyotrophic Lateral Sclerosis

2. IN THE DIFFERENTIAL DIAGNOSIS OF THIS PATIENT'S ILLNESS, INDICATE WHETHER THE FOLLOWING ARE TRUE OR FALSE:
    A. Central nervous system disease is unlikely in the absence of pyramidal or long sensory tract abnormalities or other cranial nerve deficits
    B. The abnormal chest film is probably an incidental and unrelated finding
    C. The normal reflexes and sensation are against the diagnosis of a neuropathy
    D. Proximal weakness is usually evidence of a myopathy, but may be seen in spinal cord or neuropathic disease
    E. The negative family history, the worsening of the ptosis in the afternoon, and the normal reflexes are against the diagnosis of muscular dystrophy

3. THE PROCEDURE MOST LIKELY TO CONFIRM THE DIAGNOSIS IS:
    A. Electromyography
    B. Muscle biopsy
    C. Nerve conduction velocity
    D. Injection of edrophonium
    E. None of the above

An injection of 10 mgm of edrophonium (Tensilon) was given intravenously, with dramatic improvement in ptosis, facial and limb strength.

LABORATORY DATA: Chest films showed an anterior mediastinal mass (Figs. 11 A and B). CBC, urinalysis, sedimentation rate, PBI, RAI uptake, LE prep, transaminase, latex fixation, electromyography, electrocardiogram, and muscle biopsy were all normal.

Antibodies were found in the patient's blood against skeletal muscle and thymic cells.

QUESTION:

4. THE MOST LIKELY PATHOLOGY OF THE MEDIASTINAL MASS IS:
    A. Hyperplastic thymus gland
    B. Lymphoma
    C. Thymoma
    D. Carcinoma of lung
    E. Teratoma

CASE STUDY #14

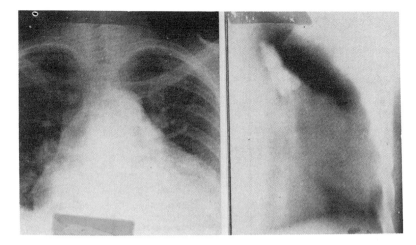

Figure 11A   Figure 11B

COURSE AND TREATMENT: She was treated with pyridostigmine (Mestinon), initially 60 mgm tid, gradually increasing to 300 mgm daily, with improvement. In June 1965 a thoracotomy was done and a large thymic tumor was found which extended over the pericardium and invaded the left lung. The tumor could only be partially removed. The thymoma consisted pathologically of lymphoid and epithelial cells. Following surgery a 3000 R course of radiation was given. She gradually became stronger. Myocarditis developed which required long term prednisone for control. Her strength continued to improve and her need for anticholinesterase medication decreased and then disappeared. A complete remission, except for occasional mild eyelid ptosis lasted for five years. She then contracted bacterial pneumonia, complicated by candida albicans septicemia and died.

QUESTIONS:

5.   NEOSTIGMINE IS OF BENEFIT IN MYASTHENIA GRAVIS BECAUSE:
      A. It inhibits the enzyme which destroys acetylcholine
      B. It prolongs the interaction between acetylcholine and the receptor
         protein
      C. Both of the above
      D. Neither of the above

      TRUE OR FALSE:

6.   Neostigmine is usually able to completely eliminate the signs and
      symptoms of myasthenia.

7.   ACTH and adrenal corticosteroids may increase myasthenic weakness.

8.   THE INDICATIONS FOR SURGERY IN A PATIENT WITH MYASTHENIA
      AND A THYMOMA ARE:
      A. To prevent local extension of the tumor
      B. The possibility of improvement of the myasthenia
      C. Both of the above
      D. Neither of the above

CASE STUDY #14

9. OPTIMAL MANAGEMENT OF A MYASTHENIC DURING AND IMMEDIATELY POST THYMECTOMY INCLUDES:
   A. No anticholinesterase drugs during surgery and in the immediate post-operative period
   B. Tracheostomy
   C. Respirator if needed
   D. Beginning medications after 3-4 days at a lower dosage than preoperatively
   E. All of the above

10. WEAKNESS IN A PATIENT WITH MYASTHENIA GRAVIS MAY BE INCREASED BY:
    A. Overdosage of anticholinesterase medication
    B. Ether
    C. Curare
    D. Ephedrine
    E. Pralidoxime (PAM)
    F. Quinidine
    G. Polymyxin
    H. Sodium lactate
    I. Gin and tonic
    J. ACTH

11. THE THYMUS:
    A. Is usually abnormal in myasthenia, most often showing hyperplasia
    B. Is a vestigial organ, of little importance, atrophying at puberty
    C. Is vital to the development of normal immunological competence
    D. During fetal life contains cells resembling striated muscle
    E. May elaborate a hormone, which stimulates immunological maturation

12. THE PROPONENTS OF THE AUTOIMMUNE ETIOLOGY OF MYASTHENIA POINT TO:
    A. The frequency of thymic pathology
    B. The common occurrence of myasthenia in families
    C. The occasional association, in the same patient, of myasthenia and other possible autoimmune diseases such as lupus erythematosus
    D. The possibility that transient neonatal myasthenia may represent passive transplacental antibody transfer
    E. The binding of antimuscle antibodies to the neuromuscular junction, the site of pathology in myasthenia

13. WHAT PERCENTAGE OF MYASTHENICS HAVE THYROTOXICOSIS?
    A. 1%
    B. 5%
    C. 25%
    D. None of these

ANSWERS AND DISCUSSION:

1. C   The ptosis, diplopia, easy fatigability, ophthalmoparesis and extremity weakness, with normal reflexes and sensation, are all typical features of myasthenia gravis.

2.   A. True, B. False, C. True, D. True, E. True
        In addition to these differential points, ophthalmoplegia is not a feature of amyotrophic lateral sclerosis or polymyositis and is uncommon in infectious polyneuritis and muscular dystrophy.

3. D   The improvement in strength in generalized myasthenia gravis with the injection of edrophonium is often impressive and striking. This response is virtually specific for myasthenia gravis.

4. C   Thymomas occur in about twenty-five percent of myasthenic individuals over age thirty-five. Thirty-three to seventy-five percent of patients with thymoma have myasthenia gravis.

CASE STUDY #14

5. C

6. False   Although improvement may be considerable, anticholinesterase therapy hardly ever completely restores the myasthenic patient to full strength.

7. True   Both ACTH and adrenal corticosteroids have been effective in the treatment of myasthenia. Both, however, may induce initial worsening followed by later improvement. Beginning steroids at low dosage and then gradually increasing the dose may diminish or eliminate the initial worsening. A myasthenic patient, especially with bulbar or respiratory involvement, should be hospitalized before beginning steroid treatment.

8. C

9. E   Some clinicians do not routinely tracheostomize myasthenic patients with only mild weakness. (19, 20)

10. ABCEF   Quinine in the tonic water of a gin and tonic may increase myasthenic GHIJ   weakness. Ephedrine has been helpful as an adjunctive drug in myasthenia.

11. ACDE

12. ACD   Familial myasthenia occurs but is rare. The antimuscle antibody has recently been found to bind to the sarcoplasmic reticulum surrounding the I-band of the sarcomere. It does not specifically accumulate at the neuromuscular junction, which is the presumed site of pathology in myasthenia gravis, suggesting that this antibody is not significant in causing the disease. Perhaps, as with anti-liver antibodies seen after carbon tetrachloride poisoning, or anti-heart antibodies following myocardial infarction or cardiac surgery, they result from tissue injury due to another cause. Thus the presence of autoantibodies is not proof that a disease is "auto-immune."

13. B

REFERENCES

1. Drachman, D., Myasthenia Gravis and the Thyroid Gland, New Eng J Med 266:330, 1962.

2. Head, J.M., Respiratory Failure after Thymectomy for Myasthenia Gravis, Ann Surg 160:123, 1964.

3. Namba, T., et al., Lymphocytes of Patients with Myasthenia Gravis, Arch Neur 21:285, 1969.

4. Osserman, K.E., Myasthenia Gravis, Grune and Stratton, New York, 1958.

5. Van de Velde, R.L., and N. Friedman, The Thymic "Myoidzellen" and Myasthenia Gravis, JAMA 198:287, 1966.

6. Wolf, S., et al., Myasthenia as an Autoimmune Disease, Ann New York Acad Sci 135:517, 1966.

7. Wolf, S.M., The Relationship between Thymoma and Myasthenia Gravis, Bull Los Angeles Neuro Soc 31:107, 1966.

CASE STUDY #14

8. Wolf, S.M., and H.S. Barrows, Myasthenia Gravis and Systemic Lupus Erythematosus, Arch Neurology 14:254, 1966.

9. Papatestas, A.E., et al., Studies in Myasthenia Gravis, Effects of Thymectomy, Am J Med 50:465, 1971.

10. Namba, T., et al., Familial Myasthenia Gravis, Arch Neurology 25:49, 1971.

11. Namba, T., and D. Grob, Effect of Serum and Serum Globulin of Patients with Myasthenia Gravis on Neuromuscular Transmission, Neurology 19:173, 1969.

12. McQuillen, M., et al., Myasthenic Syndrome Associated with Antibiotics, Arch Neurol 18:402, 1968.

13. Warmolts, J., and W.K. Engel, Benefit from Alternate Day Prednisone in Myasthenia Gravis, New Eng J Med 286:17, 1972.

14. Flacke, W., Treatment of Myasthenia Gravis, New Eng J Med 288:27, 1973.

15. Armstrong, R., Thymic Lymphocyte Function in Myasthenia Gravis, Neurology 23:1078, 1973.

16. Rosenberg, R., and J. Campbell, Myasthenia Gravis, Calif Med 118:18, 1973.

17. Seybold, M., and D. Drachman, Gradually Increasing Prednisone in Myasthenia Gravis, New Eng J Med 290:81, 1974.

18. Myasthenia Gravis, Combined Clinical Staff Conference, NINDS, Ann Int Med 81:225-246, 1974.

19. Loach, et al., Postoperative Management after Thymectomy, Brit Med J 1:309, 1975.

20. Genkins, G., et al., Studies in Myasthenia Gravis, Am J Med 58:517, 1975.

CASE STUDY #15

Wrist Drop in an Alcoholic

HISTORY: A 43 year-old man, with a history of heavy alcoholic intake, was referred for neurological evaluation because of a "stroke." He awoke one morning unable to straighten out his wrist. There was no pain, neck aching, visual, sensory, or other neurological symptoms. The night previously, he had drunk a whole bottle of whiskey and had fallen asleep in a chair.

EXAMINATION: When the right arm was held out, the hand dropped down (wrist drop) and he could not extend the fingers or the hand (Fig. 12). If the wrist was straightened by the examiner, adduction and abduction of the fingers, wrist flexion, and the grip were all seen to be of normal strength. The remainder of the neurological examination was normal except for a small patch of sensory loss present over the dorsum of the right thumb.

CASE STUDY #15

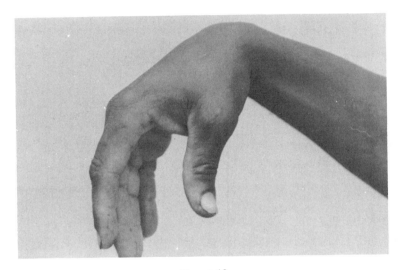

Figure 12

QUESTIONS:

1. THE LESION IS:
    A. In the opposite internal capsule
    B. In the spinal cord at the C 7-8 segmental level
    C. In the brachial plexus, since extension of both the wrist and fingers are impaired
    D. In the peripheral nerve, since other muscles innervated by the same spinal segments are not affected, and all the muscles which are weak are innervated by one peripheral nerve
    E. In the muscles, representing probably an acute distal myositis

2. THE STRUCTURE INVOLVED IS THE:
    A. Median nerve
    B. Lower trunk of the brachial plexus
    C. Pyramidal tract
    D. Radial nerve
    E. Ulnar nerve

3. IT MOST LIKELY WAS DAMAGED BY:
    A. Metabolic causes
    B. Compression
    C. Avitaminosis
    D. None of the above

CASE STUDY #15

4.   LESIONS OF THE BRACHIAL PLEXUS TYPICALLY CAUSE:
      A.   Babinski signs
      B.   Weakness of muscles innervated by more than one peripheral nerve
      C.   A glove type of hypalgesia
      D.   A dissociation between pin and touch sensation

5.   A SEGMENTAL LESION OF THE SPINAL CORD WOULD PROBABLY BE
      ASSOCIATED WITH:
      A.   Babinski signs
      B.   Weakness of muscles innervated by more than one peripheral nerve
      C.   Decreased sensation below the level of the lesion due to damage to
           the long sensory tracts
      D.   All of the above

6.   USEFUL TESTS IN THIS PATIENT'S EVALUATION MIGHT INCLUDE:
      A.   Electromyogram
      B.   Myelography
      C.   2 hour postprandial sugar
      D.   All of the above

LABORATORY DATA AND COURSE: Laboratory tests were normal except for
evidence of cirrhosis of the liver. The wrist was splinted in physiologic neutral
position and normal strength returned in about three weeks.

QUESTION:

7.   IN ADDITION TO TRAUMA, OTHER CAUSES OF ACUTE MONONEURO-
      PATHIES INCLUDE:
      A.   Diabetes mellitus
      B.   Cancer
      C.   "Collagen disease"
      D.   All of the above

ANSWERS AND DISCUSSION:

1. D

2. D   This patient has impaired function of the radial nerve, which
                 innervates the wrist and finger extensors and supplies sensation
                 to the dorsum of the thumb. A lesion of the corticospinal tract
                 in the internal capsule would produce the usual signs of contra-
                 lateral spastic paresis with hyperreflexia, pathological toe
                 signs etc.

3. B   This condition, called "Saturday night palsy," is fairly frequently
                 seen in alcoholics who, in a drunken sleep, with little change of
                 position, compress the radial nerve as it courses in the upper
                 arm against a hard surface.

4. B

5. D   The neurologic signs would depend on the extent and severity of
                 the lesion.

6. AC

7. D

REFERENCE

Merritt, H. H., A Textbook of Neurology, 5th Ed.,Lea and Febiger, Philadelphia,
1973.

CASE STUDY #16

Occipital Headache and Papilledema in a Twenty-nine Year-Old Man

HISTORY: A 29 year-old Mexican man suffered from headaches for three years prior to admission. These were occipital, aching, and worse with coughing or straining at stool. The headaches became increasingly frequent and severe, sometimes arousing him from sleep. They were sometimes associated with nausea and vomiting.

QUESTION:

1.   THE DESCRIPTION OF THE HEAD PAIN SUGGESTS:
     A.   Tic douloureux
     B.   Muscle contraction (tension) headaches
     C.   Sinus headache
     D.   None of the above

On the day of admission, he was found sitting in bed, holding his head in his hands, and complaining of violent headache. He was confused, had bitten his tongue, had been incontinent of urine, and had no memory of the events of the previous hour. There was no history of hearing loss, tinnitus, diplopia, dysphagia, dysarthria, numbness, weakness, cough or weight loss. Past medical history was unremarkable. There was no family history of diabetes, cancer, or tuberculosis.

EXAMINATION: He was afebrile, and there was no nuchal rigidity or adenopathy. Heart and lungs were normal. Bilateral papilledema was present. Horizontal nystagmus was present when he looked to either side. The neurological examination was otherwise normal. Examination of the visual fields showed enlarged blind spots. He was placed on anticonvulsant medications.

QUESTIONS:

2.   HEADACHE, VOMITING, AND PAPILLEDEMA ARE EVIDENCE OF INCREASED INTRACRANIAL PRESSURE. IT IS ALSO TRUE THAT:
     A.   A unilateral weakness of the lateral rectus muscle would lateralize the lesion to that side
     B.   Unilateral weakness of the lateral rectus muscle would not be of localizing value, as it may accompany increased intracranial pressure of many causes
     C.   Skull films might show erosion of the dorsum sella
     D.   The intracranial lesion is on the same side as the eye with the more severe papilledema
     E.   The increase in the size of the blind spots seen on the visual field examination results from swollen optic nerve heads

3.   OCCIPITAL HEADACHE, NYSTAGMUS, AND PAPILLEDEMA SUGGEST:
     A.   A subfrontal tumor
     B.   A posterior fossa tumor
     C.   Multiple lesions
     D.   Nothing definitely localizing

4.   MAJOR MOTOR SEIZURES:
     A.   May occasionally be seen with disease in the posterior fossa
     B.   Rule out a cerebellar tumor
     C.   A and B
     D.   None of the above

CASE STUDY #16

5. IN EVALUATING THIS PATIENT, USEFUL STUDIES MIGHT INCLUDE:
    A. Skull films
    B. Electroencephalogram
    C. Brain scan
    D. Computerized Tomography (EMI Scan)
    E. All of the above

6. A LUMBAR PUNCTURE IN THE PRESENCE OF INCREASED INTRA-
    CRANIAL PRESSURE:
    A. Is always contraindicated
    B. Carries a risk of precipitating uncal or cerebellar tonsillar
       herniation
    C. If done at all, should be done with a small gauge needle to decrease
       the size of the hole in the dura, and just enough fluid obtained for the
       studies necessary
    D. In general should only be done if there is some information to be
       gained which cannot be obtained another way as, for instance, the
       possibility of infection of the central nervous system
    E. Will always show that the pressure is elevated, even without a
       manometer, since the fluid will spurt out more rapidly than normal

LABORATORY: Skull and chest films and a brain scan were normal. The
electroencephalogram showed a small amount of bi-occipital slowing. Carotid
angiography showed bilateral dilation of the lateral ventricles. Ventriculography
with pantopaque (Fig. 13) showed a large mass in the right cerebellar hemisphere
displacing the aqueduct to the left and kinking it forward. Blood UDRL was
negative.

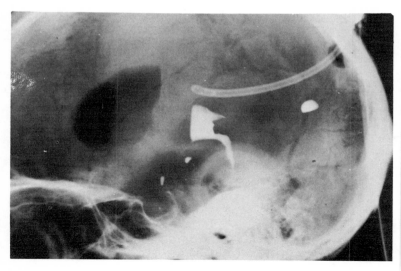

Figure 13

CASE STUDY #13

QUESTION:

7. THE MORE FREQUENTLY ENCOUNTERED CEREBELLAR TUMORS
   INCLUDE:
   A. Astrocytoma
   B. Hemangioblastoma
   C. Cysticercosis
   D. Medulloblastoma
   E. Metastases
   F. All of the above

COURSE: At craniotomy, the cerebellar hemispheres were seen to be bulging.
A solid, very hard avascular yellowish tumor was found two cm below the surface
of the right cerebellar hemisphere. It measured 2.5 x 3 cm, was easily removed
and found to be irregular and lobulated.

PATHOLOGY: In the center of the tumor, caseous necrosis was seen. Surrounding
this was a zone of granulomatous inflammation with epithelioid, round and giant cells,
the typical picture of a tuberculoma(Fig.14A and B), although no organisms could be
demonstrated.

COURSE: He was begun on isoniazid, streptomycin, and para amino salicylic
acid, and steadily improved, with disappearance of the headaches and papilledema.

COMMENT: This case illustrates the importance of including the granulomas in
the differential diagnosis of intracranial mass lesions. The tumor was most
likely tuberculous. The histopathology was typical, and there was no evidence of
syphilis, fungus or parasitic disease.

QUESTIONS:

TRUE OR FALSE:

8. Although now greatly outnumbered by the gliomas, in the last century
   tuberculomas were the most common form of intracranial tumor in
   children.

9. Rare now in the United States, intracranial tuberculomas represent up to
   20% of brain tumors in other countries.

10. In about one third of patients with intracranial tuberculomas there is no
    history of, nor evidence of, tuberculosis elsewhere in the body.

11. In the absence of tuberculous meningitis or extracranial infection, fever
    is rare with tuberculoma of the brain.

12. The spinal fluid is usually pathognomonic of an intracranial tuberculoma.

13. In the absence of tuberculous meningitis or extraneural infection, intra-
    cranial tuberculomas cannot usually be distinguished from intracranial
    neoplasms prior to surgery.

14. The treatment of choice for intracranial tuberculoma is surgical excision,
    with drug therapy in doses equivalent to those used in tuberculous menin-
    gitis.

CASE STUDY #16

Figure 14A

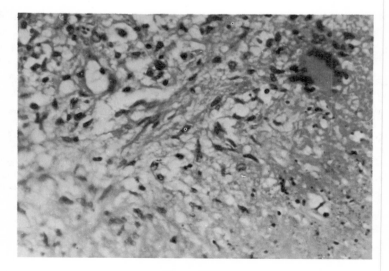

Figure 14B

CASE STUDY #16

ANSWERS AND DISCUSSION:

1. D   The pain of trigeminal neuralgia is sharp, lancinating, momentary and in the distribution of the fifth cranial nerve. Muscle contraction "tension" headaches are usually occipital or bifrontal and sometimes described as feeling like a band tied around the head. This type of headache does not interrupt sleep. Headache due to sinusitis would not be occipitally located.

2. BCE   Asymmetry of papilledema does not help in lateralizing a cerebral mass lesion.

3. B   The absence of abnormalities of cranial nerve function suggest that this posterior fossa tumor is in the cerebellum rather than in the brain stem.

4. A   Grand mal seizures are typical signatures of disease of the cerebral hemispheres, but are said by Merritt to occur in five percent of cases of cerebellar tumor. In this case one cannot exclude the possibility of coexisting cerebral disease.

5. E

6. BCD   The practice of gauging an increase in intracranial pressure by the rapidity of the fluid emerging through the needle is grossly inaccurate and misleading. The needle tip may, for example, be lodged against a nerve root, causing a slow spinal fluid drip.

7. ABDE

8. True

9. True

10. True

11. True

12. False   Cerebrospinal fluid findings are similar to those in other types of intracranial tumors with an increased protein level, and usually normal cell count.

13. True

14. True   The frequency of spontaneous healing of tuberculomas of the brain is not known, but is probably uncommon. Prior to the use of antituberculous drugs, removal of a tuberculoma almost invariably resulted in death with tuberculous meningitis. Surgical excision, with use of isoniazid, streptomycin, rifampin and ethambutol in doses equivalent to those used in tuberculous meningitis is now the treatment of choice. The overall mortality is about twenty two percent.

REFERENCES

1.   Greenfield's Neuropathology, Blackwood, W., W.H. McMenemey, A. Meyer, R.M. Norman, and D.S. Russell, Williams and Wilkins Co., 2nd Ed., 1963.

2.   Sibley, W.A., and J.L. O'Brien, Intracranial Tuberculomas; A review of Clinical Features and Treatment, Neurology 6:157, 1956.

CASE STUDY #16

3. Ramamurthi, B., and M.G. Varadarajan, Diagnosis of Tuberculomas of the Brain, J Neurosurgery 18:1, 1961.

4. Schwartz, M., R.A. Gilman, J.S. Robey, J. Settle, and L.E. Paddock, Tuberculomas of the Central Nervous System, Review and Report of Four Cases Successfully Managed with Surgery and Chemotherapy, Ann Int Med 42:1076, 1955.

5. Clinicopathological Conference, New Eng J Med 289:366, 1973.

6. Steiner, P., C. Portugaleza, Tuberculous Meningitis in Children, Am Rev of Respiratory Dis 107:22, 1973.

7. Petito, F., F. Plum, The Lumbar Puncture, New Eng J Med 290:225, 1974.

8. Wolinsky, E., New Antituberculosis Drugs and Concepts of Prophylaxis, Med Clin N Am 58:697, 1974.

9. Jacques, S., Supratentorial Tuberculoma, Bull LA Neurol Soc 39:56, 1974.

CASE STUDY #17

Proximal Extremity Weakness in an Alcoholic

HISTORY: This 45 year-old male was hospitalized because of recurrent weakness. The patient has been a heavy drinker, drinking about a fifth per day of hard liquor since his youth. Over the last several years he has noted muscle weakness which has been intermittent but progressive. These attacks last 3-4 days on the average. At times this weakness gets so severe that he is unable to rise out of a chair or comb his hair. At other times the weakness seems to be minimal. Weakness frequently is associated with muscle tenderness and pain. Weakness and pain seem to be exacerbated during periods when the patient is also vomiting. These vomiting episodes occur every few months.

In the few weeks PTA the patient has been following his usual drinking habits. About three days PTA he began to have marked increase in his muscle weakness as well as recurrent vomiting.

During a severe attack of vomiting, with upper abdominal pain radiating through the back in 1966, he was hospitalized and treated with nasogastric suction. Since that time he has complained of large, bulky, foul-smelling, foamy, floating stools. Subsequent to his attack of pancreatitis he has had numerous episodes of severe vomiting without recurrence of abdominal pain, often associated with an exacerbation of his muscle weakness and pain. The patient has been transfused for anemia, had ulcer disease at one time, and had surgery for hemorrhoids. Patient has no allergies.

Mother has diabetes and heart disease. No evidence of neuromuscular disorder of any type.

QUESTIONS:

1.   WHICH OF THE FOLLOWING ARE CONSIDERED NEUROLOGIC CONSEQUENCES OF CHRONIC ALCOHOLISM?
     A. Peripheral neuropathy
     B. Myopathy
     C. Cerebellar degeneration
     D. Seizure disorder
     E. All of the above

CASE STUDY #17

2.   WHICH OF THE FOLLOWING NEUROLOGIC DISORDERS RESULT IN
     EPISODIC WEAKNESS?:
     A. Multiple sclerosis
     B. Myasthenia gravis
     C. Duchenne muscular dystrophy
     D. Hypokalemic periodic paralysis
     E. Charcot-Marie-Tooth disease

EXAMINATION: B. P. 130/100; T. 99.8°; P. 88; R. 20.   Patient appeared to be
in no acute distress.   There was marked arcus cornealis.   Fundi showed
arteriolar narrowing with slight tortuosity and mild venous distention.   EOM's
intact.   Lungs were clear.   PMI was displaced slightly to the left.   The first
sound was intermittently split.   There was an occasional dropped beat.   There
was no organomegaly.

Mental status and cranial nerves were unremarkable.   There was generalized
weakness of all muscle groups.   Proximal muscle groups were weaker than distal,
and flexors weaker than extensors.   There was atrophy of the shoulder girdle
muscles and small muscles of the hand as well as marked atrophy of the biceps.
There was lesser generalized atrophy in the lower extremities.   No fasciculations
were seen.   Tone was normal.   There was no evidence of cerebellar deficit.
Vibratory sense was decreased in the right lower extremity below the ankle.
Sensation to pin prick was normal.   Position sense was normal.   The deep tendon
reflexes were absent throughout except for a 2+ patellar on the right and 1+ on the
left.   There were no pathological reflexes.

LABORATORY DATA: BUN 29, 44; Creatinine 1.3; K 4.5, 4.2; Na 132, 136;
Hgb 12.3, 12.2.   Myoglobin negative in urine; total bilirubin 2.4; direct bilirubin 0.8.   SGOT 1009; CPK 712.   Albumin 3.4; globulin 3.6; Urinalysis revealed
2+ protein.   Anti DNA negative.

QUESTIONS:

3.   THE PHYSICAL FINDINGS IN THIS PATIENT ARE MOST SUGGESTIVE
     OF:
     A. Myelopathy
     B. Peripheral neuropathy
     C. Myasthenia gravis
     D. Myopathy
     E. None of the above

4.   THE COMBINATION OF PROXIMAL WEAKNESS AND ATROPHY AND
     HIGH SERUM ENZYMES IN THIS PATIENT IS MOST SUGGESTIVE OF:
     A. Alcoholic myopathy
     B. Myasthenia gravis
     C. Myotonia congenita
     D. Periodic paralysis
     E. None of the above

5.   TRUE OR FALSE:
     A. Electromyographic fibrillations may be seen in myopathy
     B. CPK is primarily located within muscle fibers
     C. Myoglobinuria results from the rapid, widespread breakdown of muscle
         fibers
     D. Alcoholic myopathy is probably due to Vitamin B deficiency
     E. A muscle biopsy is indicated in this case

CASE STUDY #17

ANSWERS AND DISCUSSION:

1. E   Most of the effects of chronic alcoholism on the central nervous system and the motor unit are presumably due to vitamin B-1 deficiency. Some evidence, however, suggests that other vitamin deficiencies may be involved as well as the possibility of a direct toxic effect of the alcohol. Most prominent is the peripheral neuropathy which is frequently accompanied by painful burning dysesthesia and is usually more evident in the lower extremities than the uppers. Not infrequently, peripheral neuropathy may be associated with cerebellar degeneration. The latter is caused by a progressive and sometimes severe fall-out of Purkinje cells in the cerebellar cortex. The myopathy of alcoholism was initially reported in a group of acutely intoxicated patients with rapid onset of quadriparesis, muscle tenderness, increased serum enzymes and myoglobinuria. Subsequently, a more chronic form, with slowly progressive pelvic and shoulder girdle weakness and atrophy, has been described. Pathologic studies have shown scattered fiber necrosis, central nuclei, phagocytosis and a few inflammatory changes. Alcoholic myopathy appears not to be due to vitamin deficiency or malnutrition, per se, but rather to some direct toxic effect of alcohol on the muscle fiber.

Seizure disorder is a frequent occurrence in chronic alcoholism, especially during the withdrawal state. Thus all of these neurologic complications can be seen in the chronic alcoholic and not infrequently simultaneously.

2. ABD   Multiple sclerosis is a disorder characterized by exacerbations and remissions, except in the older age group where a slowly progressive course may occur. In fact, in a younger person, one should be very wary of making a diagnosis of MS without a history that has had at least two clear-cut episodes. Myasthenia gravis is a disease of the neuromuscular junction affecting all striated muscle, but especially the bulbar musculature. Frequent fluctuations in the degree of weakness is to be expected in the affected patient, although the episodes rarely begin abruptly. The degree of weakness in any one muscle may vary from day to day or even hour to hour. Hypokalemic periodic paralysis in its early stages typically presents with attacks of flaccid weakness, often occurring shortly after arising in the morning. These episodes remit spontaneously if untreated, but disappear much more rapidly when exogenous potassium supplement is given. In contradistinction to these episodic disorders, the weakness of Duchenne muscular dystrophy and Charcot-Marie-Tooth Disease is relentlessly progressive without significant improvement at any time.

3. D   Presence of atrophy and weakness which is symmetrical and more marked proximally than distally, is characteristic of a myopathic disorder.

4. A   The high serum enzymes in this patient suggest that widespread, rather acute muscle necrosis is occurring. Actual breakdown of muscle fibers to any significant degree is unusual in myasthenia gravis, myotonia congenita and any of the periodic paralyses. Thus the most likely diagnosis here is that of alcoholic myopathy.

5.   A. True; B. True; C. True; D. False; E. True
Fibrillations are hallmarks of denervating disease. Rarely, however, they may be seen in myopathic processes. They are especially prominent in active, acute polymyositis, but may also be seen in such disorders as Duchenne muscular dystrophy.

CASE STUDY #17

The creatine phosphokinase, because it is primarily located within muscle, is an extremely helpful indicator of muscle fiber destruction. CPK can also be elevated in hypothyroidism and, on rare occasions, if there is massive central nervous system infarction. Myoglobinuria is a non-specific phenomenon which may occur whenever there is enough muscle fiber breakdown to liberate sufficient myoglobin to cause visible discoloration of the urine. Myoglobinuria should not be thought of as a specific disease entity but rather as a symptom which can occur in the setting of any severe acute insult to the muscle fiber. A proper muscle biopsy should be carried out in any patient who has undiagnosed motor unit disease. An interesting, but as yet unexplained, metabolic abnormality occurs in the acute phase of alcoholic myopathy in most patients. This is the inability to produce lactic acid with ischemic exercise of the forearm. This occasionally occurs between attacks of myopathy when the patient is asymptomatic, but is most prominent during an acute attack. Normally an individual should double or triple his resting serum lactic acid if he exercises the forearm to exhaustion in the ischemic condition. In alcoholic myopathy, negligible elevation, if at all, is the rule. The exact reason for this is not clear and studies have shown a normal amount of glycogen within these muscle fibers and at best, only equivocal reduction of muscle phosphorylase activity. Most cases of alcohol myopathy respond satisfactorily to bedrest and supportive care. Intravenous vitamins do not alter the clinical course.

REFERENCES

1. Perkoff, G. , Alcoholic Myopathy, Ann Rev Med 22:125, 1971.

2. Song, S. , and E. Rubin, Ethanol Produces Muscle Damage in Human Volunteers, Science 175:327, 1972.

3. Munsat, T. , et al. , Experimental Acute Alcoholic Myopathy, Neurology 23:407, 1973.

4. Chui, L. , et al. , Tubular Aggregates in Subclinical Alcoholic Myopathy. Neurology 25:405, 1975.

CASE STUDY #18

Progressive Distal Weakness of the Extremities

HISTORY: A 56 year-old male noted the gradual onset of progressive weakness and numbness of both legs. Several months later, similar symptoms developed in the arms. There was no history of diabetes or alcoholism.

EXAMINATION: General physical examination was normal. All extremities were weak, predominantly distally. The deep tendon reflexes were symmetrically depressed. Plantar responses were flexor. There was a glove and stocking hypalgesia. Perception of vibration and position were impaired in the lower extremities. The cranial nerves were normal.

CASE STUDY #18

QUESTIONS:

1.   DISTAL WEAKNESS OF THE EXTREMITIES, DECREASED DEEP TENDON
     REFLEXES, AND GLOVE AND STOCKING HYPALGESIA CHARACTERIZE:
     A.   Brain stem disease
     B.   Spinal cord disease
     C.   Neuropathy
     D.   Myopathy
     E.   Either B or C

2.   CAUSES OF THIS SYNDROME INCLUDE:
     A.   Diabetes mellitus
     B.   Vitamin deficiency
     C.   Porphyria
     D.   "Collagen" disease
     E.   Uremia
     F.   All of the above

LABORATORY DATA: Normal or negative studies included complete blood count,
urinalysis, blood sugar, urine arsenic, thallium, mercury, lead, sedimentation
rate, LE preparation, urine porphobilinogen, protein bound iodine, Schilling test,
serum protein electrophoresis, chest film. Spinal fluid protein was 56mgm%;
cell count was normal.

QUESTION:

3.   THE ELECTROMYOGRAM WOULD PROBABLY SHOW:
     A.   Fibrillation and motor units of increased size
     B.   Fasciculations and motor unit potentials of decreased size
     C.   Electrical silence distally in the extremities
     D.   Myotonia
     E.   None of the above

COURSE: Because of the otherwise unexplained neuropathy, a search was made
for an occult malignancy.

X-rays of the sacrum revealed a scalloped erosion (Fig. 15). At surgery, an
encapsulated, yellow, hemorrhagic tumor was removed, which was histologically
a plasmacytoma. No other bony lesions were seen on X-ray and the bone marrow
showed no increase in plasma cells. A course of radiotherapy was given postoperatively. Strength and sensation gradually began to improve following removal
of the tumor. He had preoperatively been confined to a wheelchair, but became
fully ambulatory and remains so four years later, with impressive improvement
in all neurological functions.

This case is an example of a "remote" effect of malignancy - in this case a
plasmacytoma - on the peripheral nervous system.

QUESTIONS:

4.   CANCER MAY AFFECT THE NERVOUS SYSTEM IN MANY WAYS, THE
     MOST COMMON OF WHICH IS:
     A.   Metastasis
     B.   Vascular disease
     C.   Infections as with fungi, herpes zoster, etc.
     D.   Metabolic

CASE STUDY #18

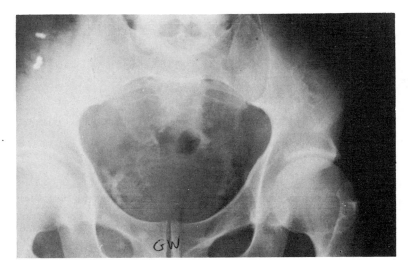

Figure 15

5.   THE VASCULAR COMPLICATIONS OF CANCER WHICH AFFECT THE
     CENTRAL NERVOUS SYSTEM INCLUDE:
     A.   Nonbacterial endocarditis with cerebral emboli
     B.   Tumor emboli
     C.   Intracranial hemorrhage,either within the tumor or as a result of
          blood dyscrasia (as low platelets from marrow invasion)
     D.   Accelerated atherosclerosis
     E.   B and C

6.   ELECTROLYTE ABNORMALITIES ASSOCIATED WITH CANCER CAN
     PRODUCE SEVERE DISTURBANCES OF NERVOUS SYSTEM FUNCTION.
     THUS LETHARGY OR COMA MAY OCCUR WITH HYPERCALCEMIA
     WHICH MAY RESULT EITHER FROM BONE METASTASES OR FROM THE
     PRODUCTION BY THE TUMOR OF A SUBSTANCE SIMILAR TO
     PARATHYROID HORMONE. HYPONATREMIA, WHICH CAN PRODUCE
     SEIZURES AND STUPOR, MAY OCCUR AS THE RESULT OF
     INAPPROPRIATE PRODUCTION OF:
     A.   ACTH
     B.   ADH
     C.   Aldosterone
     D.   None of the above

CASE STUDY #18

7. THERE IS ALSO A GROUP OF SYNDROMES OF UNKNOWN ETIOLOGY ASSOCIATED WITH NON-METASTATIC CANCER WHICH AFFECT THE NERVOUS SYSTEM, AS ILLUSTRATED BY THIS CASE. NUTRITIONAL, VIRAL, AND IMMUNOLOGIC ETIOLOGIES HAVE BEEN POSTULATED. THESE SYNDROMES INCLUDE:
   A. Dementia
   B. Multifocal leukoencephalopathy
   C. Cerebellar degeneration
   D. Myelopathy
   E. Neuropathy
   F. Tabes dorsalis
   G. Myasthenic syndrome
   H. Myopathy
   I. All except F

8. THE NEUROLOGICAL DISEASE ASSOCIATED WITH NON-METASTATIC CANCER:
   A. Always improves with treatment of the tumor
   B. May preceed the discovery of the neoplasm by months or years
   C. Both of the above
   D. Neither of the above

9. A VIRAL ETIOLOGY IN AT LEAST ONE OF THESE CONDITIONS IS SUGGESTED BY THE FINDING OF INTRANUCLEAR INCLUSIONS RESEMBLING POLYOMA VIRUS SEEN IN THE OLIGODENDROGLIA IN:
   A. Cerebral cortical degeneration
   B. Cerebellar degeneration
   C. Multifocal leukoencephalopathy
   D. All of the above

10. THE PERCENTAGE OF PATIENTS WITH CANCER WHO HAVE NEUROLOGIC DISEASE NOT ASSOCIATED WITH METASTASES IS ABOUT:
    A. 0.05%
    B. 1%
    C. 7%
    D. 65%

11. THE MOST COMMON OF THESE "DISTANT" NEUROLOGICAL SYNDROMES ASSOCIATED WITH CANCER IS:
    A. Neuromyopathy
    B. Dementia
    C. Myelopathy
    D. Myasthenic syndrome
    E. None of the above

12. THE CHANCE OF FINDING AN OCCULT CANCER IN A MALE OVER 50 WHO DEVELOPS PROXIMAL WEAKNESS IS:
    A. Less than 1%
    B. Greater than 20%

CASE STUDY #18

13. THE "MYASTHENIC SYNDROME" ASSOCIATED WITH CANCER OF THE LUNG DIFFERS FROM MYASTHENIA GRAVIS IN THAT:
   A. The myasthenic syndrome responds poorly to anticholinesterase drugs, though excessive sensitivity to curare is seen in both
   B. The patient with the myasthenic syndrome shows initial weakness with improvement in strength after repeated rapid muscle contractions, whereas the patient with myasthenia gravis shows maximal strength with the initial contraction, rapidly fatiguing with repeated effort
   C. The most common tumor in association with myasthenia gravis is thymoma; with the myasthenic syndrome it is lung cancer
   D. The deep tendon reflexes in myasthenia gravis are normal, whereas they are often decreased in the myasthenic syndrome
   E. All of the above

14. IN A CASE OF "CARCINOMATOUS" NEUROPATHY ONE WOULD EXPECT:
   A. Elevation of spinal fluid protein
   B. Spinal fluid pleocytosis
   C. Slowing of nerve conduction velocities
   D. Electromyographic evidence of denervation
   E. All of the above

   TRUE OR FALSE:

15. Remission of a neuropathy rules out underlying malignancy.

16. Mononeuropathy can occur with nonmetastatic cancer.

17. Steroids have no value in the treatment of dermatomyositis associated with cancer.

18. Vincristine, an anticancer drug, can cause a mixed sensorimotor neuropathy.

19. "Carcinomatous" neuropathy is most common with cancer of the lung.

   ANSWERS AND DISCUSSION:

1. C   This description is the classical pattern of a peripheral poly-neuropathy. Occasionally an acute polyneuropathy, as in the Guillain-Barré syndrome, may produce primarily proximal weakness.

   In most forms of myopathy, the weakness is mainly proximal. Myotonic muscular dystrophy is a prominent exception to this rule with predominantly distal weakness. Sensation is unaffected in the myopathies.

   The sensory abnormalities associated with disease of the spinal cord include either evidence of damage to specific long sensory tracts or a sensory level, below which sensation is impaired, due to a segmental cord lesion. An example of the former is combined system disease of pernicious anemia, in which the damage to the posterior columns produces decreased perception of touch, position and vibration. An example of the latter would be multiple sclerosis, or a spinal cord tumor. The deep tendon reflexes in spinal cord disease are usually increased due to damage to the corticospinal tracts.

   One theory of why, in peripheral neuropathy, the weakness and sensory loss is distal, is that the neuron manufactures nutrient substances which are transported down the nerve. In diseases of the nerve, the regions

CASE STUDY #18

furthest from the neuron, with the longest "supply line" might be affected initially and primarily.

2. F

3. A   Fibrillations are spontaneous contractions of individual muscle fibers which occur following denervation of the muscle. These contractions are not visible to the naked eye.

Motor units of increased size may be seen with lesions of the lower motor neuron or of the nerve. The explanation is thought to be that, after death of the axon supplying a motor unit, reinnervation of that muscle occurs with a regenerating branch of an adjacent axon. The resultant new motor unit is thus larger than normal size.

4. A	8. B	12. B	16. True
5. ABC	9. C	13. E	17. False
6. B	10. C	14. ACD	18. True
7. I	11. A	15. False	19. True

REFERENCES

1. Rubenstein, M.K., Carcinomatous Neuromyopathy, Calif Med 110:482, 1969.

2. Layzer, R.B., Cancer and the Nervous System, Calif Med 110:517, 1969.

3. Victor, M., B.Q. Banker, and R.D. Adams, The Neuropathy of Multiple Myeloma, J Neurol Neurosurg Psychiat 21:73, 1958.

4. Davidson, S., Solitary Myeloma with Peripheral Polyneuropathy, Calif Med 116:68, 1972.

5. Patten, J., Remittent Peripheral Neuropathy and Cerebellar Degeneration Complicating Lymphosarcoma, Neurology 21:189, 1971.

6. Walsh, J., The Neuropathy of Multiple Myeloma, Arch Neurol 25:404, 1971.

7. Walsh, J., Neuropathy Associated with Lymphoma, J Neurol Neurosurg Psychiat 34:42, 1971.

8. Posner, J., Neurological Complications of Systemic Cancer, Med Clin N Am 55:625, 1971.

9. McKendall, R., and M. Cohen, The Remote Effects of Cancer on the Nervous System: A Review, Rush-Presbyterian St. Luke's Medical Bulletin 11:92, 1972.

10. Case Records of the Massachusetts General Hospital, New Eng J Med 287: 138, 1972.

11. Satoyoshi, E., et al., Subacute Cerebellar Degeneration and Eaton Lambert Syndrome with Bronchogenic Carcinoma, Neurology 23:764, 1973.

12. Reagan, J., and H. Okazaki, Thrombotic Syndrome Associated with Carcinoma, Arch Neurol 31:390, 1974.

13. Cohen, H., and R. Rundles, Managing the Complications of Plasma Cell Myeloma, Arch Int Med 135:177, 1975.

CASE STUDY #19

Sudden Weakness of the Left Arm in a Middle-Aged Man

HISTORY: A 52 year-old man was well until three days prior to admission when he suddenly felt light headed and noted weakness of the left arm. The next morning the left leg also became weak. He denied headache, chest pain, cardiac palpitations, alterations of consciousness, visual changes. There was no history of venereal disease, diabetes, hypertension or trauma. Review of systems was unremarkable. He did not smoke. His father had died of "arteriosclerosis."

EXAMINATION: He was alert, well-developed, and cooperative. Vital signs were normal. The heart, lungs, carotid arteries, and the remainder of the general physical examination were normal. The deep tendon reflexes were increased in the left arm and leg, but the plantar responses were flexor. There was a left hemiparesis, more severe in the arm than the leg. Sensory examination was normal except for impaired ability to identify objects placed in the left hand. There was mild weakness of the lower left facial muscles. Neurological examination was otherwise normal.

QUESTIONS:

1.   THE CLINICAL STORY THUS FAR, WITH ABRUPT ONSET OF NEURO-
      LOGICAL DISEASE,SUGGESTED VASCULAR DISEASE. THE CLINICAL
      PICTURE SUGGESTS THE DIAGNOSIS OF:
      A. Transient ischemic attack
      B. Subarachnoid hemorrhage
      C. Either of the above
      D. Neither of the above

2.   THE WEAKNESS OF THE LOWER PART OF THE FACE, WITH GOOD
      PRESERVATION OF THE UPPER FACIAL MUSCLES,SUGGESTS THAT
      THE LESION:
      A. Is in the left facial nerve
      B. Is rostral to the caudal pons
      C. Is in the left facial nucleus
      D. Affects the left corticobulbar tract prior to crossing
      E. Affects the right corticobulbar tract prior to crossing

3.   INABILITY TO IDENTIFY AN OBJECT PLACED IN THE HAND AND
      MANIPULATED BY THE FINGERS, IN SPITE OF NORMAL PAIN,
      TOUCH AND POSITION SENSE IN THAT HAND,IN AN ALERT PATIENT
      WHO IS NOT CONFUSED,IS CALLED ASTEREOGNOSIS AND IS
      ASSOCIATED WITH A LESION IN THE CONTRALATERAL:
      A. Frontal lobe
      B. Parietal lobe
      C. Temporal lobe
      D. Occipital lobe

CASE STUDY #19

4.   SOME USEFUL TESTS TO OBTAIN AT THIS POINT WOULD INCLUDE:
      A.   Electromyography
      B.   Spinal tap
      C.   Brain scan
      D.   Skull films
      E.   All of the above

LABORATORY DATA: Normal tests included blood count, urinalysis, cholesterol, serology, serum triglycerides, glucose tolerance test, sedimentation rate, opthalmodynamometry, brain scan and visual fields, and electroencephalogram. Lumbar puncture revealed a protein of 20mgm%, no cells, a normal sugar and negative serology. The spinal fluid was under normal pressure. Skull and chest films were normal (Figure 16).

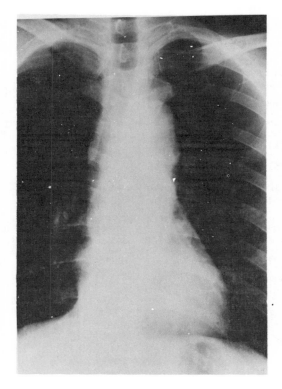

Figure 16

There was no progression of the neurological deficit for several days, and the clinical impression was that of a cerebral infarction-a completed stroke.

CASE STUDY #19

QUESTION:

5. THE MOST IMPORTANT TREATMENT TO BE GIVEN NOW WOULD BE:
    A. Anticoagulants
    B. Carbon dioxide inhalation
    C. Stellate ganglion block
    D. None of the above

A week later his left arm began to twitch. This shaking spread up the arm to the shoulder and then to the left leg, and lasted several minutes. There was no alteration of consciousness.

QUESTIONS:

6. THIS EPISODE IS MOST SUGGESTIVE OF A:
    A. TIA (transient ischemic attack)
    B. Jacksonian motor seizure
    C. Myoclonic seizure
    D. None of the above

7. IN THIS PATIENT, THE INITIAL SITE OF THE ABNORMAL CEREBRAL DISCHARGE IS:
    A. On the medial surface of the right hemisphere
    B. Over the convexity of the right hemisphere near the occipital lobe
    C. Over the convexity of the right hemisphere near the prefrontal gyrus of the frontal lobe
    D. None of the above

8. FOCAL ONSET AND "MARCH" OF THE SEIZURE ACTIVITY TO CONTIGUOUS AREAS OF THE BRAIN ARE THE CHARACTERISTICS OF JACKSONIAN SEIZURES. THE JACKSON REFERRED TO IS:
    A. Stonewall
    B. Andrew
    C. Hughlings
    D. None of the above

Because of the relative infrequency of Jacksonian seizures in cases of cerebral infarction, a right carotid angiogram was done. This showed some stretching of the arterial branches supplying the parietal lobe. A pneumoencephalogram was performed which suggested a parietal lobe mass. Craniotomy was performed. There appeared to be a softened area in the parietal lobe which was biopsied. The pathologic report was necrosis and gliosis, compatible with infarction. Postoperatively, the patient showed a left hemiplegia, hyper-reflexia, Babinski sign, anosognosia, and left sensory and visual extinction of double simultaneous stimuli. He gradually improved and was discharged with a moderate hemiparesis.

A month later, however, he presented with marked painless swelling of the face and neck, with some prominent dilated superficial veins of the upper chest and neck.

QUESTIONS:

9. THE MOST LIKELY DIAGNOSIS IS:
    A. Mumps
    B. Cellulitis
    C. Compression of the superior vena cava
    D. None of the above

CASE STUDY #19

10. THE MOST USEFUL EXAMINATION TO ORDER NOW WOULD BE:
    A. Cannulation of the parotid ducts
    B. Examination of the parotid gland by an otolaryngologist
    C. Electrocardiogram
    D. Chest film

A chest film now showed a superior mediastinal mass (Fig. 17).

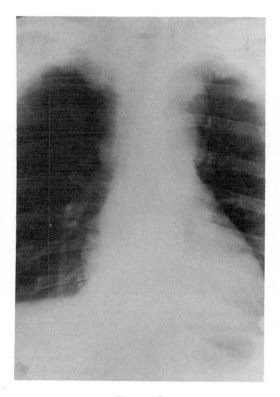

Figure 17

A scalene node biopsy was normal. The day after admission, the patient became increasingly obtunded with marked bulging of the craniotomy flap. This was considered to be due to cerebral swelling caused by obstruction to the venous drainage of the brain by the superior mediastinal mass. Because of the patient's grave condition, high doses of decadron were begun and 350 Rads were given to the mediastinal area. The next day he was much more alert. A thoracotomy was performed, and multiple large hard nodes were palpated about the mediastinum. Biopsy showed metastatic bronchogenic carcinoma. Brain scan now showed an increase of isotope uptake in the right parietal area. A repeat right carotid

CASE STUDY #19

angiogram showed an increase in the size of the right parietal mass as compared with the previous films. Several early draining veins, characteristic of malignancy, were now also seen. A course of radiotherapy to the brain and mediastinum was given, with improvement in the superior vena cava syndrome and in the hemiparesis. However, a month later there was an increase in facial edema, and multiple nodules were now seen scattered throughout the lungs. His course thereafter was gradually downhill, with neurological deterioration, eventual coma and death. Autopsy was not obtained.

QUESTIONS:

11. THE PART OF THE CENTRAL NERVOUS SYSTEM MOST COMMONLY AFFECTED BY METASTATIC CANCER IS:
    A. Cerebellum
    B. Cerebrum
    C. Spinal cord
    D. Brain stem

12. THE TWO MOST COMMON SOURCES OF CENTRAL NERVOUS SYSTEM METASTASES ARE:
    A. Carcinoma of the lung
    B. Breast carcinoma
    C. Malignant melanoma
    D. Leukemia

13. IN AUTOPSY SERIES, METASTASES ARE LIKELY TO BE MULTIPLE IN:
    A. 20% of cases
    B. 40% of cases
    C. 60% of cases
    D. More than 70% of cases

14. AMONG PATIENTS WITH METASTATIC BRAIN TUMOR, THE POOREST PROGNOSIS EXISTS IF THE PRIMARY IS IN THE:
    A. Lung
    B. Thyroid
    C. Kidney
    D. GI tract

COMMENT: This case illustrates how occasionally a malignant brain tumor may simulate vascular disease, with abrupt onset of neurological symptoms, at a time when a primary tumor site is not apparent. In this instance, the biopsy was most likely taken from the zone of necrosis and gliosis which often surrounds a metastatic tumor. A large increase in spinal fluid protein, a positive brain scan within the first week after the onset of neurological deficit, or as in this case, a focal seizure may be clues to underlying neoplastic etiology. In this patient, the subsequent appearance of the lung disease, the growth of the brain lesion, and the appearance of angiographic evidence of malignancy confirmed the true state of affairs. It is of interest that Vieth and Odom[2] noted that in only 18% of their patients with cancer of the lung metastatic to brain was the primary lesion diagnosed before the intracranial metastases.

ANSWERS AND DISCUSSION:

1. D   A subarachnoid hemorrhage begins with an apoplectic and severe
             headache, often followed by stiff neck, alteration of consciousness,
             and other neurological symptoms.

             A transient ischemic attack produces neurological symptoms
             lasting minutes to hours and then disappearing completely. The
             patient's course thus far would be compatible with cerebral

CASE STUDY #19

infarction.

2. BE   A corticobulbar tract lesion produces weakness of the lower portion of the face on the opposite side because the lower motor
nuclei innervating the upper part of the face receive corticobular
fibers from both ipsi and contralateral tracts, whereas the
nuclei supplying the lower face receive innervation which is
primarily crossed from the contralateral corticobulbar tract.

3. B

4. BCD   There is no evidence of disease of the motor unit (i. e. the motor
neuron, peripheral nerve, neuromuscular junction or muscle)
and therefore electromyography would not yield useful
information.

The brain scan is useful in differentiating a cerebral infarct from
a cerebral neoplasm. The scan in cerebral infarction is usually
positive after the first week and then reverts to negative after
about a month. In contrast. about 85% of brain tumors show
a positive scan initially and after a month the area of isotope uptake on the scan either remains the same or increases
in size. Other conditions too may show a zone of increased
isotope uptake on the brain scan-abscess of the brain, subdural
hematoma, etc.

Skull films may provide much important information-abnormal
calcification, evidence of increased intracranial pressure,
pineal shift etc.

Lumbar puncture, with examination of the cerebrospinal fluid for
cells, protein, sugar and serology, may furnish important information about intracranial pressure and the possible presence of
intracranial hemorrhage, infection, neoplasm, etc.

5. D   Most studies suggest that anticoagulants are of no value in cases
of completed stroke in lowering mortality, morbidity or pre-
venting future stroke.

The use of cerebral vasodilators as carbon dioxide in stroke is
controversial. In some cases, vasodilation may increase the
local blood flow in an ischemic area. In other cases, there is
concern that carbon dioxide, in producing generalized cerebral
vasodilation will cause blood to be shunted away from the ischemic infarcted area in which maximum vasodilation had already
existed because of local anoxia, hypercarbia, and acidosis. This
latter phenomenon has been referred to as an "internal steal."

There is little evidence that block of the stellate ganglion is
beneficial in stroke. The sympathetic nervous system plays a
very minor role in regulating the diameter of intracranial blood
vessels compared to the effects of carbon dioxide and oxygen.

6. B

7. C   A Jacksonian seizure may be motor or sensory. It is a critically
important symptom, since the location of the initial and subsequent
sites of twitching or sensory abnormality informs the clinician
of both the initial site of abnormal cerebral cortical electrical
discharge and its subsequent pathway of spread. Cerebral
stimulation studies have shown that motor and sensory function
of each half of the body is represented on the opposite pre

CASE STUDY #19

central gyrus (motor) or post central gyrus (sensory) in a typical way, as shown in the photograph (Fig. 18).

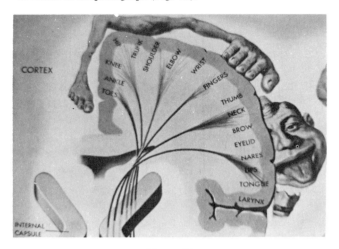

Figure 18

If the seizure activity spreads to involve both hemispheres, consciousness is lost and a grand mal seizure ensues.

8. C John Hughlings Jackson (1835-1911), a famous and prolific British neurologist, author of approximately 300 neurological publications. He is perhaps best known for his work on epilepsy and his concepts of evolutionary levels of the sensorimotor mechanisms.

9. C   12. AB

10. D   13. D

11. B   14. A

REFERENCES

1. Chason, J., F. Walker, and J. Landers, Metastatic Carcinoma in the Central Nervous System and Dorsal Root Ganglia, Cancer 16:781, 1963.

2. Vieth, R., and G. Odom, Intracranial Metastases and their Neurosurgical Treatment, J Neurosurgery 23:375, 1965.

3. Lang, E.F., and J. Slater, Metastatic Brain Tumors; Results of Surgical and Nonsurgical Treatment, Surg Clin N Amer 44:865, 1964.

4. Russell, D.S., and L.J. Rubinstein, Pathology of Tumors of the Nervous System, 3rd Ed., The Williams and Wilkins Co., Baltimore, 1971.

5. Busch, E., and E. Christensen, Treatment of Tumors Metastatic to the Central Nervous System, Treatment of Cancer and Allied Diseases, 2nd Ed., G. Pack, I. Ariel, Ed., Paul B. Hoeber, 1959.

CASE STUDY #19

6. Sciarra, D., Course of Metastatic Tumors to the Brain, Trans Am Neurol Ass'n 78:265, 1953.

7. Hazra, T., et al., Management of Cerebral Metastasis from Bronchogenic Carcinoma, Johns Hopkins Med J 130:377, 1972.

8. Haar, F., and R. Patterson, Surgery for Metastatic Intracranial Neoplasm, Cancer 30:1241, 1972.

9. Weinstein, J., et al., The Effects of Dexamethasone on Brain Edema in Patients with Metastatic Brain Tumors, Neurology 23:121, 1973.

10. Posner, J., Diagnosis and Treatment of Metastases to the Brain., Clinical Bulletin of the Memorial Sloan Kettering Cancer Center 4:47, 1974.

11. Newman, S., and H. Hansen, Frequency, Diagnosis, and Treatment of Brain Metastases in 247 Consecutive Patients with Bronchogenic Carcinoma, Cancer 33:492, 1974.

CASE STUDY #20

Progressive Unilateral Hearing Loss in a Young Woman

HISTORY: This nineteen year-old girl complained of progressively decreased hearing in the right ear of two years duration. She was able to hear speech over the telephone only with the left ear. During this time she had also noted occasional high pitched tinnitus in the right ear. For several years she had suffered from occipital headaches which had recently become worse and which occasionally awakened her from sleep. She denied dizziness, speech, swallowing or visual difficulty, or ear infections.

QUESTION:

1. THIS HISTORY MIGHT LEAD ONE TO SUSPECT:
   A. Meniere's syndrome
   B. Otosclerosis
   C. Either of the above
   D. Neither of the above

EXAMINATION: She appeared in good general health. The left plantar response was extensor. Early papilledema was present bilaterally. Visual acuity was normal. There was both vertical and horizontal nystagmus. There was no response in either eye when the right cornea was stimulated. Both eyes blinked when the left cornea was touched. The right nasolabial fold was flattened and there was moderate right lower facial weakness when she grimaced. Hearing was decreased in the right ear. The tympanic membranes were normal. The Rinne test showed air to be better than bone conduction bilaterally. The Weber test lateralized to the left.

QUESTIONS:

2. THIS PATIENT SHOWS EVIDENCE OF DAMAGE TO:
   A. The corticospinal tract
   B. Cerebellar connections
   C. Fifth cranial nerve
   D. Seventh cranial nerve
   E. All of the above

CASE STUDY #20

3. IN THE WEBER TEST, A VIBRATING 512cps TUNING FORK IS PLACED IN THE MIDDLE OF THE FOREHEAD. IN UNILATERAL MIDDLE EAR DEAFNESS (CONDUCTIVE),THE SOUND WILL BE HEARD BETTER BY THE:
   A. Healthy ear
   B. Impaired ear
   C. Either ear, with a great deal of individual variation

4. IN SENSORI-NEURAL HEARING LOSS, THE SOUND WILL LATERALIZE TO THE:
   A. Healthy ear
   B. Impaired ear
   C. Either

5. IN THE NORMAL, OR IN SENSORI-NEURAL HEARING LOSS, AIR CONDUCTION, AS COMPARED TO BONE CONDUCTION IS:
   A. Better
   B. Worse
   C. Equal

6. IN CONTRAST, IN MIDDLE EAR DISEASE, WHICH IS BETTER ?:
   A. Air conduction
   B. Bone conduction
   C. No difference

7. IN EVALUATING THIS CASE AT THIS POINT, USEFUL TESTS WOULD INCLUDE:
   A. Audiograms
   B. Caloric testing
   C. Skull films to show the internal auditory canals
   D. Carotid angiography
   E. All of the above

LABORATORY DATA: Audiological tests: Pure tone audiograms showed a high tone sensorineural loss in the right ear. The left was normal. Speech discrimination was 36% in the right ear and 100% in the left ear. The von Bekesy test was type I. No recruitment was seen on the Alternate Binaural Loudness Balance Test.

Vestibular tests: A minimal ice water caloric test was performed. 0/2 cc of ice water instilled in the left ear produced nystagmus for 140 seconds. 0/4cc of icewater in the right ear produced no response.

X-rays: skull films and laminagrams of the petrous pyramids showed erosion of the right internal auditory canal.

8. THE MOST LIKELY DIAGNOSIS IS:
   A. Brainstem glioma
   B. Acoustic neuroma
   C. Teratoma
   D. Basilar artery aneurysm
   E. None of the above

CASE STUDY #20

9.   DEFINITIVE STUDIES MIGHT INCLUDE:
     A. Pneumoencephalography
     B. Cerebellar-pontine angle pantopaque cisternography
     C. Echoencephalography
     D. Electroencephalography
     E. Carotid arteriography

COURSE: A suboccipital craniectomy was performed, and a golf ball-sized right acoustic neuroma was totally removed. The right facial nerve was sacrificed at surgery, but a subsequent hypoglossal-facial nerve anastomosis was performed, with a good result.

QUESTIONS:

10. SPINAL FLUID IN PATIENTS WITH ACOUSTIC NEUROMA USUALLY
     SHOWS:
     A. Increased protein
     B. Lymphocytic pleocytosis
     C. No abnormalities
     D. Low sugar

11. A PATIENT HAS BILATERAL ACOUSTIC NEUROMAS. ON HIS SKIN
     YOU MIGHT SEE:
     A. Spiders
     B. Eczema
     C. Café-au-lait spots
     D. A macular rash

12. IN DISTINGUISHING BETWEEN A COCHLEAR LESION (AS MENIERE'S
     SYNDROME) AND A NERVE OR RETROCOCHLEAR LESION (AS AN
     ACOUSTIC NEUROMA):
     A. A low speech discrimination score (as in hearing the difference be-
         tween deck and peck) is often associated with a retrocochlear lesion
     B. Recruitment, a phenomenon in which the difference between the
         hearing of the normal and defective ear decreases with increasing
         loudness of the sound, is characteristic of cochlear disease
     C. A type 3 von Bekesy pattern is often seen with acoustic neuroma
     D. Although all the above are true, no one of these special auditory tests
         is definitive or entirely accurate in the differential diagnosis between
         cochlear and retrocochlear lesions; however, a similar pattern in
         several of the tests is highly significant

13. TRUE VERTIGO IS COMMON IN:
     A. Labrynthitis
     B. Meniere's syndrome
     C. Acoustic neuroma
     D. All of the above

ANSWERS AND DISCUSSION:

1. D   Meniere's syndrome is characterized by recurrent episodes of
               acute vertigo. Otosclerosis could begin at this age with un-
               ilateral tinnitus and hearing loss, but would not be associated
               with severe headaches.

2. E

3. B

CASE STUDY #20

4. A

5. A

6. B   In the Rinne test, the vibrating tuning fork is applied to the mastoid process until the sound is no longer heard, after which the still vibrating fork is held next to the external auditory canal. In the patient with normal hearing, or a sensorineural loss, the sound will still be heard, showing that air is better than bone conduction. In the patient with middle ear disease, the sound will not still be heard, since bone conduction of sound through the skull to the inner ear, bypassing the defective middle ear, is better than air conduction which requires the function of the tympanic membrane and ossicle chain of the middle ear.

7. ABC   The lesion is in the cerebellopontine angle in the posterior cranial fossa. Except in cases of posterior fossa tumors, when it is important to know the size of the lateral ventricles (as outlined by the thalamo-striate veins) to determine the degree of obstructive hydrocephalus, carotid angiography is performed to evaluate supratentorial lesions in the anterior and middle cranial fossae.

8. B   Brainstem gliomas typically present with cranial nerve and long tract abnormalities without evidence of increased intracranial pressure. Any of the other possibilities could present as a cerebellopontine angle mass blocking cerebrospinal fluid flow and producing increased intracranial pressure, but the occurrence of hearing loss as the first symptom as well as the X-ray findings favor acoustic neuroma as the diagnosis.

9. AB   Either of these tests have been used to outline the tumor mass with air in the first procedure, with dye in the latter.

10. A   Acoustic neuromas over one cm in diameter usually are associated with elevated spinal fluid protein levels. However, the smaller, particularly the intracanalicular, tumors may not elevate the protein.

11. C   4% of acoustic neuromas are bilateral. Other stigmata of Von Recklinghausen's neurofibromatosis, such as café-au-lait spots on the skin are usually present in these cases.

12. ABCD are all true.

13. AB   Acute severe vertigo such as one might see in Meniere's syndrome, labrynthitis, or basilar artery disease is unusual in acoustic neuroma. A vague constant sense of imbalance is much more common.

REFERENCES

1.   Third Workshop on Microsurgery of the Ear, March 27-31, 1967, as reported in Arch Otolaryng (Jan.) 1969 and (Feb.) 1969.

2.   Monograph II, Acoustic Neuroma, Arch Otolaryng (Dec.) 1968.

3.   House, H. P., F. H. Linthicum and E. W. Johnson, Current Management of Hearing Loss in Children, Am J Dis Child 108:677, 1964.

CASE STUDY #20

4. Nelson, J.R., The Minimal Ice Water Caloric Test, Neurology 19:577, 1969.

5. Nager, G., Acoustic Neurinomas, Arch Otolaryng 89:68, 1969.

6. Johnson, E., Audiologic Diagnosis of Acoustic Neuromas, Arch Otolaryng 89:96, 1969.

7. Valvassori, G., Diagnosis of Acoustic Neuromas, Arch Otolaryng 89:101, 1969.

8. Pool, J.C., and A.A. Pava, Acoustic Nerve Tumors, Early Diagnosis and Treatment, 2nd Ed., Charles C Thomas, Springfield, 1970.

9. Ojemann, R., et al., Evaluation and Surgical Treatment of Acoustic Neuroma, New Eng J Med 287:895, 1972.

CASE STUDY #21

Generalized Weakness in a Child

HISTORY: This 7 year-old patient was the only living child of this marriage. Throughout the pregnancy, especially during the last two months, small amounts of bloody vaginal discharge occurred. During the third trimester, weekly medical visits were made, and at times the fetal heart was hard to hear. Throughout the pregnancy recurrent urinary tract infections were treated with various antibiotics and tranquilizers of unknown types. In retrospect, fetal movement seemed considerably less than the following normal pregnancy by a different husband.

The fetal membranes ruptured 12 hours before an unremarkable 1-1/2 hour delivery under gas anesthesia. No forceps were used. Immediately after birth the patient was noted to be silent, flaccid, cyanotic, and in respiratory difficulty. Assisted respiration was instituted. She remained in an incubator for three weeks and gradually improved, although at no time did her mother consider her normal.

During her early weeks she was hypotonic and diffusely weak, ate poorly, and required multiple formula changes. No specific impairment of deglutition was noted. At two months she began to hold her head up, appeared healthy, but was still somewhat hypotonic and weak. At four months she began to have sudden apneic spells with cyanosis, occasionally associated with jerking movements of one or more extremities. On a few occasions generalized and akinetic seizures occurred without prior apnea. Because of these spells, she was briefly hospitalized at eight months, at which time a left-sided focal motor seizure was observed. She was discharged on a regimen of phenobarbital with a diagnosis of convulsive disorder secondary to perinatal asphyxia. At 11 months, she was rehospitalized because of vomiting, diarrhea, and pneumonitis. Retardation of motor function, hypotonia, and areflexia were noted. An electroencephalogram was diffusely slow. She was given 0.5 mg neostigmine without improvement in strength.

From age 1, slow progression of weakness occurred. Photographs document the appearance of ptosis at about 10 months. Facial weakness was also observed at this time. She sat at 9 months and walked at 18 months, but with poor and unsteady gait and frequent falls. "Turning in" of the left foot was noted when she began to walk and increased in severity to produce a marked equinovarus deformity. Language and intellectual development were normal. She was an alert, cheerful child with average intellectual abilities. Mild dysphagia was present. Impairment of eye movements was noted after age 3. She was toilet trained at age 2-1/2, but occasional urinary incontinence continued.

CASE STUDY # 21

There was no skin rash, pigmenturia, or muscle pain. Other than occasional mild respiratory infections, she was in good general health. Mild fluctuations in weakness were observed, especially during respiratory infections.

PHYSICAL EXAMINATION: The patient was a thin, pale child with facial weakness and left talipes equinovarus deformity. Blood pressure 90/60 mm Hg, pulse 80/min and regular, respirations 20/min, height 100 cm, weight 15 kg, head circumference 49.5 cm and normocephalic. There was an increase of normal lumbar lordosis, scapular winging, and mild pectus excavatum. She walked with a waddling gait circumducting the left leg. She was unable to do deep knee bends or step on an 8-inch stool without assistance. The skin and mucous membranes were clear. The heart and lungs were normal. The liver edge was palpable two fingerbreadths below the right costal margin. At times the spleen tip was palpable.

There was marked bilateral ptosis and weakness of all facial muscles producing an expressionless facies with pouting of the lips and an open mouth. The muscles of mastication and deglutition were minimally weak. No tongue fasciculations or atrophy were noted. The voice was high-pitched but did not fatigue. Ocular movements were impaired in a conjugate manner, equally in all directions of gaze, to about 50% of normal range of motion. Rapid head turning did not increase the range of eye motion. No nystagmus was present. Pupillary responses and fundi were normal.

There was generalized thinness of all limbs in a symmetrical and nonfocal manner. No myotonia or fasciculations were present. The muscles were not tender. The deep tendon reflexes were absent throughout. No abnormal reflexes were present. There was symmetrical and generalized muscle weakness in all striated muscles including neck, extremities, and axial muscles. A slight proximal preponderance was present with an estimated 75% loss of power proximally and 50% distally. No abnormal fatigability was noted with repetitive activity, and edrophonium tests on three occasions were negative. Sensory examination was normal. Autonomic function was unremarkable.

LABORATORY DATA: Complete blood count, erythrocyte sedimentation rate, urinalysis, protein bound iodine, T-3 uptake, stool guaiacs, and cerebrospinal fluid were normal. The following serum studies were also within normal limits: electrolytes, glutamic oxaloacetic transaminase, glutamic pyruvic transaminase, lactate dehydrogenase, creatine phosphokinase, aldolase, amylase, alkaline phosphatase, creatinine, creatine, cholesterol, lactic acid, pyruvic acid, bilirubin, protein electrophoresis. The 24-hour urine levels for 17-hydroxy and ketogenic steroids, creatine, creatinine and amino acids were within normal limits.

Admission chest film was normal except for the absence of ossification of the first center of the body of the sternum. Skull, cervical spine, and lumbosacral spine films were unremarkable. X-rays of the left ankle revealed talipes equinovarus deformity with demineralization and thinning of the cortex. Hip X-ray films showed normal results. An electrocardiogram revealed nonspecific ST and T wave changes. An EEG was abnormal because of poorly organized 4-6 cps basic frequency with occasional nonfocal 3 to 4 cps activity. Nerve conduction times were withing normal limits.

An electromyogram revealed rather prominent abnormalities. Two studies were done approximately two months apart and revealed essentially similar findings in all muscle groups tested. Most motor units were abnormally low in voltage and short in duration with polyphasia, i.e. "myopathic." There were frequent positive sharp waves and fibrillatory activity. Frequent myotonic discharge was seen. The findings were symmetrical and present both proximally and distally.

CASE STUDY #21

QUESTION:

1. WHICH OF THE FOLLOWING CONDITIONS MIGHT BE CONSIDERED IN
   THE DIFFERENTIAL DIAGNOSIS?:
   A. Multiple sclerosis
   B. Werdnig-Hoffman Disease
   C. Nemaline myopathy
   D. Centronuclear (myotubular) myopathy
   E. Guillain-Barré Syndrome
   F. Glycogen storage disease
   G. Hurler's Syndrome
   H. Arthrogryposis multiplex congenita
   I. Duchenne Muscular Dystrophy
   J. Benign Congenital Hypotonia

SUBSEQUENT COURSE: On the fifth hospital day she developed an acute and
severe pneumonitis with marked left hilar infiltrates, acute respiratory distress,
fever, increased white blood cell count, tachycardia, and tachypnea. In addition
there was a striking increase in muscle weakness. She was unable to swallow
secretions, requiring tracheostomy. Her eye movements became limited to only
a few degrees of conjugate gaze in the lateral plane. Only feeble distal upper
and lower extremity movements could be carried out. With supportive care,
frequent suctioning, oxygen, intravenous cephalothin, sodium iodide, and fluid
and electrolyte replacement, a gratifying response occured withing 48 hours.
As the pneumonia improved, so did her muscle strength. On two occasions,
while changing her tracheotomy tube, cardiac arrest occured which responded
to mouth-to-mouth resuscitation and closed chest massage in less than one minute. Later pneumonia recurred, and once again there was a striking increase in
the amount of extremity and extraocular muscle weakness. No correlation
between increased weakness and serum electrolyte alteration was found, nor
did the weakness respond to edrophonium.

One night at age 8-4/12, her mother was awakened by the sound of the patient's
suction machine. The patient was found in bed having apparently died while
attempting to suction her secretions, something she had always been able to do
without difficulty in the past. An autopsy was carried out. A representative
slide of her striated muscle is illustrated (Fig. 19).

QUESTIONS:

2. A MUSCLE BIOPSY ON THE PATIENT IS ILLUSTRATED IN THE
   PHOTOGRAPH. THIS BIOPSY REVEALS:
   A. No significant alteration
   B. Polymyositis
   C. Centrally nucleated fibers ("myotubular" or "centronuclear" myopathy)
   D. Muscular Dystrophy

3. MYOTONIA CONGENITA (THOMPSEN'S DISEASE) IS BEST CHARACTER-
   IZED AS A DISORDER:
   A. Of glycogen metabolism
   B. Resulting in difficulty relaxing a contracted muscle
   C. With episodes of weakness
   D. With progressive distal wasting of muscles

CASE STUDY #21

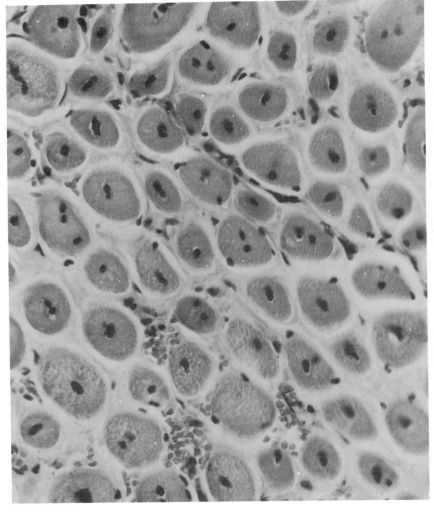

Figure 19

CASE STUDY #21

4. THE CONGENITAL NON-PROGRESSIVE MYOPATHY SYNDROME
   INCLUDES SUCH DISORDERS AS:
   A. Centronuclear myopathy
   B. Central core disease
   C. Duchenne muscular dystrophy
   D. Nemaline myopathy

5. SECONDARY CAUSES OF MUSCLE WASTING INCLUDE MALNUTRITION,
   TRAUMA, AND WHICH OF THE FOLLOWING?:
   A. Immobilization of a limb by a cast
   B. Damage to peripheral nerves
   C. Damage to anterior horn cell
   D. Damage to corticospinal tracts

6. INDICATE WHICH DISORDERS MAY LEAD TO INFANTILE HYPOTONIA:
   A. Cerebral palsy
   B. Glycogen storage diseases
   C. Guillain-Barré Syndrome
   D. Acute bacterial meningitis

ANSWERS AND DISCUSSION:

1. BCDEFJ   This child presented with diffuse weakness and flaccidity, the
            so-called "floppy child" syndrome. There was no evidence of
            central nervous system involvement as judged by normal
            intellectual development and the absence of upper motor neuron
            signs on physical examination. There was no evidence of other
            organ system involvement, and the disease process appeared to
            be limited to the motor unit. The EEG was abnormal in a non-
            specific manner, and the electromyogram revealed a myopathic
            pattern mixed with elements suggestive of denervation, i.e.,
            positive sharp waves and fibrillations. The extraocular
            muscles were also involved in this process as were the muscles
            of respiration. Muscle sclerosis is essentially non-existent in
            this age group and the absence of involvement of the central
            nervous system would make this diagnosis untenable. Arthro-
            gryposis multiplex congenita is a descriptive syndrome which
            should be used to indicate individuals born with joint deformities;
            it should not be used as a specific nosologic entity. Congenital
            joint deformities can occur with either neurogenic or myopathic
            disease of any variety and occasionally can be seen with
            primary disorder of the joint itself. Duchenne muscular
            dystrophy never becomes symptomatic within the first year
            of life. Although enzyme alterations do occur in the neonatal
            period, clinical manifestations are extremely rare in Duchenne

CASE STUDY #21

dystrophy. The term "benign congenital hypotonia" has replaced "amyotonia congenita" as a descriptive term for children born hypotonic, usually strong, and who have a benign course. This term constitutes a variety of known and unknown neuromuscular disorders and dysfunction of the central nervous system, rather than a specific nosologic entity. When long term follow-up is done on patients with the benign congenital hypotonia syndrome, a large percentage turn out to have various forms of central nervous system dysfunction, e. g., "cerebral palsy." A fair percentage have benign forms of Werdnig-Hoffman disease and a large proportion are never accurately diagnosed. Motor unit disease beginning in the neonatal period can occur with anterior horn cell involvement (Werdnig-Hoffman Disease), central nervous system dysfunction (Tay-Sachs Disease), disease of the peripheral nervous system (Guillain-Barré syndrome), primary disorder of the muscle fiber (nemaline myopathy), or processes which may affect the motor unit at several different levels (glycogen storage diseases). An accurate diagnosis often depends on proper evaluation of a muscle biopsy.

2. C   Myotubular or centronuclear myopathy is one of a group of disorders which begin in the neonatal period and are usually non-progressive in course. In this condition, the muscle involvement is symmetrical affecting limbs and trunk. In occasional patients, cranial nerve muscles are involved. The primary pathological alteration in centronuclear myopathy is centrally nucleated muscle fibers. This is somewhat analogous to the myotubular stage of embryogenesis which has led some to postulate that this disorder represents an arrest of normal maturation. Other evidence suggests that this is a peculiar pathological response to an as yet undefined insult. The primary pathologic alteration in polymyositis is one of round cell, inflammatory infiltration, both between and within muscle fibers, as well as perivascular cuffing. Regenerative activity is usually pronounced, especially in the more acute phases. The pathology of muscular dystrophy is one of scattered individual fiber necrosis, variation in fiber size, and replacement of muscle tissue by fat and connective tissue.

3. B   Myotonia congenita is one of the myotonic disorders which is relatively benign in course and manifestations. These patients present in childhood with enlarged muscle, and slowness and difficulty carrying out motor activity due to the myotonia. Muscle wasting and weakness is extremely rare. The course is usually non-progressive, and rarely is there a great deal of functional limitation. These patients may receive relief by using pharmacological agents which stabilize the muscle membrane, such as diphenylhydantoin. The primary defect in the myotonic disorders appears to be an unstable muscle membrane which results in repetitive discharge of muscle fibers.

CASE STUDY #21

4. ABD

5. ABCD

6. ABCD

REFERENCES

1. Munsat, T.L., L.R. Thompson, and R.F. Coleman, Centronuclear ("Myotubular") Myopathy, Arch Neurol 20:120, 1969.

2. Engel, W.K., G.N. Gold, and G. Karpati, Type 1 Fiber Hypotrophy and Central Nuclei, Arch Neurol 18:435, 1968.

3. Bethlem, J., et al., Centronuclear Myopathy, European Neurology 1:325, 1968.

4. Sher, J.H., A.B. Rimalovski, T.J. Athanassiades, and S.M. Aronson, Familial Centronuclear Myopathy, Neurology 17:727, 1967.

5. Munsat, T., Congenital Myopathies, in The Striated Muscle, Chapter 21, Williams and Wilkins Co., Baltimore, 1973.

6. Saper, J., Benign Congenital Myopathy, Am J Med 57:157, 1974.

CASE STUDY #22

 A Young Woman with Headaches, Vomiting, and Blurred Optic Disc Margins

HISTORY: A 23 year-old woman was well until six months previously when she began to suffer from severe bitemporal headaches, which occurred daily, were not relieved by aspirin, were steady, and sometimes associated with vomiting. There was no history of seizures, trauma, visual difficulty or other neurological symptoms. Menstrual periods were normal.

EXAMINATION: She was an obese, alert, pleasant young woman. Physical and neurological examinations were normal except for bilateral blurring of the optic disc margins with retinal vein engorgement and retinal hemorrhages.

QUESTIONS:

1. THE DIFFERENTIAL DIAGNOSIS INCLUDES:
   A. Hypoparathyroidism
   B. Hypoadrenalism
   C. Anemia
   D. None of the above

CASE STUDY #22

2. IF THE PATIENT HAD SEVERE ACNE, YOU MIGHT:
    A. Doubt any relationship to her papilledema
    B. Suspect cavernous sinus thrombosis
    C. Question about excessive vitamin A intake
    D. Inquire about antibiotic usage

There was no history of antibiotic, vitamin, hormonal or other drug use. Blood
count, urinalysis, calcium,electrolytes, serology were all normal.

QUESTION:

3. IMPORTANT STUDIES TO OBTAIN INITIALLY WOULD INCLUDE:
    A. Urine arylsulfatase
    B. Skull films
    C. Posterior fossa myelography
    D. Echoencephalogram if an undisplaced pineal were not visualized on
        the skull films
    E. Spinal tap
    F. Brain scan
    G. Urine homovanillic acid
    H. Electroencephalogram
    I. Visual fields

Skull films showed demineralization of the dorsum sella. Brain scan was normal.
Echoencephalogram did not show any shift of midline structures. Visual fields
showed enlarged blind spots. Visual acuity was normal. Electroencephalogram
showed small amounts of bitemporal 5cps slowing.

4. AT THIS POINT, BILATERAL CAROTID ANGIOGRAMS WERE DONE.
    CAROTID ANGIOGRAPHY IS OF VALUE TO:
    A. Show ventricular size
    B. Show any shift of midline structures
    C. Outline most cerebellar masses
    D. Rule out subdural hematomas

The carotid angiograms were normal, as was pneumoencephalography (Figs. 20,
21).

A spinal tap showed an opening pressure of 210, protein 19 mgm%, no cells and
normal sugar.

5. THE MOST LIKELY DIAGNOSIS IS:
    A. "Normal" pressure hydrocephalus
    B. Pseudopapilledema
    C. Pseudotumor cerebri
    D. Pseudohypoparathyroidism

She was given a course of treatment with dexamethasone for three weeks, with
gradual improvement of the papilledema and disappearance of the headaches.
She has subsequently been followed for four years and has remained entirely well.

6. CHARACTERISTICS OF THE SYNDROME ILLUSTRATED BY THIS CASE
    INCLUDE ALL OF THE FOLLOWING, EXCEPT:
    A. Papilledema
    B. Third nerve palsy
    C. Stupor
    D. Sixth nerve palsy
    E. Increased protein content in the spinal fluid
    F. Normal pneumoencephalogram

CASE STUDY #22

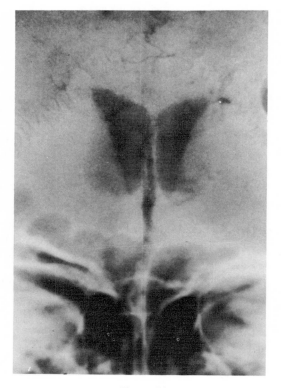

Figure 20

7.   THE SYNDROME IS USUALLY SELF LIMITING, WITH RECURRENCE:
    A. Very frequent
    B. Frequent
    C. Not uncommon
    D. Rare

8.   IF YOU WERE A NEUROLOGIST IN THE ARCTIC CIRCLE AND AN
    ESKIMO CAME TO CONSULT YOU WITH HEADACHES, PAPILLEDEMA
    AND NO OTHER NEUROLOGICAL ABNORMALITIES, YOU MIGHT SUS-
    PECT HE HAD EATEN TOO MUCH:
    A. Tuna fish, with excessive mercury
    B. Polar bear liver, with excessive vitamin A
    C. Walrus, with excessive vitamin D
    D. Eggs, with excessive cholesterol

CASE STUDY #22

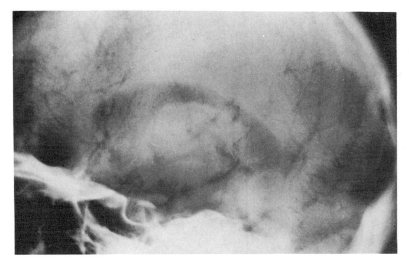

Figure 21

9. ONE THEORY OF CAUSE OF THIS SYNDROME IS IMPAIRMENT OF
    ABSORPTION OF CEREBROSPINAL FLUID BACK INTO THE BLOOD;
    THE PRIMARY SITE(S) OF THIS REABSORPTION IS/ARE THE:
    A. Thoracic duct
    B. Arachnoid villi
    C. Chorioid plexus
    D. None of the above

10. ALTHOUGH UNCOMMON, A SERIOUS COMPLICATION OF THIS SYN-
    DROME IS:
    A. Deafness
    B. Seizures
    C. Mental deficiency
    D. Blindness

11. USEFUL METHODS OF TREATMENT OF THIS CONDITION HAVE IN-
    CLUDED:
    A. Glycerol
    B. Repeated spinal taps
    C. Dexamethasone
    D. Rice Diet with weight reduction
    E. Subtemporal decompression if medical measures fail and there is
       threatened loss of vision
    F. All of the above

CASE STUDY #22

ANSWERS AND DISCUSSION:

1. ABC   This patient poses two problems. First, is true papilledema present,
         and secondly if so, what is its cause. The characteristics of papilledema,
         as present in this patient, include blurring of the optic disc margins,
         elevation of the optic disc, and increase in the ratio or retinal venous to
         arterial diameter (usually 3:2), erythema of the discs, retinal hemor-
         rhages and exudates, increased size of the blind spots on the visual field
         examination, with preservation of vision in the early stages, although
         later visual loss and post papilledema optic atrophy may ensue.

         The differential diagnosis of papilledema includes optic neuritis which
         can produce a similar fundoscopic picture. Optic neuritis can be distin-
         guished because of the sudden profound visual loss which occurs.

         Central retinal vein thrombosis occurs in an more elderly age group and
         is characterized by widespread retinal and preretinal hemorrhages.

         Pseudopapilledema is an anomalous elevation of the optic disc resembling
         papilledema but unassociated with visual field defect, hemorrhage,
         exudates, venous congestion, symptoms of increased intracranial pres-
         sure or signs of neurological disease.

         The most common causes of increased intracranial pressure with papil-
         ledema, even in the absence of lateralizing neurological signs, are intra-
         cranial mass lesions-neoplasm, abscess, hemorrhage - and these must
         be ruled out with appropriate studies.

         Hypocalcemia, hypoadrenalism and anemia have all, though rarely, been
         associated with a syndrome of increased intracranial pressure. The
         underlying pathogenic mechanism is not understood.

2. CD   Vitamin A toxicity has caused a syndrome of increased intracranial pres-
         sure which was reversible when the vitamin was discontinued. A few
         cases of increased intracranial pressure have also been reported in
         young children receiving tetracycline.

3. BDF   Skull films might give important information about shift of midline
   HI   structures, or localizing findings such as erosions, hyperostosis, etc.

         Since the midline echoencephalogram correlates with the position of the
         pineal gland, it would be an important and safe test to obtain if the pineal
         gland were not calcified.

         At this point a spinal tap should not be done. The provisional diagnosis
         is of an intracranial mass lesion producing papilledema, and the risk of
         precipitating cerebral herniation is not counterbalanced by the urgent
         necessity to examine the cerebrospinal fluid, as would exist with the
         suspicion of meningitis.

         Brain scan and electroencephalogram can of course furnish valuable
         localizing information. This is true of the visual field examination too.
         An inferior quadrantanopsia for instance would indicate a contralateral
         parietal lobe lesion, a superior quadrantanopsia contralateral temporal
         lobe disease.

4. ABD

5. C   This is a syndrome of increased intracranial pressure in which mental
         alertness is preserved, no focal neurological signs exist (except at times
         for a lateral rectus palsy which can occur with increased intracranial
         pressure of any cause) and in which intracranial mass lesions, obstruc-

CASE STUDY #22

tion of the cerebral ventricles, intracranial infection, hypertensive encephalopathy and chronic carbon dioxide retention have been excluded by appropriate studies including lumbar puncture, brain scan, arteriography, and pneumoencephalography. Some clinicians feel that a normal computerized tomogram may obviate the need for angiography or pneumoencephalography when the rest of the clinical and laboratory picture is typical for pseudotumor.

There are diverse etiologies of this syndrome, some of which include venous sinus thrombosis, hypocalcemia, anemia, and vitamin A, tetracycline, adrenal steroid and oral contraceptive administration, and disseminated lupus erythematosus.

Follow up examinations are extremely important in this syndrome to rule out an evolving neoplasm in spite of initially negative studies.

The syndrome of "normal" pressure hydrocephalus includes dementia, gait abnormality, normal spinal fluid pressure, and ventricular enlargement, due to extraventricular obstruction to cerebrospinal fluid flow.

6. BCE   9. B

7. D   10. D

8. B   11. F

REFERENCES

1. Bercaw, B., and M. Greer, Transport of Intrathecal RISA in Benign Intracranial Hypertension, Neurology 20:787, 1970.

2. Feldman, M., and N. Schlezinger, Benign Intracranial Hypertension Associated with Hypervitaminosis A, Arch Neurol 22:1, 1970.

3. Lysak, W., and H. Svien, Long Term Follow Up on Patients with Diagnosis of Pseudotumor Cerebri, J Neurosurg 25:284, 1966.

4. Fishman, R. A., Benign Intracranial Hypertension, Cecil-Loeb Textbook of Medicine, 13th Ed., P. B. Beeson, and W. McDermott, W. B. Saunders Co., 1971.

5. Greer, M., Benign Intracranial Hypertension, I. Mastoiditis and Lateral Sinus Obstruction, II. Following Corticosteroid Therapy, III. Pregnancy, IV. Menarche, V. Menstrual Dysfunction, Neurology 12:472, 1962; 13:439, 1963; 14:569, 1964; 14:688, 1964.

6. Paterson, R., N. DePasquale, and S. Mann, Pseudotumor Cerebri, Medicine 40:85, 1961.

7. The Use and Abuse of Vitamin A, Editorial, Canadian Pediatric Society, Canad Med Ass'n J 104:521, 1971.

8. Silberberg, D., and A. Laties, Increased Intracranial Pressure in Disseminated Lupus Erythematosus, Arch Neurology 29:88, 1973.

9. Newborg, B., Pseudotumor Cerebri Treated by Rice/Reduction Diet, Arch Intern Med 133:802, 1974.

10. Boddie, H., et al., Benign Intracranial Hypertension, Brain 97:301-326, 1974.

11. Johnston, I., and A. Paterson, Benign Intracranial Hypertension, Brain 97:289-300, 1974.

12. Mikkelson, B., et al., Vitamin A Intoxication Causing Papilledema and Simulating Acute Encephalitis, Acta Neuro Scand 50:642, 1974.

13. Weisberg, L., The Syndrome of Increased Intracranial Pressure Without Localizing Signs: A Reappraisal, Neurology 25:85, 1975.

CASE STUDY #23

Ptosis of the Eyelids and Progressive Limb Weakness

HISTORY: This 54 year-old woman (Fig. 22) was referred because of weakness in both arms over the past five years. She stated that she has been having increasing difficulty picking up and holding grocery packages and lifting her grandchildren. When taking long walks, during the past year, she has experienced easy fatiguability. She is able to climb stairs and get in and out of a car without difficulty.

QUESTION:

1.   THIS TYPE OF COMPLAINT MIGHT BE DUE TO:
    A.   Cerebellar incoordination
    B.   Parkinsonism
    C.   Primary muscle disease
    D.   Peripheral neuropathy

The patient stated that since childhood, she had "droopy eyes," and that this has been increasingly more prominent. In addition, she feels that her eye movements are limited and this has also been noted by relatives and friends. She has never had diplopia nor has she had difficulty chewing or dysphagia. She had no sensory complaints, pigmenturia, muscle pain or exposure to neurotoxins.

QUESTION:

2.   WHICH OF THE FOLLOWING WOULD EXPLAIN IMPAIRMENT OF EYE MOVEMENT WITHOUT CONCOMITTANT DIPLOPIA?
    A.   Impaired visual acuity in one eye
    B.   Third nerve palsy
    C.   Myasthenia gravis
    D.   Very slow evolution of the ophthalmoparesis

The family history was of interest. The patient's parents originally both came from a small town in northern Germany. Her father was killed in an accident at age 21. Old photographs of him showed minimal but definite bilateral ptosis at age 18. He was a strong man, however, with no evidence of weakness in trunk or limbs. The patient's younger and only sister, now age 48, has had an entirely similar problem with bilateral "lid drooping" since her late teens. She has had two operations for the ptosis but neither was effective for more than a few months. One of the patient's children,a male age 30 and unmarried, also had "droopy eyes" and possibly some atrophy of muscles about the shoulder girdle.

QUESTION:

3.   WHICH MODE OF INHERITENCE BEST DESCRIBES THE PATTERN IN THIS FAMILY?
    A.   Autosomal recessive
    B.   Sex-linked recessive
    C.   Autosomal dominant
    D.   Sex-linked dominant

PHYSICAL EXAMINATION: Blood pressure 140/85, pulse 72 - regular.

The patient was of borderline intelligence. Her liver was enlarged two finger-breadths below the right costal margin. The patient had difficultly arising from a squatting position and stepping up on a chair with either foot.

CASE STUDY #23

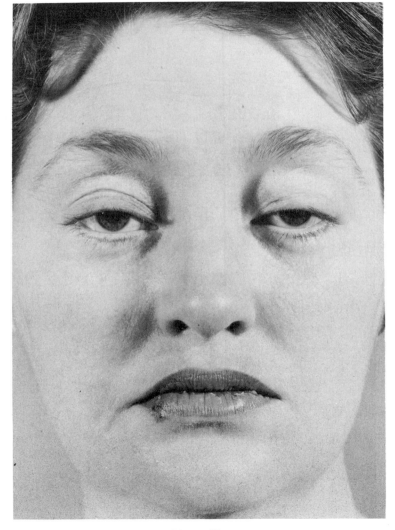

Figure 22

CASE STUDY #23

Examination of the cranial nerves revealed brisk pupillary reflexes bilaterally. The fundi were benign. There was moderate bilateral ptosis (Fig. 22).

QUESTIONS:

4. WHICH OF THE FOLLOWING LESIONS MAY CAUSE PTOSIS?:
    A. Optic neuropathy
    B. Oculomotor nerve (III)
    C. Horner's Syndrome
    D. Primary muscle disease
    E. Parietal lobe damage

5. WHICH OF THE FOLLOWING DISEASE ENTITIES OFTEN CAUSE BI-LATERAL PTOSIS?:
    A. Myasthenia gravis
    B. Multiple Sclerosis
    C. Ocular muscular dystrophy
    D. Amyotrophic lateral sclerosis

Extraocular movements were impaired, but conjugately, in all directions of gaze, expecially horizontally. Gaze was limited to 20o movement upwards, 15° downward and 5-10° horizontally. At no time, however, was dissociative gaze noted. The range of eye motion was not improved with rapid head turning (oculocephalic reflex). There was marked weakness of all facial muscles bilaterally (see photograph) with flattening of the normal facial lines, inability to smile and difficulty blowing out her cheeks. There was minimal wasting of temporalis and masseter muscles bilaterally. She was able to swallow normally. There was moderate weakness of neck flexors, supraspinatus, infraspinatus and deltoids. Other muscles were normally strong. Wasting about the shoulder girdle was apparent. The reflexes were 2+ active bilaterally with no abnormal reflexes present. There was no cerebellar deficit. The sensory examination was entirely normal.

QUESTION:

6. THIS PATTERN OF NEUROLOGIC INVOLVEMENT IS MOST SUGGESTIVE OF:
    A. Intramedullary brain stem disease
    B. Extramedullary brain stem disease
    C. Neuropathy
    D. Primary muscle disease

The patient was given 2 mg of Tensilon IV to rule out mysthenia gravis. The only observed effect was increased tearing. Muscle strength did not improve.

QUESTION:

7. INDICATE THE APPROPRIATE RESPONSE:
    A. This rules out myasthenia gravis
    B. The purity of the Tensilon is suspect
    C. Additional Tensilon should be given
    D. An EMG is indicated

LABORATORY DATA: CBC, Urinalysis, ESR-normal; Serum Na-137, K-4.8, Cl-100, Co2 -28; Serum Creatinine-0.8; SGOT -52 (8-40) Aldolase - 18(6-12); SGPT - 45 (5-35) CPK 49.5 (20-50); EKG-normal; EEG-short bursts of non-focal 5-7 cps activity;

CASE STUDY #23

Skull films-normal. Pineal not calcified. EMG-Deltoid, biceps, triceps, quadriceps, and gastrocnemius muscles were sampled bilaterally. At rest no spontaneous discharge was observed. With low grade contraction, individual motor units were found to be decreased in duration and voltage as well as polyphasic. No fibrillatory or sharp wave activity was observed. Theses changes were present in all muscles sampled, but especially the deltoids and quadriceps. Lumbar puncture revealed an opening pressure of 120 mm, crystal clear and colorless fluid. There were three lymphocytes per cu. mm. Protein-44 mg%. VDRL-non-reactive.

QUESTIONS:

8.   THESE FINDINGS ARE BEST EXPLAINED BY:
       A. Myasthenia gravis
       B. Myotonic muscular dystrophy
       C. Ocular muscular dystrophy
       D. Wernicke's encephalopathy
       E. Multiple sclerosis

9.   TRUE OR FALSE:
       A. The next procedure to be done should be a muscle biopsy
       B. Nerve conduction times are helpful in differentiating muscle disease from CNS disease
       C. CPK is more specific than SGOT for disease of muscle
       D. In myopathy the reflexes are usually enhanced
       E. Positive Babinski reflexes are frequently seen in peripheral neuropathies

ANSWERS AND DISCUSSION:

1. ABCD   These complaints are relatively non-specific. In patients with parkinsonism and cerebellar dysfunction, easy fatiguability, and "weakness, "are frequent complaints, although on examination, little weakness, if any, is observed. When these complaints are related to either primary muscle disease or peripheral neuropathy, it is usually easy to confirm the presence of impaired muscle function on examination. Primary muscle disease presents with weakness, more prominent proximally, and is usually manifested by difficulty getting in and out of a chair and climbing stairs due to pelvic girdle involvement. When the disease affects primarily the peripheral nervous system, the more distal muscles are characteristically involved which gives rise to a foot drop gait, tripping easily, and impairment of fine skill movements of the hands, such as buttoning or sewing.

2. AD   In an adult who acutely develops loss of normal conjugate eye movements, diplopia almost always occurs. This may not be the case in the patient who has had long-standing strabismus and has learned to suppress one of the visual images that is presented to the cortex. Diplopia may also be absent if the extraocular muscle weakness develops very slowly over many years, whereby, presumably the patient "learns" to suppress one image. Conceivably, diplopia would also not occur if the eye movement impairment was conjugate, so that binocular vision was maintained. This probably occurs very rarely. Third nerve palsy and myasthenia gravis characteristically result in complaints of diplopia very early.

CASE STUDY #23

3. C   The fact that the patient's father had evidence of ptosis is very suggestive that he, too, had a form of the same neuromuscular problem. This type of parent to child transmission is most consistent with a dominant trait which, since both sexes are involved, would most likely be autosomal, i. e. not involving either of the sex chromosomes. Autosomal recessive traits are usually manifested in one generation only. The parent is rarely clinically involved, although biochemical or structural alterations may be detected, depending on the disease entity.

4. BCD   Disease of the optic nerve or cerebrum will not result in ptosis. Ptosis can occur with a lesion anywhere from the third nerve nucleus to the muscle fibers. With third nerve involvement the ptosis may be quite profound, resulting in a completely closed eye. Ptosis may be due to weakness of the levator palpebrae muscle which may be caused either by interruption of its nerve supply, block at the neuromuscular junction, (myasthenia gravis) or damage to the muscle fibers themselves, (a primary or secondary myopathy). The ptosis that occurs in Horner's syndrome is presumably due to damage to the sympathetic pathways which ultimately innervate a small percentage of muscle fibers in the upper lid. Here, the ptosis is almost always relatively mild, never completely closing the eye. Frequently it is accompanied by other manifestations or interruption of sympathetic innervation such as ipsilateral small pupil, loss of sweating, and at times an appearance of enophthalmos.

5. AC   Multiple sclerosis is primarily a disease of the central nervous system and only infrequently results in Horner's syndrome or third nerve damage. Although amyotrophic lateral sclerosis results in anterior horn cell disease, which is widespread in the limbs and trunk, it rarely, if ever, affects the motor nuclei to the extraocular muscles. Thus, full extraocular movement is usually maintained throughout the course of the disease. Myasthenia gravis characteristically involves the extraocular muscles, and almost all patients with myasthenia gravis will at some time complain of diplopia. This symptom is frequently an early and presenting one in myasthenia and any patient with a long-standing diagnosis of myasthenia who does not have involvement of ocular movement should be suspect. Ocular muscular dystrophy is one of the dystrophic myopathies which is relatively infrequent. It is inherited in an autosomal dominant manner and occurs more in patients of French-Canadian extraction. Although there may be striking impairment of extraocular movement, patients rarely complain of diplopia, since the disease evolves so slowly. Ptosis and facial weakness occur early. The disease progresses very slowly over many years, with the life span shorter only rarely. In later years, involvement of the proximal upper extremities and pelvic girdle may occur. Dysphagia is also fairly common in this syndrome.

6. D

7. C   An adequate Tensilon (edrophonium) test for suspected myasthenia gravis consists of an initial injection of 2 mgs. If this does not produce a noticeable result, then an additional 8 mgs should be given before concluding that the test is negative. An unequivocal, striking response to Tensilon is diagnostic of myasthenia gravis. Equivocal or minimal responsiveness can

CASE STUDY #23

be seen in many other neurologic conditions. One should be careful about placebo reactors. It is possible to make the test somewhat more objective by measuring specific parameters such as the ability to hold the limbs out for a measured period of time, measurement of the degree of ocular movement or ptosis, ability to count without developing nasal speech, etc. In addition, if there is any question of placebo responsiveness, the test should be carried out in a double-blind manner using intravenous saline or atropine as a placebo. In this patient, an additional 8 mgm of tensilon produced no improvement.

8. C

9.   A. True; B. False; C. True; D. False; E. False

COMMENT: The syndrome of progressive ophthalmoplegia is of diverse etiology and may be caused by disease involving the central or peripheral nervous system, the neuromuscular junction or the muscle fibers.

REFERENCES

1. Magora, A., and H. Zauberman, Ocular Myopathy, Arch Neurol 20:1, 1969.

2. Rosenberg, R., D. Schotland, R. Lovelace, and L. Rowland, Progressive Ophthalmoplegia, Arch Neurol 19:362, 1968.

3. Bray, G.M., M. Kaarsoo, and M.D. Ross, Ocular Myopathy with Dysphagia, Neurology 15:678, 1965.

4. Perman, A.F., G.A. Lillington, and R.W. Jamplis, Progressive Muscular Dystrophy with Ptosis and Dysphagia, Arch Neurol 10:39, 1964.

5. Drachman, D., Ophthalmoplegia Plus, Arch Neurol 18:654, 1968.

6. Brust, J., et al., Ocular Myasthenia Gravis Mimicking Progressive External Ophthalmoplegia, Neurology 24:755, 1974.

CASE STUDY #24

Deafness and Facial Weakness in a Middle-Aged Woman

HISTORY: A 56 year-old woman was in excellent health until 6 weeks previously when she began to note decreased hearing and a persistent, annoying sense of fullness in the left ear. Two weeks later, because of these complaints, she consulted an otolaryngologist who found fluid behind the left tympanic membrane. This fluid was aspirated and cultured, but was sterile. Two weeks afterwards her lower face pulled to the right. There was no dysphagia, dysarthria, headache, numbness or weakness of the extremities, or dizziness. Audiograms revealed a mixed conductive and neurosensory hearing loss on the left.

QUESTION:

1. THE HISTORY SUGGESTS INVOLVEMENT OF:
   A. The right cerebral hemisphere   C. Cranial nerves 5 and 7
   B. The left cerebral hemisphere   D. Cranial nerves 7 and 8

EXAMINATION: She was alert and cooperative. There was weakness of the left upper and lower facial muscles; hearing was decreased in the left ear. The Weber test lateralized to the left, but air was greater than bone conduction bilaterally. The left portion of the palate was lower at rest than the right, and moved more poorly on contraction with attempted phonation. Sensation was diminished in the left oropharynx. Lingual movements were normal.

CASE STUDY #24

QUESTIONS:

2. THE MOTOR AND SENSORY ABNORMALITIES OF THE PALATE AND
    PHARYNX ARE DUE TO INVOLVEMENT OF CRANIAL NERVES:
    A. 9 and 11
    B. 9 and 10
    C. 10 and 11
    D. 10 and 12

3. THE ABSENCE OF DECREASED SENSATION IN THE LIMBS, OR OF
    PYRAMIDAL TRACT ABNORMALITY OR INCOORDINATION, SUGGESTS
    THAT:
    A. The lesion is cerebral
    B. The lesion involves only corticobulbar fibers
    C. The disease process is extra-axial, i. e. outside the brainstem
    D. Myasthenia gravis would be an important diagnostic possibility

4. IN CONSIDERING THE DIFFERENTIAL DIAGNOSIS:
    A. Progressive bulbar palsy should be considered since this can produce
        a mixed sensory and motor cranial nerve involvment
    B. Stroke in evolution secondary to vertebral artery thrombosis is a
        likely diagnosis
    C. A glomus jugulare tumor may damage the lower cranial nerves
        asymmetrically
    D. Chronic granulomatous meningitis along the base of the skull could
        produce this picture

5. USEFUL LABORATORY TESTS TO ORDER AT THIS POINT WOULD
    INCLUDE:
    A. Carotid angiogram
    B. Base views of the skull
    C. FTA-ABS
    D. Lumbar puncture
    E. Electromyogram

LABORATORY DATA: Skull films, including base views and views of the internal
auditory canals, were normal, as were brain scan and electroencephalogram.
Blood count, urinalysis, 2 hour post prandial blood sugar, and serology were also
normal. X-rays of the mastoids showed sclerosis on the left, suggesting chronic
mastoiditis. Lumbar puncture showed 14 wbc/cu. mm. with 1 polymorphonuclear
and 13 mononuclears. Protein was 62 mgm %, sugar 57 mgm % and the serology
was negative.

COURSE: Examination now showed a red left eardrum and antibiotics were begun.
Three days later she began to complain of double vision and increasing difficulty
swallowing. Examination now showed inability of the left eye to abduct when looking to the left, and left facial weakness (Fig. 23). When the left cornea was
stimulated with a wisp of cotton, only the right eye blinked. When the right
cornea was stimulated, only the right eye blinked. Hearing was decreased in the
left ear. The left side of the palate was weak. There was decreased sensation
over the left pharynx and the gag reflex was diminished on the left. The left
sternomastoid muscle was weak and the tongue protruded to the left (Fig. 24).

CASE STUDY #24

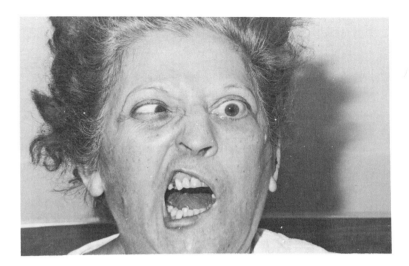

Figure 23

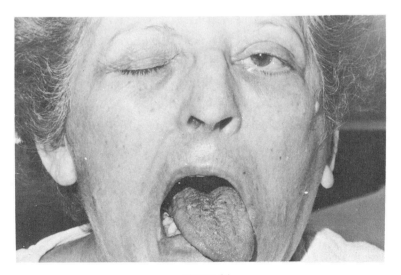

Figure 24

CASE STUDY #24

QUESTIONS:

6. WEAKNESS OF THE LEFT STERNOCLEIDOMASTOID MUSCLE WOULD
   PRODUCE DIFFICULTY IN TURNING THE HEAD TO THE:
   A. Right
   B. Left

7. A LESION OF THE 12th NERVE WHICH CAUSES THE TONGUE TO
   DEVIATE TO THE LEFT IS ON THE:
   A. Right
   B. Left

8. THE AFFERENT AND EFFERENT ARCS OF THE GAG REFLEX ARE:
   A. 5th and 10th cranial nerves
   B. 5th and 7th cranial nerves
   C. 7th and 10th cranial nerves
   D. 9th and 10th cranial nerves
   E. 9th and 12th cranial nerves

9. THE ABNORMAL CORNEAL REFLEX PATTERN DESCRIBED ABOVE IS
   DUE TO A LESION OF:
   A. The right 5th cranial nerve
   B. The left 5th cranial nerve
   C. The right 6th cranial nerve
   D. The left 6th cranial nerve
   E. The right 7th cranial nerve
   F. The left 7th cranial nerve

The patient thus showed a rapidly progressive involvement, over several weeks,
of cranial nerves 6 through 12 on the left. At this point a definitive diagnostic
procedure was done-can you guess it?

Examination of the nasopharynx revealed an abnormal appearing area which was
biopsied. The pathological report was of cords and nests of moderately well-dif-
ferentiated epidermoid carcinoma. A course of radiotherapy was begun.

QUESTIONS:

10. THIS PATIENT'S OTITIS WAS PROBABLY SECONDARY TO:
    A. Unrelated causes
    B. Blockage of the nasopharyngeal opening of the eustachian tube by the
       tumor
    C. Tumor in the middle ear

11. SYMPTOMS OF A NASOPHARYNGEAL TUMOR MAY INCLUDE:
    A. Hearing loss
    B. Diplopia
    C. Epistaxis
    D. Hoarsness
    E. Swelling of cervical lymph nodes

12. NASOPHARYNGEAL CANCER IS ESPECIALLY COMMON AMONG:
    A. Jews
    B. Chinese
    C. Egyptians
    D. Indians

CASE STUDY #24

13. RADIOTHERAPY IS THE TREATMENT OF CHOICE, AND PROGNOSIS IS IMPROVED IF THE TUMOR IS DIAGNOSED EARLY AND IS LIMITED TO THE PRIMARY SITE. THE OVERALL 5 YEAR SURVIVAL IS ABOUT:
    A. 2-5%
    B. 15-20%
    C. 40-50%
    D. 70-80%

ANSWERS AND DISCUSSION:

1. D   The twisting of the lower part of the face to the right is due to weakness of the left side of the face. The facial muscles are innervated by the 7th cranial nerve. The neurosensory hearing loss results from eighth nerve impairment. Unilateral hearing loss does not occur with a cerebral lesion, since hearing from each ear is represented in the temporal lobes of both hemispheres.

2. B   The pharynx receives sensory innervation from the 9th, motor innervation from the 10th cranial nerve.

3. C   There are none of the hallmarks of cerebral disease, i.e. seizures, aphasia, visual field cuts, etc.

    A lesion within the brainstem usually produces long tract motor and sensory and reflex abnormalities.

    Myasthenia gravis does not produce decreased hearing.

4. CD   Progressive bulbar palsy involves the lower cranial motor nuclei. Sensory abnormalities do not occur. Brainstem infarction is not probable because of the lack of long tract abnormalities.

5. BCD   Base views of the skull might demonstrate bone erosion. The FTA would be of use in ruling out meningovascular syphillis. Examination of the cerebrospinal fluid might furnish helpful clues about the possibilities of central nervous system infection or neoplasm.

6. A   The sternomastoid muscle arises from the sternum and inserts into the mastoid portion of the temporal bone. Its contraction turns the head to the opposite side.

7. B   After a 12th nerve lesion, when the tongue is protruded, its tip deviates toward the side of the paralysis due to the contraction of the genioglossus muscle on the sound side.

8. D

9. F   The pattern of responses of the corneal reflex in the presence of 5th or 7th nerve lesions is given below. The lesion in each case is on the right, in this hypothetical illustration.

	Stimulation of	Contraction of the	
		Right Eye	Left Eye
Right V lesion	Right cornea	0	0
	Left cornea	+	+
Right VII lesion	Right cornea	0	+
	Left cornea	0	+

CASE STUDY #24

> The 6th nerve innervates the lateral rectus muscle which abducts the eye and has no relationship to the corneal reflex.

10. B

11. ABCDE

12. B

13. B

REFERENCES

1. Hara, H. J., Cancer of the Nasopharynx, Laryngoscope 79:1315, 1969.

2. Dawes, J. D. K., D. G. Harkness, H. F. Marshall, and P. J. Van Miert, Malignant Disease of the Nasopharynx, J Laryng Otol 83:211, 1969.

3. Chan, P., and J. Stein, Cancer of the Nasopharynx, Calif Med 110:375, 1969.

4. Thomas, J., and A. Waltz, Neurological Manifestations of Nasopharyngeal Malignant Tumors, JAMA 192:103, 1965.

5. Choa, G., Nasopharyngeal Carcinoma, J Laryngology and Otology 88:145, 1974.

CASE STUDY #25

Progressive Weakness and Muscle Wasting

HISTORY: A 51 year-old woman was well until one year previously when she noted gradually increasing weakness of both arms and twitching in various muscles of all of her extremities. She denied arm pain, neck aching, or paresthesiae. There was a history of heavy alcoholic intake. There was no family history of neuromuscular disease.

EXAMINATION: She was alert, cooperative and severely weak, so that she could not lift her arms above her head (Fig. 25).

In the upper extremities the weakness was equally profound distally and proximally. The weakness of the legs was more severe proximally. There was atrophy of the interossei and deltoids (Figs. 26 and 27).

Scattered fasciculations were seen in both pectoral muscles. Sensation and coordination were normal. Examination of the cranial nerves was normal, except for bilateral atrophy and fasciculations of the tongue (Fig. 28).

The deep tendon reflexes were normal, and the plantar responses were flexor.

QUESTIONS:

1. IN CONSIDERING THE AREA OF THE NERVOUS SYSTEM CLINICALLY AFFECTED BY THE DISEASE, SOME IMPORTANT FEATURES ARE:
   A. Only motor function is affected
   B. There is evidence of pyramidal tract dysfunction
   C. The weakness involves all limbs
   D. The tongue is bilaterally wasted
   E. Fasciculations are pronounced
   F. All of the above

CASE STUDY #25

MATCH THE SITE OF PATHOLOGY PRODUCING DISTURBANCES IN MOTOR FUNCTION WITH THE MOST APPROPRIATE SYMPTOMS AND SIGNS USUALLY ASSOCIATED (THERE MAY BE MULTIPLE CORRECT CHOICES):

2. ___ Corticospinal tract

3. ___ Basal ganglia

4. ___ Cerebellum

5. ___ Anterior horn cells

6. ___ Peripheral nerves

7. ___ Neuromuscular junction

8. ___ Muscles

A. Spasticity
B. Rigidity
C. Tremor
D. Muscle atrophy
E. Fasciculations
F. Glove and stocking distribution of sensory loss
G. Primarily proximal weakness of arms and legs
H. Babinski signs
I. Decreased deep tendon reflexes
J. Increased deep tendon reflexes
K. Cogwheeling
L. Ataxia
M. Usually distal weakness
N. Dysdiadokokinesis
O. Normal deep tendon reflexes
P. Rapid increase in weakness with successive muscle contractions
Q. Initial weak contraction with increase in strength noted with rapid successive contraction
R. Normal strength

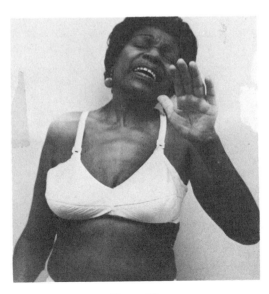

Figure 25

CASE STUDY #25

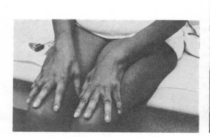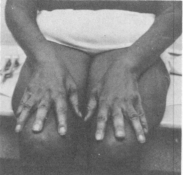

Figure 26 and Figure 27

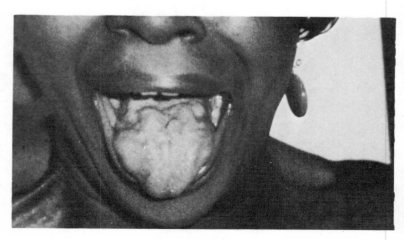

Figure 28

CASE STUDY #25

9. THE MOST IMPORTANT LABORATORY TEST OR PROCEDURE TO OBTAIN AT THIS POINT WOULD BE:
    A. Myelogram
    B. Pneumoencephalogram
    C. Vertebral angiogram
    D. Serum phosphofructokinase
    E. None of the above

LABORATORY DATA: Electromyogram of all muscles tested in the right upper and both lower extremities showed large numbers of fibrillation potentials, and occasional fasciculations. Giant polyphasic motor units were frequently seen with muscle contraction.

Biopsy of the left deltoid muscle showed clumps and groups of atrophic shrunken fibers.

Nerve conduction velocities in all extremities were normal.

The transaminase, creatine phosphokinase and lactic dehydrogenase were normal.

Other normal tests included complete blood count, fasting blood sugar, 2 hour postprandial blood sugar, LE cell preparation, VDRL, urine heavy metal determinations, cerebrospinal fluid, electrocardiogram, X-rays of the chest and entire spine, barium enema, intravenous pyelogram, upper GI series.

QUESTIONS:

10. FASCICULATIONS ARE:
    A. Contractions of a motor unit
    B. Visible to the examiner's eye
    C. Always evidence of neurological disease
    D. A but not B or C
    E. Neither A, B, nor C

11. FIBRILLATIONS ARE:
    A. Visible to the examiner's eye
    B. Contractions of individual muscle fibers
    C. Always abnormal
    D. Almost always associated with denervation, but may be seen occasionally with myopathies such as polymyositis
    E. Of much lower voltage and shorter duration than fasciculations

12. MUSCLE BIOPSY SHOULD NOT BE PERFORMED IN MUSCLES WHICH HAVE RECENTLY BEEN ELECTROMYOGRAPHICALLY TESTED, SINCE THE PATHOLOGIST MAY REPORT THE FALSE DIAGNOSIS OF:
    A. Dystrophy
    B. McArdle's syndrome
    C. Myositis
    D. None of the above

13. THE MOST LIKELY DIAGNOSIS IN THIS PATIENT IS:
    A. Myasthenic syndrome
    B. Wernicke syndrome
    C. Amyotrophic lateral sclerosis
    D. Muscular dystrophy
    E. Charcot-Marie-Tooth disease
    F. Compression of the cervical spinal cord
    G. Refsum's disease

CASE STUDY #25

14. DEFINITIVE TREATMENT FOR THIS ILLNESS IS:
     A. Guanidine
     B. Thiamine
     C. Vitamin E
     D. Diet low in phytanic acid
     E. There is no effective treatment
     F. Pancreatic extract

COURSE: Over the following month, the extremity weakness gradually increased and she began to complain of increasing dyspnea, slurred speech and difficulty in bringing up sputum and saliva. She was readmitted to the hospital, and showed considerable respiratory difficulty with intercostal muscle weakness. She was afebrile and the lungs were clear to percussion and auscultation. On the night of admission, nasal oxygen was administered. The next morning the patient was found to be stuporous, responding only to severe painful stimuli.

QUESTION:

15. THE MOST LIKELY EXPLANATION OF THE STUPOR IS:
     A. CVA
     B. Oxygen administration to a patient whose respiratory center was probably depressed by chronic hypercarbia due to inadequate ventilation
     C. Systemic alkalosis
     D. Drug overdosage in a depressed patient with a chronic central nervous system disease

The oxygen was discontinued. Blood gases were obtained, which showed a pCO_2 of 138 mm Hg, and a pO_2 of 55 mm Hg. Arterial pH was 7.13.

QUESTIONS:

16. THE BEST THERAPY WOULD BE:
     A. Rapid infusion of bicarbonate intravenously
     B. Mechanical ventilatory assistance
     C. Both of above
     D. Neither of above

17. A RAPID INTRAVENOUS INFUSION OF SODIUM BICARBONATE:
     A. Would be useful and important therapy
     B. Might cause increasing stupor
     C. Might cause increasing spinal fluid acidosis even as the blood pH was returning to normal
     D. Should not be given

She was given intermittent positive pressure breathing assistance fifteen minutes of each hour around the clock, with marked improvement in mental state, pH, and blood gases. She was placed in an Emerson respirator in the hospital's special nursing unit.

QUESTIONS:

18. PROGNOSIS IS:
     A. Good if respiratory infections can be prevented
     B. Good if prophylactic antibiotics are given
     C. Unpredictable
     D. Very poor

CASE STUDY #25

19. THE FAMOUS ATHLETE WHO DIED OF THIS DISEASE IS:
    A. Babe Ruth
    B. Jack Johnson
    C. Lou Gehrig
    D. Red Grange

20. THE PATHOLOGIC CHANGES IN THIS DISEASE OCCUR IN:
    A. Muscle
    B. Neuromuscular junction
    C. Nerve
    D. Anterior horn cells
    E. Corticospinal tracts

21. THE DIFFERENTIAL DIAGNOSIS OF THIS DISEASE INCLUDES:
    A. Syringomyelia
    B. Spinal cord tumor
    C. Syphilis
    D. Spondylosis
    E. Thoracic outlet syndrome
    F. Peripheral neuropathy
    G. All of the above

22. THE AVERAGE DURATION OF LIFE IN THIS DISEASE, AFTER APPEAR-
    ANCE OF SYMPTOMS, IS ABOUT:
    A. 3 months
    B. 3 years
    C. 6 years
    D. 15 years

23. A CLINICAL PICTURE SIMILAR TO ALS HAS BEEN REPORTED WITH:
    A. Chronic mercury poisoning   D. Gastrectomy
    B. Hypoglycemia   E. Lead poisoning
    C. Occult cancer

ANSWERS AND DISCUSSION:

1. ACDE   Weakness with atrophy of muscle occurs with disease of the
               motor unit-i. e. the anterior horn cell, peripheral axon, and
               muscle. Peripheral nerve disease is usually associated with
               sensory loss. Prominent fasciculations are much more common
               in anterior horn cell disease than in neuropathy or myopathy.

2. AHJ

3. BCKR

4. CLNR

5. DEMI

6. DIMF

7. OPQ   In myasthenia gravis, O and P are correct. In the myasthenic
               syndrome associated with cancer, Q is true, and the deep
               tendon reflexes may be depressed.

8. GI

CASE STUDY #25

9. E   Electromyography, nerve conduction velocity determinations, muscle biopsy and serum enzyme levels such as transaminase, creatine
phosphokinase, and lactic dehydrogenase have traditionally been the
most useful laboratory tests in separating and distinguishing between
motor, neuron, peripheral nerve and muscle disease, as in the diagram below.

	EMG	Nerve conduction	Enzymes	Biopsy
Motor Neuron Disease	denervation	normal	normal	neurogenic pattern of atrophy
Peripheral Nerve "	denervation	slowed	normal	"
Muscle disease	myopathic	normal	elevated	myopathic

In recent years, however, some of these distinctions between neurono-
pathy, neuropathy and myopathy have become blurred. "Myopathic"
changes in muscle biopsies (variation in fiber size, central nuclei,
degenerative and regenerative changes in the muscle, endomysial
fibrosis) have been reported in neuronal diseases as poliomyelitis,
amyotrophic lateral sclerosis and Kugelberg-Welander syndrome. Increases in serum enzymes, and "myopathic" electromyographic patterns, have also been seen in neuronal disease. On the other hand,
some consider that diseases where the site of pathology has been considered to be in the neuromuscular junction, as myasthenia gravis,
or the muscle fiber, as the muscular dystrophies, may be neurogenic
diseases. Thus, although the characteristics given in the table are
generally useful in clinical practice, our traditional and classical
concepts of neurogenic and myopathic disease are currently being re-
evaluated, challenged and redefined.

10. AB   Fasciculations, unassociated with weakness or atrophy, may be seen
in normal persons, or in metabolic disorders such as tetany or salt
deprivation.

11. BCDE

12. C   Because of the needle-induced inflammation.

13. C   Amyotrophic lateral sclerosis is a progressive disease with degeneration of pyramidal tracts and the lower motor neurons in the brain and
spinal cord. The cause is unknown. Either lower motor neuron signs
of flaccid weakness with atrophy or corticospinal tract abnormalities
of spasticity, hyperactive and pathological reflexes may predominate,
or various mixtures may occur.

The myasthenic syndrome occurs with cancer and consists of weakness with strength increasing on rapid successive muscle contractions.
It is thought to be due to a defect of acetylcholine release. Severe
wasting and fasciculations are not features of this syndrome.

Muscular dystrophy is a hereditary disease and is distinguished from
amyotrophic lateral sclerosis by the proximal muscle weakness (except for myotonic dystrophy in which the weakness is distal), rarity
of fasciculations, increased serum enzymes and myopathic changes
on the electromyogram and muscle biopsy.

Charcot-Marie-Tooth disease is a hereditary peripheral neuropathy
with abnormal sensation as well as distal extremity weakness.

Cervical cord compression may produce weakness and wasting of the
upper limb muscles, but also results in pyramidal tract abnormalities and impairment of sensation below the level of the lesion.

CASE STUDY #25

14. E

15. B   Apnea and stupor may result from oxygen administration in a patient with chronic depression of the respiratory center, which becomes relatively insensitive to the usual driving force of CO_2 tension.

The main driving force to the respiratory center then becomes anoxia. When oxygen is given, the anoxic drive for rhythmic breathing movements disappears with resultant apnea, stupor and coma.

16. B

17. BCD   The treatment of systemic acidosis with rapid infusions of intravenous bicarbonate may result in stupor or delirium because of the paradoxical development of cerebrospinal fluid acidosis in the face of an improving blood pH. When intravenous bicarbonate is given, a portion of it forms carbonic acid, and thence carbon dioxide and water. $H^+ + HCO3^- \rightleftarrows H2CO3 \rightleftarrows CO2 + H2O$. The bicarbonate ion diffuses slowly into the cerebrospinal fluid, but carbon dioxide exchanges rapidly between blood and CSF. The increase in CSF pCO_2 may lower the pH of the spinal fluid with resulting neurological deterioration in spite of a rising blood pH. The most rational therapy would be to correct the hypoxia and hypercarbia with mechanical respiratory assistance.

18. D

19. C

20. DE

21. G   Syringomyelia usually produces sensory loss in addition to muscle weakness. A spinal cord tumor also may produce atrophy and wasting of muscle by compression, invasion or impairment of the blood supply of anterior horn cells, but sensory impairment and pyramidal tract abnormalities are usually present below the level of the lesion. Meningovascular syphilis affecting the spinal cord would be expected to produce both sensory and motor deficits, as well as spinal fluid pleocytosis and a positive serology. Cervical spondylosis may cause impingement on nerve roots causing weakness and wasting of the muscles of the arm. Neck and arm pain are frequent, however, and cervical spine films will show the typical osteoarthritic changes.

Pain, sensory symptoms and signs, and evidence of vascular impairment in the arm are some of the features which may separate the thoracic outlet syndromes from ALS. Most peripheral neuropathies cause sensory abnormality, do not produce prominent fasciculation, or result in weakness and wasting of the tongue.

22. B

23. ABCDE

REFERENCES

1. Merritt, H.H., A Textbook of Neurology, 5th Ed., Lea and Febiger, 1973.

2. Elizan, T., K.M. Chen, K.V. Mathai, D. Dunn, and L.T. Kurland, Amyotrophic Lateral Sclerosis and Parkinsonism-Dementia Complex, Arch Neurol 14:347, 1966.

3. Kantarjian, A.D., A Syndrome Clinically Resembling Amyotrophic Lateral Sclerosis Following Chronic Mercurialism, Neurol 11:639, 1961.

4. Bulger, R., R. Schrier, W. Arend, and A. Swanson, Spinal Fluid Acidosis and the Diagnosis of Pulmonary Encephalopathy, New Eng J Med 274:433, 1966.

CASE STUDY #25

5. Welch, K., and D. Goldberg, Serum Creatine Phosphokinase in Motor Neuron Disease, Neurology 22:697, 1972.

6. Engel, W.K., Myopathic EMG-Nonesuch Animal, New Eng J Med 289:485, 1973.

7. Bobowick, A., and J. Brody, Epidomiology of Motor Neuron Diseases, New Eng J Med 288:1047, 1973.

8. Boothby, J., et al., Reversible Forms of Motor Neuron Disease, Arch Neurology 31:18, 1974.

9. Brown, W., and N. Jaatoul, Amyotrophic Lateral Sclerosis, Arch Neurol 30:242, 1974.

10. Achari, A., and M. Anderson, Myopathic Changes in Amyotrophic Lateral Sclerosis, Neurology 24:477, 1974.

11. Norris, F., et al., The Administration of Guanidine in Amyotrophic Lateral Sclerosis, Neurology 24:721-728, 1974.

12. Rowland, L.P., Are the Muscular Dystrophies Neurogenic? Annals NY Acad Sciences 228:244-260, 1974.

13. Engel, W.K., Brief, Small, Abundant Motor Unit Action Potentials, Neurology 25:173, 1975.

CASE STUDY #26

A Woman Who Couldn't Open Her Eye

HISTORY: A 55 year-old woman in good health began to complain of blurred vision. Three days later, she awoke unable to open her left eye. She was admitted to the hospital for investigation.

EXAMINATION: Neurological examination was negative except for the ocular findings. There was complete ptosis of the left upper eyelid (Fig. 29A). When the left upper eyelid was elevated passively, the left eye was found to be deviated outward (Fig. 29B).

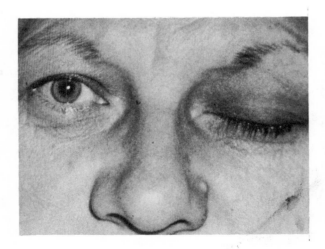

Figure 29A

CASE STUDY #26

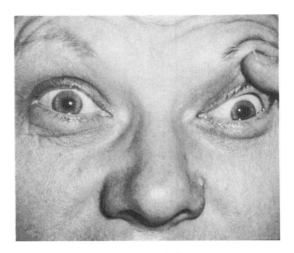

Figure 29B

When she attempted to look to the right, she was unable to adduct the left eye beyond the midline (Fig. 29C).

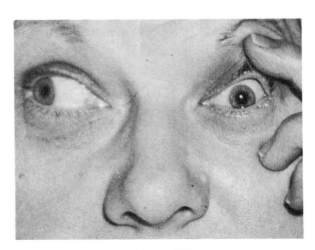

Figure 29C

CASE STUDY #26

In addition, she was unable to elevate or depress the left eye. The left pupil was larger than the right and it did not react to light, directly or consensually, or to accommodation. The right pupil reacted briskly to all stimuli. Visual acuity was 20/20 in both eyes. Visual fields were full. The fundi were normal. Corneal sensation was intact.

QUESTIONS:

1. IF THE RIGHT PUPIL REACTS TO LIGHT BOTH DIRECTLY AND CONSENSUALLY, AND THE LEFT PUPIL IS TOTALLY NONREACTIVE, THE LESION IS DUE TO:
   A. Interruption of the afferent arc of the left pupillary reflex
   B. Interruption of the efferent arc of the left pupillary reflex
   C. Interruption of the afferent or efferent arc of the right pupillary reflex
   D. None of the above

2. THE LEFT EYE IS DEVIATED OUTWARD DUE TO WEAKNESS OF:
   A. Superior oblique muscle
   B. Medial rectus muscle
   C. Inferior oblique muscle
   D. Lateral rectus muscle

   WITH RESULTANT OVERACTION OF:
   E. Superior oblique muscle
   F. Medial rectus muscle
   G. Inferior oblique muscle
   H. Lateral rectus muscle

   TRUE OR FALSE:

3. The lesion is probably not in the brain stem since there are no associated long tract motor, sensory or reflex abnormalities.

4. All of the abnormalities cannot be explained on the basis of a single lesion.

5. The fixed, dilated pupil eliminates myasthenia gravis as the cause of the opthalmoplegia

6. The lesion is probably located in the 4th and 6th cranial nerves.

7. The lesion is located in the 3rd nerve.

8. The pupil is dilated and fixed because of interruption of parasympathetic fibers located in the third nerve.

9. The pupil is dilated because of unopposed activity of the sympathetic fibers innervating the pupil.

10. If both sympathetic and parasympathetic innervations to the pupil are interrupted, as in a lesion high in the brain stem, the pupil is usually fixed in mid-dilation.

11. A third nerve palsy due to diabetes is usually associated with a fixed, dilated pupil.

12. A third nerve palsy due to compression by an aneurysm is commonly associated with a fixed, dilated pupil.

CASE STUDY #26

13. THE SYMPATHETIC PATHWAY TO THE PUPIL IS SPARED WHEN THE THIRD NERVE IS DAMAGED SINCE:
   A. It extends from the hypothalamus through the brain stem to the spinal cord
   B. It exits from the spinal cord at the eighth cervical and first thoracic segments, and it ascends in the cervical sympathetic chain
   C. It accompanies the internal carotid artery intracranially
   D. It reaches the eye in the first division of the fifth cranial nerve
   E. All of the above

14. DIAGNOSTIC POSSIBILITIES IN THIS CASE INCLUDE:
   A. Aneurysm
   B. Tumor
   C. Lues
   D. Chronic meningitis
   E. All of the above

15. APPROPRIATE INITIAL TESTS MIGHT INCLUDE:
   A. FTA absorption test
   B. X-rays of skull
   C. Pneumoencephalogram
   D. Spinal tap
   E. Brain scan
   F. Blood sugar

16. IF ALL INITIAL TESTS ARE NEGATIVE (AS THEY WERE IN THIS CASE), THE FOLLOWING ADDITIONAL TEST IS INDICATED:
   A. Posterior fossa myelogram
   B. Left carotid arteriogram
   C. Both of the above
   D. Neither of the above

COURSE: A left carotid arteriogram was performed (Fig. 30).

QUESTION:

17. THE LOCATION OF THE ANEURYSM IS:
   A. In the anterior cerebral artery
   B. At the origin of the posterior communicating artery from the internal carotid artery
   C. In the basilar artery
   D. In the middle cerebral artery

TREATMENT: A craniotomy was performed. A clip was placed around the neck of the aneurysm. Recovery was uneventful. There was partial return of function of the left third nerve.

CASE STUDY #26

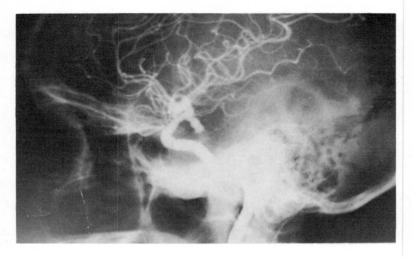

Figure 30

ANSWERS AND DISCUSSION:

1. B

2. BH

3. True

4. False

5. True   Myasthenia gravis does not affect pupillary function.

6. False   The trochlear (4th) nerve innervates the superior oblique muscle. A lesion of this nerve produces impairment of ocular rotation downward and inward. The abducens (6th) nerve innervates the lateral rectus muscle, which rotates the eye outward. A lesion affecting the 6th nerve will result in an inward deviation of the eye, unlike the outward deviation noted in this patient.

7. True

8. True   Inability to elevate the upper eyelid is due to weakness of the levator palpebrae superioris. Inability to elevate the eye is the result of weakness of the superior rectus and inferior oblique muscles; inability to depress the eye is due to paresis of the inferior rectus muscle. The fixed dilated pupil is due to interruption of parasympathetic fibers innervating the sphincter of the pupil. The third cranial nerve controls all of these functions.

9. True

CASE STUDY #26

10. True Conversely, if a lesion is located in the lower brain stem (e.g. pons), the pupil is usually miotic. This is the result of unopposed activity by the parasympathetic fibers which leave the brain stem at a higher level in company with the third nerve. In such a low brainstem lesion, would you predict that the pupillary reflex would be impaired?

11. False Third nerve palsies due to diabetes mellitus are usually characterized by pupillary sparing. The pupil is equal in size to its fellow and it is normally reactive.

12. True

13. E

14. E

15. ABDEF A pneumoencephalogram should be considered a major diagnostic procedure. It is associated with a significant morbidity rate. It should not be considered an "initial" test. Furthermore, when an aneurysm is an important diagnostic possibility, an arteriogram rather than a pneumoencephalogram is the appropriate contrast study to be performed.

16. B

17. B

REFERENCES

1. Walsh, F.B., and W.F. Hoyt, Clinical Neuro-Ophthalmology, 3rd Ed., Williams and Wilkins, Baltimore, 1969.

2. Green, W., et al., Neuro-Ophthalmologic Evaluation of Oculomotor Nerve Paralysis, Arch Ophthalmol 72:154, 1964.

3. Dailey, E., Evaluation of Ocular Signs and Symptoms in Cerebral Aneurysms, Arch Ophthalmol 71:463, 1964.

CASE STUDY #27

A Child with a Learning Problem

HISTORY: A seven year-old boy was referred for neurological evaluation because of learning difficulty.

Since his second year, the child had been hyperactive, always in motion, touching and pulling whatever he could, frequently breaking objects around the house. He had difficulty getting along with other children, and was often fighting. He was impulsive and easily frustrated, with frequent temper tantrums when not given his way. Both teachers and parents had noted that the child seemed to be able to concentrate on any task or subject for only a very short time. His intelligence, however, was felt to be normal. The boy had been adopted, and the family, pregnancy, and birth history were unknown. There was no history of seizures, head trauma or serious illness.

EXAMINATION: The boy was alert but could not keep still, constantly squirming, fidgeting, and reaching for objects. He showed some clumsiness in rapid successive movements and had considerable difficulty in reading and copying diagrams. Speech, vision, hearing, and the remainder of the neurological examination were normal. He seemed of normal intelligence.

CASE STUDY #27

QUESTIONS:

1. THE MOST LIKELY DIAGNOSIS OF THIS CHILD'S ILLNESS IS:
    A. Cerebral palsy
    B. Minimal brain damage syndrome of childhood
    C. Childhood Huntington's chorea
    D. None of the above

2. THE DIFFERENTIAL DIAGNOSIS INCLUDES:
    A. Organic disease of the central nervous system
    B. Psychiatric illness
    C. Both of the above

    MATCH THE CHARACTERISTICS WITH THE APPROPRIATE DISEASE
    INVOLVED IN THE DIFFERENTIAL DIAGNOSIS OF THIS CASE:

3. ___ Pervasive impairment of   A. Juvenile lipidosis
         interpersonal relationships,
         bizarre behavior   B. Mental retardation
4. ___ Frequent lapses of attention
5. ___ Seizures, hemiparesis   C. Petit mal
6. ___ Global impairment of
         intellectual function   D. Subacute sclerosing
7. ___ Early decrease of vision,   panencephalitis
         abnormalities of retina
8. ___ Myoclonic seizures, high   E. Brain tumor
         spinal fluid gamma globulin
9. ___ Normal vision and intelligence   F. Hearing impairment
         impaired speech
                                          G. Childhood schizophrenia

10. USEFUL LABORATORY TESTS IN THIS CASE MIGHT INCLUDE:
    A. Psychometric testing
    B. Audiometric testing
    C. Electroencephalogram
    D. Visual testing
    E. All of the above

LABORATORY DATA: Stanford-Binet testing showed an IQ of 125. Electroencephalogram, skull films, auditory and visual testing, protein bound iodide,
urine amino acid screening were all normal.

QUESTIONS:

11. THE TREATMENT OF THIS SYNDROME INCLUDES:
    A. Avoidance of excessive excitement and stimulation
    B. Drug therapy
    C. Firm consistent discipline
    D. All of the above

CASE STUDY #27

12. USEFUL DRUGS INCLUDE:
    A. Methylphenidate
    B. Phenobarbital
    C. Dextroamphetamine
    D. All of above

COURSE: The parents were reassured about the absence of progressive central nervous system disease. Goals of consistency, firmness in discipline, and avoidance of excessive stimulation were also discussed with the parents. On a regimen of dextroamphetamine, 5 mgm three times daily, the child has shown considerable improvement.

ANSWERS AND DISCUSSION:

1. B

2. C   The term minimal brain damage has been applied to children in
             whom overall general intelligence is within the normal range,
             but who have disturbances of perception, conceptualization,
             language function, and impulse and emotional control and reg-
             ulation. These children often have severe learning difficulties
             in school in spite of good verbal abilities and overall normal
             level of intellectual functioning. Hyperactivity, restlessness and
             destructiveness are common. The attention span is character-
             istically short and the child is easily distracted. The child is
             often impulsive, emotionally labile, and forgetful. Awkwardness,
             clumsiness and hyperactivity are frequently the only abnormalities
             on neurological examination. This disorder is estimated to
             affect at least 5% of the entire child population, making it one of
             the most common neurological disorders of childhood. Genetic,
             emotional factors as well as ante or perinatal brain injury have
             been etiologically implicated.

             In the differential diagnosis, hearing and visual impairment,
             mental retardation, seizures, progressive cerebral diseases
             (such as neoplasms, lipidosis, subacute sclerosing panencephal-
             itis), schizophrenia, childhood adjustment reactions, and socio-
             cultural deprivation are to be considered.

             Cerebral palsy is associated with gross motor deficit. Hunting-
             tons chorea may occur in childhood; this is quite rare. This
             disease is inherited as a dominant trait.

3. G

4. C

5. E

6. B

7. A

8. D

9. F

10. E   Electroencephalographic abnormalities in the form of mild
             dysrhythmias are frequently reported in children with this syn-
             drome and are often of little assistance in evaluation or prognosis.

CASE STUDY #27

Suspicion of seizures or progressive CNS disease requires EEG evaluation. In practice, parents often arrive at the office convinced by school authorities that the neurological evaluation is incomplete without an EEG and so one is ordered for the peace of mind of both the doctor and the parents.

11. D

12. AC Children with this syndrome react paradoxically to certain groups of drugs, becoming even more hyperactive and unmanageable with barbiturates and more tranquil and less hyperactive with stimulant drugs as methylphenidate and dextroamphetamine.

REFERENCES

1. Schain, R. J., Minimal Brain Dysfunction in Children, A Neurological Viewpoint, Bull Los Angeles Neuro Soc 33:145, 1968.

2. Menkes, M. M., J. S. Rowe, and J. H. Menkes, A Twenty Five Year Follow-Up Study on the Hyperkinetic Child with Minimal Brain Dysfunction, Pediatrics 39:393, 1967.

3. Paine, R. S., Syndromes of Minimal Cerebral Damage, Ped Clin N A 15:779, 1968.

4. Towbin, A., Organic Causes of Minimal Brain Dysfunction, JAMA 217:1207, 1971.

5. Groover, R., The Hyperkinetic Child, Psych Annals 2:36, 1972.

6. Howell, M., G. Rever, and M. Scholl, Hyperactivity in Children, Clin Ped 11:30, 1972.

7. Cohn, R., Minimal Brain Dysfunction, JAMA 218:887, 1971.

8. Kinsbourne, M., Diagnosis and Treatment of School Problems, Pediatrics 52:697, 1973.

9. Schain, R., The Neurological Evaluation of Children with Learning Disorders, Calif Med 118:24-32, 1973.

10. Sroufe, L., and M. Stewart, Treating Problem Children with Stimulant Drugs, New Eng J Med 289:407, 1973.

11. Conference on Minimal Brain Dysfunction, New York Academy of Sciences, Annals of New York Academy of Sciences, Volume 205, February 1973.

12. Berlin, I., Minimal Brain Dysfunction, JAMA 229:1454, 1974.

13. Greenberg, L., et al., Side Effects of Dextroamphetamine Therapy of Hyperactive Children, West J Med 120:105-109, 1974.

14. Sleator, E., et al., Hyperactive Children, JAMA 229:316, 1974.

CASE STUDY #28

Coma and Nuchal Rigidity

HISTORY: The patient was a 16 year-old female who was in her usual state of good health until 3 days prior to hospitalization when she began to complain of malaise, anorexia, and intermittent diarrhea. On the morning of admission, she developed pressure-like frontal headaches, stiffness of the neck, and fever of 103. She vomited on three occasions prior to admission. One half hour before admission she became unresponsive. Four days before admission, she had been visited by a friend who was in a local Marine Corps boot camp. She had no exposure to individuals with known infectious disease or significant animal contacts, nor had she ever been outside of the country.

PHYSICAL EXAMINATION: Temperature 104.2, pulse 160, respiration 100/min. blood pressure 100/60. She was unresponsive to verbal commands, restless and resistive to examination. The head was normocephalic with no evidence of trauma. The posterior pharynx was erythematous without exudate. There was moderately severe nuchal rigidity. No adenopathy was present. Cardiac examination revealed no abnormalities. The skin was clear with no petechiae or rash. The liver and spleen were not enlarged.

Neurological examination revealed the fundi to be benign. The cranial nerves were normal throughout. There was no focal weakness. The deep tendon reflexes were 2+ and equal bilaterally. There was a positive Babinski on the right. She responded by withdrawal and resistiveness to painful stimuli.

QUESTIONS:

1. THE DIAGNOSTIC CONSIDERATIONS INCLUDE:
    A. Subarachnoid hemorrhage
    B. Viral encephalitis
    C. Bacterial meningitis
    D. All of above

2. RAPID DETERIORATION OF CONSCIOUSNESS IS FREQUENTLY SEEN IN:
    A. Multiple sclerosis
    B. Meningococcal meningitis
    C. Subdural hematoma
    D. Lead neuropathy
    E. All of above

3. NUCHAL RIGIDITY MAY BE SEEN WITH:
    A. Subarachnoid hemorrhage
    B. Meningitis
    C. Fracture of the cervical spine
    D. All of above

LABORATORY DATA: The following laboratory studies were obtained shortly after admission: Skull films were normal. Blood sugar 117 mgs%, BUN 13, Potassium 2.9, Sodium 139, Bicarbonate 13. Urinalysis-specific gravity 1.006, pH 7, Albumin-trace, sugar negative, acetone negative, 2-4 WBC, 20-30 RBC, no organisms were seen. Hemoglobin 14.6 gms, WBC 16,600 with 80% polys, 15% lymphs, 3% monocytes, 2% eosinophils. Electrocardiogram was within normal limits. EEG showed diffuse 5-7 cycle per second activity.

Shortly after admission, lumbar puncture was carried out. This revealed an opening pressure of 280 mm. The spinal fluid was grossly cloudy and contained 29,400 WBC's, 98% of which were polys. Spinal fluid protein was 450 mgs%, spinal fluid sugar was 15 mgs%. On gram stain, numerous gram negative

CASE STUDY #28

diplococci were observed. Blood cultures were obtained and at 36 hours these grew out Neisseria Meningitidis. Immediately after L. P. the patient was placed on intravenous Ampicillin. Within the next four days, significant improvement occurred. On the 5th day following admission, she was much more alert with only minimal evidence of an organic mental syndrome. The next day, however, she had a generalized major motor seizure and was placed on anticonvulsants. Further seizures occurred throughout the next week. Repeat EEG did not demonstrate any focal abnormality and brain scan was within normal limits. She was discharged approximately three weeks after admission, asymptomatic, on anticonvulsants, with a normal neurological examination.

QUESTIONS:

4. THE TWO MOST COMMON CAUSES OF ADULT BACTERIAL MENINGITIS ARE:
   A. Meningococcus
   B. Pneumococcus
   C. Fungal
   D. H. influenza

5. SPINAL FLUID SUGAR MAY BE DEPRESSED IN:
   A. Bacterial meningitis
   B. Meningeal carcinomatosis
   C. Fungal meningitis
   D. All of above

6. WHICH OF THE FOLLOWING IS NOT A COMMON SEQUELA OF BACTERIAL MENINGITIS?
   A. Seizure disorder
   B. Communicating hydrocephalus
   C. Peripheral neuropathy
   D. Deafness

7. FOR THE PATIENT WITH BACTERIAL MENINGITIS OF UNCERTAIN CAUSE THE ACCEPTED FORM OF THERAPY IS:
   A. Cephalothin
   B. Ampicillin intravenously
   C. Penicillin intramuscularly
   D. Any of the above

8. TRUE OR FALSE:

   A. Viral meningoencephalitis frequently causes a depressed CSF sugar.

   B. Subarachnoid hemorrhage may rarely lower CSF sugar.

   C. In most patients meningitis begins without clear-cut evidence of exposure to an infected person.

   D. Viable organisms may be found in the rash of meningococcemia.

   E. H. influenza meningitis is most common in children.

   F. In penicillin-allergic patients the antibiotic of choice for bacterial meningitis is chloramphenicol.

ANSWERS AND DISCUSSION:

1. D   In the patient who presents with meningeal irritation, fever, and organic mental syndrome, any process affecting the meninges and the adjacent cerebral cortex should be considered. Subarachnoid hemorrhage, viral, bacterial and fungal meningoen-

CASE STUDY #28

cephalitis and neoplasia should all be considered.

2. BC

3. D   In patients who have sustained a fractured cervical spine, considerable
nuchal rigidity may be present. In these patients, however, pain can be
elicited with rotational and lateral flexion movements of the cervical
spine, whereas nuchal rigidity due to meningeal irritation from a subarachnoid hemorrhage or infectious process usually results in limitation
of cervical spine movement only in the anterior plane, in forward flexion.

4. AB

5. D   Depression of spinal fluid sugar is usually a very important and helpful
laboratory finding. The spinal fluid sugar is approximately 2/3rds of
blood sugar levels. It is advisable to determine the blood sugar about
1-1/2 - 2 hours before performing a spinal tap. This is approximately the
time interval for equilibration of sugar across the blood-CSF barrier.
Profound depressions of spinal fluid sugar are seen in bacterial meningitis and on occasion in fungal meningitis. Subarachnoid hemorrhage,
sarcoidosis, and meningeal carcinomatosis may also depress spinal
fluid sugar levels.

6. C   Communicating hydrocephalus is one of the more serious sequelae of
bacterial meningitis. It is especially prominent in children, but may
occur in adults as well. It may be present without prominent elevation
of spinal fluid pressure as measured by lumbar puncture. These patients present with a progressive organic dementia and may have difficulty with gait and controlling micturition. Early detection of these
patients is important since ventriculojugular or other shunts may prevent advanced and irreversible cerebral damage. The management of
post meningitis seizure disorder is similar to idiopathic seizure disorders.

7. B   In the patient diagnosed as having bacterial meningitis, immediate
therapy should be carried out even before a specific organism is identified. At the present time, most authorities favor intravenous Ampicillin, which for the most part has replaced "triple therapy" of gantrisin,
penicillin, and chloramphenicol. When a specific organism has been
identified, changes in the antibiotic regimen may be necessary.

8.   A. False   D. True
B. True   E. True
C. True   F. True

REFERENCES

1. Carpenter, R.R., and R.G. Petersdorf, The Clinical Spectrum of Bacterial
Meningitis, Amer J Med 33:262, 1962.

2. Swarz, M.N.,and P.R. Dodge, Bacterial Meningitis - A Review of Selected
Aspects, New Eng J Med 22:725, 779, 842, 898; 1965.

3. Petersdorf, R., and D. Harter, The Fall in Cerebrospinal Fluid Sugar in
Meningitis, Arch Neur 4:21, 1961.

4. Buchan, G., and E. Alvord, Diffuse Necrosis of Subcortical White Matter
Associated with Bacterial Meningitis, Neurology 19:1, 1969.

5. Sahs, A., and R. Joynt, Meningitis, in Clinical Neurology V 2, A.B. Baker,
and L.H. Baker, Ed., Harper and Row, 1971.

CASE STUDY #28

6. Bacterial Meningitis, A Symposium, Pediatrics 52:586-600, 1973.

7. Nankervis, G., Bacterial Meningitis, Med Clin N Am 58:581, 1974.

CASE STUDY #29

Paraparesis in a Middle-Aged Man After Lifting a Heavy Weight

HISTORY: This 50 year-old male was in good health and worked as a gas station attendant until approximately three weeks before admission, when, while lifting a case of oil cans, he experienced the rather sudden onset of low back pain with difficulty in "straightening up." His productivity at work was impaired in the ensuing several days, but he was able to walk reasonably well. About one and one-half weeks before admission, the pain increased considerably and began to involve the right buttock as well as the midline low back. It was described as aching, present most of the time, but fluctuating in severity. When coughing or sneezing, the pain was significantly intensified, but did not radiate down the leg. About this time, he began to experience difficulty voiding voluntarily. He was unable to initiate the urinary stream without difficulty and began to experience urinary incontinence. Also at this time, he became constipated, requiring heavy doses of cathartics for bowel movements.

EXAMINATION: There was mild percussion tenderness at the lumbosacral interspace, but no significant impairment of straight leg raising was noted. The bladder was palpable up to the umbilicus. Rectal sphincter tone was very poor. Strength in the upper extremities was normal. The following percent of normal muscle strength was found in the lower extremities: left iliopsoas 10%, quadriceps 75%, gastrocnemius-soleus 10%, tibialis anterior and peronei 10%. On the right, the values were essentially the same, except that there was somewhat greater strength in the iliopsoas and hamstrings. There was decreased position and vibratory sensation in the distal right lower extremity with mild pin and touch impairment about the rectum. Cerebellar and cranial nerve functions were normal. Upon admission he was catherized and 2200 cc of urine was obtained. The BUN was 52, blood sugar 244. Urinalysis and serum electrolytes were normal. Lumbar spine films showed minimal osteoarthritic changes. WBC was 24,200 with a shift to the left. Electromyography revealed occasional fibrillatory activity in the tibialis anterior, gastrocnemius and lateral hamstrings bilaterally.

QUESTIONS:

1. ON THE BASIS OF THE FINDINGS SO FAR, THE LESION MOST LIKELY INVOLVES:
   A. Pyramidal tract fibers arising from the medial portion of the cerebral hemispheres, producing a paraparesis
   B. The entire width of the brainstem at a pontine level
   C. The cervical cord
   D. The thoracic spinal cord
   E. The lumbosacral roots of the cauda equina

2. THE MAIN DIAGNOSTIC POSSIBILITIES INCLUDE:
   A. Tumor compressing the cauda equina
   B. Multiple sclerosis
   C. Herniated disc compressing the cauda equina
   D. Herniated disc compressing the thoracic spinal cord
   E. Amyotrophic lateral sclerosis

CASE STUDY #29

3. THE MOST IMPORTANT TEST TO DO AT THIS POINT WOULD BE:
   A. Spinal fluid gamma globulin
   B. Bone marrow aspiration
   C. Myelography
   D. Pneumoencephalogram

A myelogram was carried out revealing epidural lesions at L4-5 and L5-S1 (Fig. 31A, B). It was felt that these were consistent with disc disease. A laminectomy was performed and, after opening the dura, the cauda equina was seen to be displaced by a large mass at the L4-5 interspace. The mass was a large herniated nucleus pulposus. During the ensuing postoperative weeks, he was treated with intensive physical therapy and rehabilitation, and eventually became able to ambulate with assistance.

QUESTIONS:

4. RUPTURE OF AN INTERVERTEBRAL DISC IS MOST COMMON AT:
   A. C5-6 and C4-5
   B. T1-2 and T3-4
   C. L1-2 and L2-3
   D. L4-5 and L5-S1

5. THE MOST COMMON REFLEX ABNORMALITY IN LUMBAR DISC DIS-
   EASE IS:
   A. Increase of all deep tendon reflexes
   B. Decrease of all deep tendon reflexes
   C. Absent abdominal reflexes
   D. Positive Babinski sign
   E. Absent ankle reflex

6. THE MOST FREQUENT MOTOR DEFICIT IN A RUPTURED DISC IS:
   A. Spastic paraparesis
   B. Peripheral neuropathy
   C. Mononeurtitis
   D. Weakness in the distribution of the compressed root
   E. None of the above

7. THE CEREBROSPINAL FLUID PROTEIN IN A HERNIATED DISC SYN-
   DROME IS USUALLY:
   A. Normal
   B. Elevated
   C. Depressed
   D. May be any of the above depending on the clinical circumstances

8. THE CSF CELL COUNT IN A HERNIATED DISC SYNDROME IS USUALLY:
   A. Normal
   B. Elevated
   C. Depressed
   D. May be any of the above depending on clinical circumstances

CASE STUDY #29

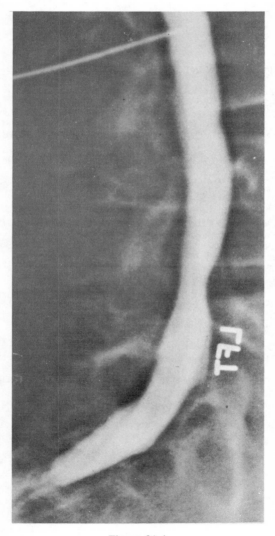

Figure 31 A

CASE STUDY #29

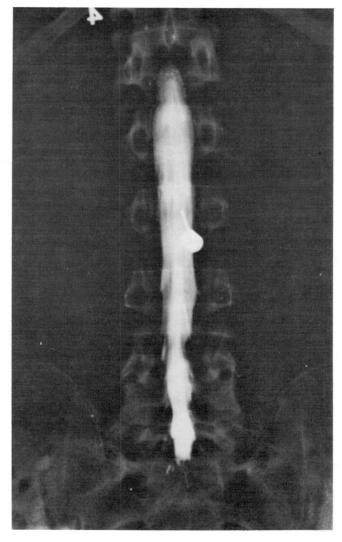

Figure 31 B

CASE STUDY #29

ANSWERS AND DISCUSSION:

1. E   Weakness of the legs, decrease in the deep tendon reflexes, and impaired bladder and bowel function all may result from damage to the lumbosacral roots.

     A cerebral lesion causing a paraparesis would cause spastic paresis with hyperreflexia, Babinski signs and the other typical abnormalities of impaired corticospinal tract function.

     The patient has no abnormalities of cranial nerve function which would suggest brain stem damage.

     The absence of pyramidal tract abnormalities in the legs, sensory level or abnormalities of the upper extremities are against the diagnosis of a cervical cord lesion.

     In an acute thoracic cord lesion (as might occur following trauma, hemorrhage, etc.) one might see, in the stage of spinal shock, a flaccid paraparesis with bowel and bladder impairment, but one would expect impaired sensation below the thoracic sensory level and an evolution of the paraparesis to a spastic, hyper-reflexic type.

2. AC   Compression of the lumbosacral roots by either tumor or disc would be an important diagnostic possibility. The onset of symptoms following lifting of a heavy weight favors the latter etiology.

     Multiple sclerosis very rarely begins this late in life and it affects various portions of the central nervous system so that long tract, corticospinal and sensory abnormalities are usually present.

     Amyotrophic lateral sclerosis is a slowly progressive disease of the lower motor neurons and pyramidal tracts producing com-binations of upper and lower neuron signs in the limbs, and various muscles innervated by cranial nerves.

3. C   The most important diagnostic task is to establish whether there is evidence of surgically remediable compression of the spinal cord, and myelography is the definitive test for this.

4. D   Disc protrusion at the L4-5 or L5-S1 level is the most frequent site of involvement. Thoracic disc protrusions are very rare, but may produce a difficult syndrome to diagnose clinically. In the cervical area, lesions at C6-7 and C7-T1 are most common, but occur less frequently than lumbar disc protrusions. Low back pain with radicular radiation into the lower extremity is the hallmark of lumbar disc protrusion.

5. E   Due to compression of the S1 root as it traverses the L5-S1 interspace.

6. D   When a disc ruptures through the annulus fibrosis and compresses the adjacent motor and/or sensory nerve root, neurologic deficit in the distribution of that root occurs. Because the L5 root is frequently affected, patients commonly have weakness in the extensor hallucis longus or tibialis anterior on that side; with compression of the S1 root the ipsilateral ankle jerk usually disappears very

CASE STUDY #29

early. With multiple or large disc protrusions, several nerve roots can be involved with a cauda equina syndrome such as occurred in this patient. At a cervical or thoracic level, in addition to root involvement, the spinal cord may be compressed and upper motor neuron signs can occur. This does not happen with lumbar disc protrusion because the spinal cord ends at about the L1 vertebral level.

7. A

8. A   The cerebrospinal fluid in disc disease usually remains normal. On rare occasions, with acute or massive herniation, there may be a slight elevation in protein or cell count. The cellular response is usually lymphocytic and in the range of 10-15 lymphocytes/cu mm. Rarely does the protein rise significantly. When such occurs, a lesion other than disc rupture should be suspected.

REFERENCES

1.   Bradford, F. K., and R. G. Spurling, The Intervertebral Disc, with Special Reference to Rupture of the Annulus Fibrosus with Herniation of the Nucleus Pulposus, Charles C Thomas, Springfield, Illinois.

2.   Yoss, R. E., et al., Significance of Symptoms and Signs in Localization of Involved Root in Cervical Disc Protrusion, Neurology 7:673, 1957.

3.   Love, J. G., and M. N. Walsh, Protruded Intervertebral Disk, Surg Gyn Ob 77:497, 1943.

CASE STUDY #30

A Young Boy with Abnormal Movements

HISTORY: A nine year-old boy who had been in excellent health previously was referred for neurological evaluation because of a peculiar posturing of his right leg when he walked.

For three months his parents had noted an unusual posturing of his hands when he played the piano, and a dragging inturning of his right leg when he walked. A maternal grandfather was said to have had a shaking tremor, and an uncle died of an unknown type of "muscle disease."

EXAMINATION: The boy was alert and bright. The deep tendon reflexes were equal, and there were no pathological reflexes. As he extended his arms, the right rotated involuntarily internally at the shoulder, and flexed at the wrist. The right foot was rotated inward, assuming an equinovarus position.

COURSE: When seen three months later he was much worse. Severe slow twisting movements of his body and all extremities contorted him into bizarre postures (Figs. 32 A, B)

CASE STUDY #30

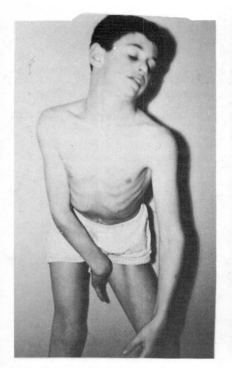
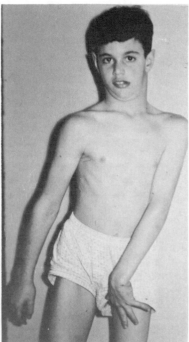

Figure 32 A   Figure 32 B

QUESTIONS:

1. THESE ABNORMAL MOVEMENTS AND POSTURES DISAPPEARED DUR-
    ING SLEEP AND WERE WORSE WITH EMOTIONAL STRESS. DOES THIS
    PROVE A HYSTERICAL ILLNESS?:
    A. Yes, since one would expect an organic dyskinesia to be constantly
        present
    B. No, since organic dyskinesias may vary in intensity with stress or
        disappear during sleep
    C. Can't tell since there is insufficient information

    TRUE OR FALSE:

2. Although a history of birth injury or asphyxia would be important to elicit
    in the differential diagnosis, this boy probably does not suffer from a form
    of cerebral palsy, since he is mentally normal, has no history of develop-
    ment retardation, nor evidence of pyramidal tract dysfunction.

CASE STUDY #30

3. Syphilis can produce this clinical picture.

4. A brownish ring around the corneas would be an important diagnostic clue.

5. Drug ingestion could produce this clinical picture and must be ruled out.

6. LABORATORY TESTS WHICH MIGHT BE USEFUL IN THE INITIAL EVALUATION INCLUDE:
    A. Myelography
    B. Skull films
    C. Serum ceruloplasmin
    D. Serum folic acid
    E. FTA-ABS
    F. Slit lamp examination of the eyes

LABORATORY DATA: Skull films, electroencephalogram, calcium, ceruloplasmin, blood sugar, serology, slit lamp examinations, and the spinal fluid were all normal. There was no history of drug ingestion.

QUESTIONS:

7. THE MOST LIKELY DIAGNOSIS IS:
    A. Juvenile Huntington's chorea
    B. Viral encephalitis
    C. Multiple sclerosis
    D. Dystonia musculorum deformans
    E. Juvenile lipidosis

8. THE HIGHEST INCIDENCE OF THIS DISEASE IS IN:
    A. Japanese
    B. Norwegians
    C. Palestinian Arabs
    D. Jews of Eastern European descent
    E. South Africans

COURSE: He continued to worsen and became unable to use his left hand for any coordinated movements. He remained intellectually normal. Valium produced only slight benefit. Surgery was performed.

QUESTION:

9. THE OPERATION WAS:
    A. Cordotomy
    B. Cerebellar resection
    C. Placement of a lesion in the ventral lateral nucleus of the thalamus
    D. Placement of a lesion in the anterior nucleus of the thalamus
    E. None of above

COURSE: Following a right cryothalamotomy, the twisting movements of the left side were much improved. Postoperatively a persistent left Babinski sign was present.

CASE STUDY #30

QUESTION:

10. THE BABINSKI SIGN SIGNIFIES DAMAGE TO THE:
   A. Rubrospinal tract
   B. Spinothalamic tract
   C. Corticospinal tract
   D. Thalamic-parietal radiations
   E. Reticulospinal tract

A year later, the same operation was performed on the left side, again with contra-lateral improvement in the involuntary movements. After the operation his speech was thickened and slurred and he noted difficulty in swallowing. There were bi-lateral Babinski signs.

QUESTION:

11. THE DYSARTHRIA IS DUE TO:
   A. Coincidental myasthenia
   B. A lesion of the corticobulbar tracts bilaterally above the level of the medul-la, causing an upper motor neuron paralysis of pharynx and palate, termed a pseudobulbar palsy
   C. Damage to brainstem nuclei
   D. None of above

Some deterioration in his condition occurred, but he then seemed to stabilize. He is still disabled by severe contortions of his trunk and limbs when he walks, but is much better than prior to surgery. Courses of amantadine and L-DOPA were given without benefit.

ANSWERS AND DISCUSSION:

1. B

2. True

3. True

4. True   This is a description of a Kayser-Fleischer ring, seen in nepatolen-ticular degeneration (Wilson's disease). This disease is most impor-tant to suspect and rule out in any case of abnormal movement dis-order since it is treatable.

5. True   The phenothiazine drugs can produce a variety of abnormal "extra-pyramidal" movements, as can reserpine and the butyrophenones.

6. BCEF   Myelography is not indicated since there is no evidence of spinal cord disease. Skull films may give clues to various dyskinesia-causing diseases. Bilateral basal ganglia calcification, for instance, would suggest the possibility of hypoparathyroidism. Brain tumor may also (rarely) present with abnormal movements suggesting extrapyramidal disease. Serum ceruloplasmin is almost always elevated in Wilson's disease, but may be normal in patients with this condition in the pres-ence of severe liver damage. The slit lamp examination should re-veal a Kayser-Fleischer ring in an untreated case of symptomatic Wilson's disease. The FTA is the most specific test for syphilitic infection.

7. D   Dystonia musculorum deformans is an uncommon disease, inherited in either autosomal recessive or dominant patterns, and character-ized by abnormal postures and movements, most commonly involving neck, trunk and extremities.

   In Huntington's chorea, the abnormal choreic movements are quicker than in dystonia. Psychiatric disturbances and dementia are promi-nent features of this disease. It is dominantly inherited and therefore a history of parental involvement is more commonly obtained.

CASE STUDY #30

The viral encephalitides are associated with a variety of neurological symptoms and signs including seizures, mental changes, weakness, spasticity, etc. Our traditional concept of viral encephalitis as an acute illness, however, with fever, evidence of meningeal irritation and cerebrospinal fluid pleocytosis, has been altered by elucidation of diseases such as subacute sclerosing panencephalitis, a viral encephalitis due to a peculiar form of measles virus infection characterized by gradual onset of dementia, myoclonus and neurological deterioration. Other "slow virus" diseases are Kuru and Jakob-Creutzfeldt disease. The absence of a history of remission and exacerbation, evidence of disseminated disease of the central nervous system, and of long tract motor, sensory and reflex abnormalities exclude multiple sclerosis as a diagnostic possibility in this case.

Dystonia has been reported in juvenile lipidosis, but the absence of visual, intellectual, or other neurological abnormalities besides the dyskinesia is against this possibility.

8. D

9. C   Cooper,[2] on the basis of his experience with the surgical treatment of 164 cases of dystonia, feels that cryothalamotomy is the present treatment of choice for dystonia.

The ventrolateral nucleus of the thalamus receives input from both the basal ganglia, via fibers from the globus pallidus, as well as from the cerebellum via the brachium conjunctivum-rubrothalamic pathway. Lesions in this thalamic nucleus have been of benefit in various types of "extrapyramidal" disease such as parkinsonism and dystonia, as well as in some cases of cerebellar intention tremor.

10. C

11. B

REFERENCES

1. Zeman, W., P. Dyken, Dystonia Musculorum Deformans; Zeman, W., C.C. Whitlock, Handbook of Clinical Neurology, P.J. Vinken, G.W. Bruyn, Ed., North Holland Publishing Co., 1968.

2. Conference on the Torsion Dystonias, R. Eldridge, Ed., Neurology, Vol. 20, Part 2 (Nov.) 1970.

3. Sciarra, D., B.E. Sprofkin, Symptoms and Signs Referable to Basal Ganglia in Brain Tumor, Arch Neurol Psychiat 69:450-461 (Apr.) 1953.

4. Eldridge, R., et al., Levodopa in Dystonia, Lancet 2:1027, 1973.

5. Drug Therapy: Neurologic Syndromes Associated with Antipsychotic Drug Use, New Eng J Med 289:20, 1973.

6. Geller, M., et al., Dystonic Symptoms in Children, Treatment with Carbamazepine, JAMA 229:1755, 1974.

7. Marsden, C., M. Harrison, Idiopathic Torsion Dystonia, Brain 97:793, 1974.

CASE STUDY #31

An Infant with a Large Head

HISTORY: Neurological consultation was requested for a newborn infant born with an unusually large head. The baby was born after 33 weeks gestation and weighed 4 lbs., 10 oz. The head circumference was 35.5 cm. The mother had been healthy during her pregnancy, and there was no family history of megal-encephaly.

EXAMINATION: A well-developed premature infant, crying vigorously and moving all extremities. The head was enlarged, the anterior fontanel widely open and full. There was no intracranial bruit. The Moro reflex was present and the neurological examination was normal.

QUESTION:

1.   THIS BABY MAY HAVE:
       A. Hydrocephalus
       B. Subdural hematomas
       C. Hydranencephaly
       D. Any of the above, which all cause macrocrania

2.   EXAMINATION DID NOT SHOW PAPILLEDEMA. THIS IS PROBABLY
       BECAUSE:
       A. The intracranial pressure must be normal
       B. The optic nerves are immature
       C. Both of the above
       D. Neither of the above

Bilateral subdural taps were negative. Skull films (Fig. 33) showed marked enlargement of the cranial vault.

3.   THE DEFINITIVE DIAGNOSTIC PROCEDURE WOULD NOW BE:
       A. Carotid angiography
       B. Vertebral angiography
       C. Electroencephalography
       D. Ventriculography
       E. None of the above

Ventriculography was performed. Huge enlargement of the lateral ventricles was seen (Fig. 34).

Other films revealed stenosis of the Sylvian aqueduct. The cortical thickness was about 1.5cm.

A ventriculo-atrial shunt was placed and the child did well for several days. At 8 days after the surgery the head circumference was 37.8cm, an excessive growth of 2.3cm in two weeks. A chest film showed that the cardiac tip of the shunt had turned transversely. The baby was taken to the operating room and the atrial shunt was revised. The baby's head then grew at a normal rate until age seven months when the head circumference was noted to increase five cm. in five weeks. The head circumference was now 46.5cm. (Figs. 35 A, B).

The child showed opisthotonic posturing. Another ventriculogram was done which again showed ventricular enlargement, but the cortical thickness had increased. Again the child was taken to surgery. The neck was explored and the cardiac tip removed, but it was impossible to place a new cardiac tip because of thrombosis and collapse of the internal jugular vein. Accordingly, a McBurney incision was made in the abdomen and a catheter placed into the peritoneal cavity. This was connected to the ventricular portion of the shunt. This ventriculoperitoneal shunt appeared to function satisfactorily and the child was discharged.

CASE STUDY #31

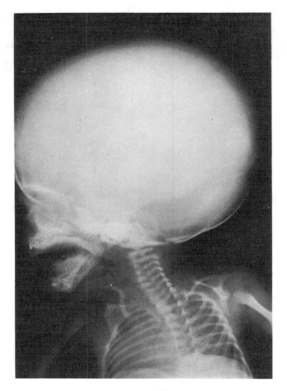

Figure 33

When seen in the clinic at age 9 months the child looked well and the head circumference was 47 cm. He had not yet been able to sit by himself. 3 weeks
later, the baby was noted to be irritable. lethargic and the head circumference
was 49 cm. He was re-hospitalized. Ventriculography showed a right subdural
collection as well as enlarged ventricles. Repeated subdural taps were performed
over several days, with removal of small amounts of grossly bloody fluid.
Subsequently carotid angiograms showed no evidence of the subdural hematoma.
As the ventriculo-peritoneal shunt seemed not to be functioning, he was again
taken to surgery and the shunt was revised. Since then, the revised ventriculo-
peritoneal shunt has been performing well. Developmentally, however, the child
does not hold his head up, roll over, or sit by himself at age thirteen months.

CASE STUDY #31

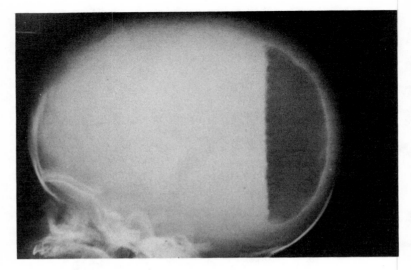

Figure 34

QUESTIONS:

4.   IF THE PARENTS ASKED YOUR PROGNOSIS FOR NORMAL INTELLEC-
      TUAL DEVELOPMENT OF THIS CHILD, YOUR REPLY WOULD BE:
      A. Enthusiastic
      B. Optimistic
      C. Hopeful
      D. Pessimistic

5.   A NORMAL INFANT USUALLY ROLLS HIMSELF OVER AT ABOUT:
      A. 2 months
      B. 3 months
      C. 5 months
      D. 9 months

6.   HE USUALLY SITS BY HIMSELF AT AGE:
      A. 3 months
      B. 6 months
      C. 9 months
      D. 12 months

7.   ENLARGED LATERAL VENTRICLES:
      A. Always mean an increase of cerebrospinal fluid pressure
      B. May occur in "degenerative" disease of the brain, such as Alzheimer's
          disease
      C. Are often seen with cerebellar tumors
      D. A and C

CASE STUDY #31

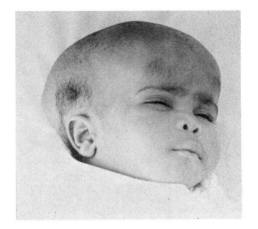

Figure 35A

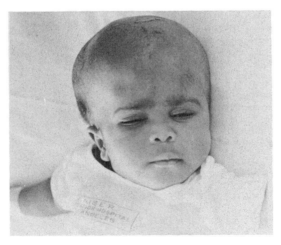

Figure 35B

CASE STUDY #31

8. STENOSIS OF THE AQUEDUCT OF SYLVIUS:
    A. Produces dilation of the third ventricle
    B. Is a common cause of infantile hydrocephalus
    C. May present initially in adulthood as a syndrome of increased intra-
        cranial pressure
    D. All of the above

9. THE CEREBROSPINAL FLUID:
    A. Is mostly produced by the ventricular chorioid plexus
    B. Contains a higher concentration of protein in the lumbar than in the
        ventricular area
    C. Is formed entirely by passive diffusion
    D. All of the above

10. THE HEAD MAY TRANSILLUMINATE IN INFANTILE HYDROCEPHALUS,
    BUT ALSO IN:
    A. Hydranencephaly
    B. Subdural effusions
    C. Porencephaly
    D. All of the above

11. THE CHANCE OF A HYDROCEPHALIC CHILD DEVELOPING WITHOUT
    MENTAL OR PHYSICAL HANDICAP IS GREATEST:
    A. With surgery
    B. Without surgery
    C. With long term treatment with diuretics
    D. No difference between A and B

12. IN THE NATURAL COURSE OF INFANTILE HYDROCEPHALUS, ABOUT
    34% WILL SPONTANEOUSLY ARREST. THIS COMPARES TO AN
    ARREST RATE FOLLOWING SURGERY OF ABOUT:
    A. 25%
    B. 35%
    C. 55%
    D. 85%

13. THE "COCKTAIL PARTY SYNDROME" NOTED IN HYDROCEPHALICS
    REFERS TO:
    A. Excessive drinking
    B. Preference for martinis
    C. Glib and superficial chatter
    D. None of the above

14. COMPLICATIONS OF SHUNTING SURGERY INCLUDE:
    A. Bacteremia
    B. Meningitis
    C. Obstruction of the shunt
    D. Thrombosis of the jugular vein or superior vena cava
    E. Myocardial perforation
    F. All of the above

15. IT HAS BEEN SHOWN THAT VENTRICULAR DILATION IN HYDRO-
    CEPHALUS OCCURS PRIMARILY AT THE EXPENSE OF THE WHITE MAT-
    TER. IN THE NARROWED WHITE MATTER THERE IS A DECREASE OF:
    A. Lipid
    B. Water
    C. Sodium chloride
    D. Protein
    E. All of the above

CASE STUDY #31

16. A DRUG WHICH LOWERS THE RATE OF CEREBROSPINAL FLUID
    FORMATION AND WHICH HAS BEEN FOUND USEFUL IN THE MEDICAL
    TREATMENT OF CHRONIC SLOWLY PROGRESSIVE HYDROCEPHALUS
    IS:
    A. Cytosine arabinoside
    B. Acetazolamide
    C. Diphenylhydantoin
    D. Nitrazepam

ANSWERS AND DISCUSSION:

1. D   It is important to remember that not all infants with large heads
have hydrocephalus. Familial megencephaly, (with or without
mental retardation), subdural hematomas, porencephalic cysts,
hydranencephaly, intracranial tumors, and some forms of
cerebral lipidosis may all cause cranial enlargement.

2. D   Ventricular obstruction in older children whose cranial nerve
sutures are almost fused may result in papilledema, but in
infants and young children the increase in head size usually
produces enough decompression to prevent the appearance of
papilledema. Even among adults, however, increased intracranial pressure may be present without papilledema.

3. D   Ventriculography is done to show the size of the ventricles and
the possible site of obstruction.

4. D   Because of the evidence of severe psychomotor developmental
retardation.

5. C

6. B

7. BC   Ventricular enlargement may result from increased intraventricular pressure as would occur with a cerebellar tumor
blocking the fourth ventricle, or may result from atrophy of
cerebral tissue, producing the so-called hydrocephalus ex-
vacuo, as in Alzheimer's disease or Huntington's chorea.

8. D

9. AB   About 25-50% of the cerebrospinal fluid is derived from the
choroid plexus and the remainder from the brain. Cerebrospinal
fluid formed within isolated ventricles from which all the choroid
plexus has been removed has the same composition as that
obtained from normal ventricles. The composition of cerebrospinal fluid depends on diffusion of some substances and
active transport of others.

10. D

11. A

12. C

13. C

14. F

15. AD

16. B

CASE STUDY #31

REFERENCES

1. Ransohoff, J.R., K. Shulman, R.A. Fishman, Hydrocephalus, J Pediat 56: 399, 1960.

2. Paine, R.S., Hydrocephalus, Pediat Clin N A 4:779, 1967.

3. Schain, R.J., Carbonic Anhydrase Inhibitors in Chronic Infantile Hydrocephalus, Am J Dis Children 117:621, 1969.

4. Fishman R.A., M. Greer, Experimental Obstructive Hydrocephalus, Arch Neur 8:156, 1963.

5. Foltz, E., D. Shurtleff, Five Year Comparative Study of Hydrocephalus in Children with and without Operation, J Neurosurg 20:1064, 1963.

6. Matson, D., Hydrocephalus in Clinical Neurosurgery, Williams and Wilkins, 1966.

7. Huttenlocher, P., Treatment of Hydrocephalus with Acetazolamide, J Ped 66:1023, 1965.

8. Laurence, K.M., Neurological and Intellectual Sequelae of Hydrocephalus, Arch Neur 20:73, 1969.

9. Weller, R., K. Shulman, Infantile Hydrocephalus: Clinical, Histological, and Ultrastructural Study of Brain Damage, J Neurosurg 36:255, 1972.

10. Young, H., et al., The Relationship of Intelligence and Cerebral Mantle in Treated Infantile Hydrocephalus, Pediatrics 52:39, 1973.

11. Epstein, F., et al., Neonatal Hydrocephalus Treated by Compressive Head Wrapping, Lancet 1:634, 1973.

12. Holtzer, G., S. DeLange, Shunt-Independent Arrest of Hydrocephalus, J Neurosurgery 39:698, 1973.

13. Shurtleff, D., et al., Hydrocephalus, Am J Dis Child 125:688, 1973.

14. Raimondi, A., P. Soare, Intellectual Development in Shunted Hydrocephalic Children, Am J Dis Child 127:664, 1974.

CASE STUDY #32

A Housewife with a Convulsion, Hypertension and Tachycardia

HISTORY: A 22 year-old housewife was admitted to the hospital because of a convulsion. A month previously, she had given birth to her first child. She had not wished the pregnancy, and became very depressed postpartum. She sought psychiatric help, and was given Amytal for night time and Valium for daytime sedation. On these drugs, she complained of drowsiness and confusion, and "pains all over." On the day before admission, she ingested five Darvons, four Valium, two Emperin with codeine, and a Percodan tablet. Her husband described her as a "hypochondriac" with a cabinet full of many medications, which she would take with any mild pain or discomfort. The evening before admission she fell in the bathroom striking her head but not losing consciousness. The next morning she had a major motor seizure, without aura or Todd's phenomenon. She began to complain of constant periumbilical pain. Past medical history was noncontributory except for occasional episodes of abdominal pain following alcohol ingestion.

The general physical examination during the first few days of hospitalization was normal except for moderate systolic and diastolic hypertension, a sinus tachycardia with a rate of 140, and generalized muscle tenderness over the entire body, especially the abdomen, without rigidity, organomegaly, or palpable masses. Neurological examination was normal. She was severely depressed.

CASE STUDY #32

QUESTION:

1. AS WITH ANY PATIENT WITH A SEIZURE BEGINNING IN ADULT LIFE,
    SOME OF THE LABORATORY TESTS YOU WOULD REQUEST INCLUDE:
    A. Fasting blood sugar
    B. Blood calcium
    C. Spinal tap and electroencephalogram
    D. X-rays of chest and skull
    E. All of the above

COURSE: All of the above mentioned laboratory tests were normal. A psychiatric
consultant felt that the patient suffered from a psychoneurosis with conversion,
depressive, and phobic features. The seizures were initially considered to be
secondary to drug overdosage and withdrawal. At a medical staff meeting, an
internist, hearing of this patient with a seizure, depression, abdominal pain,
tachycardia and hypertension suggested a test which established the correct
diagnosis.

QUESTION:

2. THE TEST WHICH ESTABLISHED THE CORRECT DIAGNOSIS WAS:
    A. A positive test for Bence Jones protein confirming the diagnosis of
        multiple myeloma
    B. A muscle biopsy revealing arteritis, confirming the suspicion of
        periarteritis nodosa
    C. A positive LE prep, confirming the diagnosis of systemic lupus
    D. A positive Watson-Schwartz test, establishing the diagnosis of acute
        porphyria
    E. A positive VDRL and FTA-ABs confirming the diagnosis of syphillis
    F. An amytal interview confirming the diagnosis of conversion hysteria

The urine showed a strongly positive reaction for porphobilinogen, as well as
markedly elevated values of urine uro and coproporphyrins.

QUESTION:

    TRUE OR FALSE:

3. Porphobilinogen is a red compound which gives the urine of patients with
    porphyria its typical color.

4. Increased urinary coproporphyrins are specifically diagnostic of acute
    intermittent porphyria.

5. In acute intermittent porphyria, diagnostic abnormalities in the urine are
    increased porphobilinogen and aminolevulinic acid.

6. The adding of Ehrlich aldehyde (Watson-Schwartz test) to urine containing
    porphobilinogen produces a red compound which, in contrast to that pro-
    duced by urobilinogen, is insoluble in chloroform.

7. Porphyrins are vital metabolic substances present in hemoglobin, myo-
    globin, cytochrome.

8. Porphyrins may be seen in normal urine.

CASE STUDY #32

COURSE: The various medications which she was receiving were discontinued, and she was given chlorpromazine. In the next few days, she became stuporous and developed a right hemiparesis. Serum sodium was 107 meq/l; chloride 71.

QUESTIONS:

9. AT THIS POINT YOU MIGHT:
    A. Be concerned about coexisting Addison's disease because of the severe hyponatremia
    B. Suspect that the hemiparesis was related to the hyponatremia
    C. Bet that the urine specific gravity would be high
    D. Doubt any relationship between the hyponatremia and the underlying porphyria

10. THE URINE OSMOLALITY WAS GREATLY INCREASED, AND THE SERUM OSMOLALITY DIMINISHED, A CONDITION WHICH HAS BEEN REPORTED REPEATEDLY AS A COMPLICATION OF ACUTE PORPHYRIA AND IS DUE TO:
    A. Decreased secretion of aldosterone
    B. Decreased secretion of hydrocortisone
    C. Repeated vomiting
    D. Inappropriate secretion of antidiuretic hormone

COURSE: She was treated for the hyponatremia with fluid restriction and gradually recovered. She was warned about the role of drugs in precipitating attacks, and has remained well since.

QUESTIONS:

11. NEUROLOGICAL ABNORMALITIES IN ACUTE INTERMITTENT PORPHYRIA MAY INCLUDE:
    A. Coma   D. Quadriplegia
    B. Seizures   E. Aphasia
    C. Peripheral neuropathy

12. PSYCHIATRIC ABNORMALITIES ARE FREQUENT, AND MAY INCLUDE:
    A. Confusional state   D. Psychosis
    B. Personality change   E. Delirium
    C. Anxiety   F. Depression

13. ACUTE INTERMITTENT PORPHYRIA CAN BE DISTINGUISHED FROM OTHER DISEASES ASSOCIATED WITH NEUROLOGICAL SYMPTOMS AND RED-BROWN URINE, SUCH AS MYOGLOBINURIA OR HEMOGLOBINURIA, SINCE:
    A. Porphyria is the only one associated with severe pain
    B. Only in porphyria is the test for urine porphobilinogen strongly positive
    C. Both of the above

14. THE TREATMENT OF ACUTE PORPHYRIA INCLUDES:
    A. Glucose and insulin   C. Griseofulvin
    B. Chlorpromazine   D. All of the above

15. ACUTE ATTACKS OF PORPHYRIA MAY BE PRECIPITATED BY:
    A. Drugs
    B. Hormones (estrogens, progestagens)
    C. Fasting
    D. Infections
    E. Any of the above

CASE STUDY #32

16. DRUGS WHICH MAY PRECIPITATE ACUTE ATTACKS OF PORPHYRIA:
    A. Include barbiturates, sulfonamides, dilantin, alcohol, librium
    B. Should be given as a provocative test if the diagnosis is doubtful
    C. Probably do so by increasing the activity of hepatic aminolevulinic
       acid synthetase
    D. All of the above

    MATCH THE DISEASES WHICH CAN MIMIC PORPHYRIA WITH THESE
    FREQUENTLY SEEN PORPHYRIC SYMPTOMS:

17. ___ Tachycardia, weakness, nervousness   A. Addison's disease
18. ___ Severe abdominal pain, nausea,   B. Periarteritis nodosa
        vomiting   C. Cholecystitis
19. ___ Weakness and hyponatremia   D. Thyrotoxicosis
20. ___ Hypertension and neuropathy

ANSWERS AND DISCUSSION:

1. F   Although drug abuse, including alcoholism, is a common cause
        of seizures beginning in adult life, the patient whose fits begin
        in adulthood has a high risk of having a structural or metabolic
        lesion. Hypoglycemia and hypocalcemia are to be ruled out
        with the appropriate tests, and screening for brain tumor is
        done with the neurological examination, skull films, electro-
        encephalogram, lumbar puncture, visual fields, brain scan and
        computerized tomogram, with the decision about contrast studies
        depending on the initial clinical and laboratory data.

2. D   Abdominal symptoms, including pain, nausea, vomiting, occur
        in 95% of patients with acute intermittent porphyria. Mental
        and emotional symptoms ranging over a wide spectrum of
        psychiatric illness are also common, as is involvement of both
        the peripheral and central nervous system. Hypertension,
        tachycardia, and exacerbations of illness due to a variety of
        drugs are further ingredients in this vivid clinical picture.

3. False Porphobilinogen is colorless, but when urine containing this
        substance is exposed to light, the urine darkens due to formation
        of uroporphyrin.

4. False Coproporphyrin is normally present in urine and feces and is
        increased in a variety of pathological states, including lead and
        other heavy metal poisoning, liver disease and some of the
        anemias.

5. True
6. True
7. True
8. True
9. BC
10. D
11. ABCDE
12. ABCDEF
13. B

-170-

CASE STUDY #32

14. AB   Griseofulvin may exacerbate acute intermittent porphyria.

15. E

16. AC   Provocative tests should not be used because of the risk to the patient.

17. D

18. C

19. A

20. B

1. Dean, G., The Porphyrias, Brit Med Bull 25:48, 1969.

2. Nielsen, B., and N. Thorn, Transient Excess Urinary Excretion of Anti-diuretic Material in Acute Intermittent Porphyria with Hyponatremia and Hypomagnesemia, Am J Med 38:345, 1965.

3. Kaufman, L., and H. Marver, Biochemical Defects in Two Types of Human Hepatic Porphyria, New Eng J Med 283:954, 1970.

4. Denny-Brown, D., and D. Sciarra, Changes in the Nervous System in Acute Porphyria, Brain 68:1, 1945.

5. Carney, M.W.P., Hepatic Porphyria with Mental Symptoms, Lancet 2:100, 1972.

6. Stein, J., and D. Tschudy, Acute Intermittent Porphyria. A Clinical and Biochemical Study of 46 Patients, Medicine 49:1-16, 1970.

7. International Conference on Porphyrin Metabolism and the Porphyrias, S African Med J 45:25, September 1971.

8. Marver, H., and R. Schmid, The Porphyrias in The Metabolic Basis of Inherited Disease, Edited by Stanbury, J., Wyngaarden, J., Fredrickson, D., 3rd Ed., McGraw-Hill, New York, 1972, p. 1087-1140.

CASE STUDY #33

Recurrent Neurological Illness in a Young Girl

HISTORY: A 19 year-old girl was well until two years previously, when she abruptly became blind in the left eye. Her vision gradually improved over the next few months.

QUESTION:

1.   THIS EPISODE IS MOST SUGGESTIVE OF:
     A. Temporal arteritis
     B. Brain tumor
     C. Optic neuritis
     D. None of the above

Three months before, she noted numbness and tingling of the right leg which lasted two weeks. A month ago, she noted hearing loss in the right ear, which became normal after three weeks. During the past few months she also complained of tingling sensations in the left arm.

CASE STUDY #33

EXAMINATION: Completely normal except for a positive Gunn pupil sign on the left (swinging flashlight test - In this test a light is flashed back and forth from one eye to the other; dilation of the pupils when the light is shined on the "bad" eye is a positive test and may be the only residual abnormality of an old retrobulbar neuritis. The test is based on the fact that with unilateral retinal or optic nerve lesions, differences in the pupillary responses occur when each eye is stimulated. "As the light shifts from the "good" to the "bad" eye the direct light stimulus is no longer sufficient to maintain the previously evoked degree of pupillary constriction: thus both pupils redilate. ")[7]

The patient's vision, fundi and visual fields were normal. She seemed oddly unconcerned about her illness.

COURSE: Two months later, she complained of blurred vision. When she looked to the right, one could see weakness of adduction of the left eye, with nystagmus of the right (abducting) eye.

QUESTIONS:

2.   THIS FINDING IS CALLED:
      A. Gaze paresis
      B. Opsoclonus
      C. Ocular dysmetria
      D. Internuclear ophthalmoplegia

3.   IT IS DUE TO A LESION IN:
      A. The optic nerve
      B. The optic tract
      C. The brainstem in the pretectal area
      D. The brainstem in the median longitudinal fasciculus

Two months afterwards, she developed weakness and clumsiness of the left leg. Examination now showed normal extraocular movements, a left hemiparesis, left facial weakness, hyperactive deep tendon reflexes in the left extremities, and a left Babinski sign.

QUESTIONS:

4.   THESE LEFT SIDED FINDINGS ARE DUE TO A LESION IN THE:
      A. Corticospinal tract
      B. Rubrospinal tract
      C. Spinothalamic tract
      D. Reticulospinal tract

5.   IN CONSIDERING THE CASE THUS FAR:
      A. All of the abnormalities can be explained on the basis of a single
          diencephalic lesion
      B. Neurosyphilis is a possible cause of this clinical picture
      C. The neurological findings cannot be explained by a single lesion and
          are evidence of multiple lesions in different areas of the central
          nervous system
      D. The temporal pattern of the disease does not suggest a tumor

6.   THE MOST LIKELY DIAGNOSIS IS:
      A. Behcet's syndrome
      B. Cerebral emboli
      C. Schilder's disease
      D. Multiple sclerosis
      E. Encephalitis

CASE STUDY #33

7. PATHOLOGICALLY, YOU WOULD PREDICT THAT THE BRAIN WOULD SHOW AREAS OF:
   A. Infarction
   B. Demyelination
   C. Granulomata
   D. Hemorrhage

8. THE DIFFERENTIAL DIAGNOSIS WOULD INCLUDE:
   A. Arteritis
   B. Syphillis
   C. Sarcoid
   D. Low pressure hydrocephalus
   E. All of the above

LABORATORY DATA: Blood count, urinalysis, calcium, serology, LE preparations, sedimentation rate, skull and chest films, were all normal, as was the spinal fluid. The electroencephalogram was mildly and diffusely slower than normal.

Over the next few months, the weakness of her left side improved, but then she developed a right hemiparesis. A course of ACTH was given. She again gradually improved. When last seen, her strength was normal, but both plantar responses were extensor, and rapid successive movements of the right hand were clumsily done.

QUESTIONS:

9. THE CAUSE OF MULTIPLE SCLEROSIS IS UNKNOWN, AND MANY THEORIES HAVE BEEN PROPOSED, INCLUDING SPIROCHETAL INFEC-TION, FAT IN THE DIET, TOXINS, VASCULAR OCCLUSION. CURRENT-LY, THE TWO MOST POPULAR THEORIES ARE THAT IT IS AN AUTO-IMMUNE DISEASE OR THAT IT MAY BE CAUSED BY A "SLOW" VIRUS. OTHER HUMAN NEUROLOGICAL DISEASES PROBABLY CAUSED BY "SLOW" VIRUSES INCLUDE:
   A. Multifocal leukoencephalopathy
   B. Kuru
   C. Jacob-Creutzfeldt
   D. Subacute sclerosing panencephalitis
   E. All of the above

10. AN ELEVATION OF CEREBROSPINAL FLUID GAMMAGLOBULIN SUP-PORTS THE DIAGNOSIS OF MULTIPLE SCLEROSIS, BUT IS BY NO MEANS SPECIFIC. SOME OTHER CONDITIONS WHICH MAY PRODUCE THIS FINDING ARE:
    A. Neurosyphillis
    B. Hypergammaglobulinemia
    C. Isolated optic neuritis
    D. Landry-Guillain-Barré syndrome
    E. All of the above

TRUE OR FALSE:

11. Although multiple sclerosis is typically characterized by remissions and exacerbations, it may occasionally present as a progressive disease.

12. Multiple sclerosis is more common in tropical than in temperate climates.

CASE STUDY #33

13.   Epidemiological studies have shown that those who move, as adults, from a high to a low risk area of multiple sclerosis, develop the low risk indigenous to the area.

14.   Several studies have shown that patients with multiple sclerosis have higher titers to measles virus than do controls.

15.   ACTH therapy dramatically improves the overall course of multiple sclerosis.

ANSWERS AND DISCUSSION:

1. C   Optic neuritis is the most likely cause of abrupt unilateral visual loss in this young girl. Temporal arteritis also produces unilateral sudden blindness, but in the age group over 50. Unilateral visual loss can occur with a variety of brain tumors-optic gliomas, meningiomas, pituitary adenomas,but the visual loss is gradual and progressive,except perhaps in the rare instance of hemorrhage into a tumor.

2. D

3. D

4. A

5. BCD   This patient shows evidence of disseminated central nervous system disease, with lesions at least in the optic nerve and brainstem. The site of the pyramidal tract lesion is not certain, but must be rostral to the mid pons level, since corticobulbar fibers to the facial nuclei are affected. On which side is the pyramidal tract lesion?

Temporally, the pattern is of remissions and exacerbations, rather than of gradual progression which would be the typical temporal profile of an intracranial neoplasm.

6. D

7. B

8. ABC   Arteritis, lues and sarcoid may all produce disseminated CNS lesions. "Low pressure" hydrocephalus results in dementia, gait disturbance and incontinence,and not a remitting pattern of scattered CNS lesions.

9. E

10. E   Optic neuritis occurs during the course of the disease in about 1/3 of patients with multiple sclerosis. Percy et. al (6) have shown that in cases of idiopathic optic neuritis the chance of progression to multiple sclerosis (during an average follow-up period of 18 years) was 17%.

11. True Usually this is true when the disease presents with spinal cord involvement in middle age.

12. False The reverse is true.

13. False

14. True

CASE STUDY #33

15. False   In the cooperative study, [2] short-term high dosage use of ACTH has-
            tened the evidences of improvement of symptoms and signs, but the
            ultimate extent of improvement was not greater than that of the
            placebo-treated group.

REFERENCES

1. Schneck, S.A., and H.N. Claman, CSF Immunoglobulins in Multiple Sclerosis and Other Neurologic Diseases, Arch Neuro 20:132, 1969.

2. Rose, A.S., et al., Cooperative Study in the Evaluation of Therapy in Multiple Sclerosis: ACTH vs. Placebo, Neurology 20:1 (part 2), 1970.

3. Sciarra, D., and S. Carter, Longevity in Multiple Sclerosis, Arch Neur Psych 62:1, 1949.

4. Brody, J., J. Sever, and T. Henson, Virus Antibody Titers in Multiple Sclerosis Patients, Siblings and Controls, JAMA 216:1441, 1971.

5. Percy, A., F. Nobrega, H. Okazaki, E. Glattre, and L. Kurland, Multiple Sclerosis in Rochester, Minnesota, Arch Neur 25:105, 1971.

6. Percy, A., A. Nobrega, and L. Kurland, Optic Neuritis and Multiple Sclerosis, Arch Ophthal 87:135, 1972.

7. Walsh, F., and W. Hoyt, Clinical Neuro-Ophthalmology, 3rd Ed., Williams and Wilkins Co., Baltimore, 1969.

8. Carter, S., D. Sciarra, and H.H. Merritt, The Course of Multiple Sclerosis as Determined by Autopsy Proven Cases, Ass Res Nerv Dis Proc 28:471, 1950.

9. Poser, C., J. Presthus, and O. Horsdal, Clinical Characteristics of Autopsy Proved Multiple Sclerosis, Neurology 16:791, 1966.

10. Seil, F., Multiple Sclerosis: Current Etiological Concepts, Calif Med 116:25, 1972.

11. Weiner, L., et al., Viral Infections and Demyelinating Diseases, New Eng J Med 288:1103, 1973.

12. Haire, M., et al., Measles and Other Virus-Specific Immunoglobulins in Multiple Sclerosis, Brit Med J 3:612, 1973.

13. Alter, M., et al., Optic Neuritis in Orientals and Caucasians, Neurology 23:631, 1973.

14. Olsson, J-E., and H. Link, Immunoglobulin Abnormalities in Multiple Sclerosis, Arch Neurol 28:392, 1973.

15. Leibowitz, U., and M. Alter, Changing Frequency of Multiple Sclerosis in Israel, Arch Neurol 29:107, 1973.

16. Weiner, L., Pathogenesis of Demyelination Induced by a Mouse Hepatitis Virus, Arch Neurol 28:298, 1973.

17. Moore, M., et al., Multiple Sclerosis, Postgraduate Medicine 53:75, 1973.

18. Rose, A., Multiple Sclerosis, J Neurosurgery 41:279, 1974.

19. Ghatak, N., et al., Asymptomatic Demyelinated Plaque in the Spinal Cord, Arch Neurol 30:484, 1974.

CASE STUDY #33

20. Sexauer, J., and F. Fekety, Pulmonary Infections Complicating Treatment of Multiple Sclerosis, Arch Neurol 30:293, 1974.

21. Raine, C., et al., Acute Multiple Sclerosis, Arch Neurol 30:39, 1974.

CASE STUDY #34

Chorea Beginning at Age Fifty-one

HISTORY: A 51 year-old male began to complain of purposeless, uncontrollable movements of his hands and feet. The initial neurological examination showed just some slight fidgeting of all extremities, but was otherwise normal. When he was examined two years later, there were definite continuous, restless, choreic movements of the limbs, with frequent facial grimacing (Figs. 36A and B). Skull films and an electroencephalogram were normal.

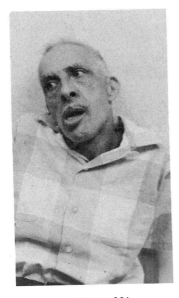

Figure 36A

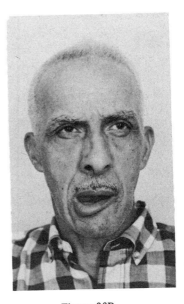

Figure 36B

CASE STUDY #34

QUESTIONS:

1. FURTHER INFORMATION WHICH WOULD BE HELPFUL IN ESTABLISH-
   ING A DIAGNOSIS WOULD INCLUDE:
   A. Family history of jaundice D. History of tranquillizer ingestion
   B. Family history of suicide   E. History of duodenal ulcer
   C. History of thyroidectomy

2. IMPORTANT FURTHER CLUES TO THE DIAGNOSIS FROM THE PHYSICAL
   EXAMINATION WOULD INCLUDE:
   A. Dementia   C. Jaundice
   B. A Chvostek sign   D. Anisocoria

3. SOME LABORATORY TESTS YOU MIGHT ORDER WOULD BE:
   A. Serum calcium   D. Slit lamp examination
   B. Serum iron   E. All of the above
   C. Serum ceruloplasmin

The patient subsequently revealed that his mother, and many relatives on her side
for many generations, had developed in adulthood, dementia, psychosis, and abnormal movements. The patient's mother had three times attempted suicide. She
had suffered from chorea, delusions of grandeur and persecution, and dementia.

LABORATORY DATA: Normal tests included calcium, magnesium, VDRL, fta-
abs, ceruloplasmin, slit lamp examination.

COURSE: During the next five years the chorea gradually worsened, but intellectual functions remained unchanged. Recently he has begun to be increasingly
moody and irascible.

QUESTIONS:

4. THE MOST PROBABLE DIAGNOSIS IS:
   A. Sydenham's chorea   C. Huntington's chorea
   B. Seronegative neurosyphilis D. Alzheimer's disease

5. THE PERCENTAGE OF THIS PATIENT'S CHILDREN WHO WOULD BE
   EXPECTED TO SHOW THIS DISORDER, IF HE MARRIED A WOMAN
   WITH A NORMAL GENOTYPE, WOULD BE:
   A. 25% of both sexes   C. 50% of both sexes
   B. 50% of the males   D. 50% of the females

6. THIS DISEASE IS SEEN:
   A. Primarily in blacks   C. In almost every country in the world
   B. Predominantly in Jews D. Primarily in tropical climates

7. PSYCHIATRIC ABNORMALITIES SEEN IN THIS DISORDER INCLUDE:
   A. Irritability   D. Dementia
   B. Paranoia   E. Hallucinations
   C. Delirium tremens

8. PATHOLOGICALLY, ONE WOULD EXPECT TO SEE:
   A. Obstructive hydrocephalus
   B. Hydrocephalus due to brain atrophy (hydrocephalus ex vacuo)
   C. Excess cerebral copper
   D. Atrophy most marked in the basal ganglia and cerebral cortex

9. THE BIOCHEMICAL ABNORMALITY IN THIS DISEASE IS:
   A. Thiamine deficiency   D. Unknown
   B. Pyridoxine deficiency   E. Copper excess
   C. Manganese excess

CASE STUDY #34

10. CHOREA MAY BE SEEN IN THESE TREATABLE CONDITIONS:
   A. Hypoparathyroidism
   B. Neurosyphilis
   C. Wilson's disease
   D. Hypomagnesemia
   E. Reserpine and phenothiazine in-
      toxication
   F. Lupus erythematosus
   G. Hyperthyroidism
   H. Dilantin intoxication
   I. Brain tumor
   J. Levodopa administration
   K. Oral contraceptives
   L. All of the above

11. INDICATE WHETHER THE FOLLOWING DRUGS WOULD BE EXPECTED
   TO IMPROVE OR WORSEN CHOREA:
   A. Levodopa
   B. Reserpine
   C. Alphamethylparatyrosine
   D. Chlorpromazine
   E. Haloperidol
   F. Physostigmine
   G. Benztropine
   H. Amphetamine

12. AN ESSENTIAL PART OF THE TREATMENT PROGRAM IS:
   A. Genetic counselling
   B. L-DOPA
   C. Thalamotomy
   D. All of the above

ANSWERS AND DISCUSSION:

1. ABCD   A family history of icterus in a choreic patient might suggest the pos-
         sibility of hepatolenticular degeneration. Familial psychiatric dis-
         ease might occur both in Wilson's disease and in Huntington's chorea.
         Chorea in a patient with a history of thyroidectomy would suggest the
         possibility of hypocalcemia due to surgical damage or removal of the
         parathyroids. The phenothiazine group of drugs can cause a variety
         of abnormal movements - tremor, chorea, dystonia, etc.

2. ABC   For reasons as described above.

3. ACD   The ceruloplasmin is elevated in almost all cases of Wilson's dis-
         ease. The slit lamp examination reveals a Kayser-Fleischer ring in
         virtually all cases of untreated Wilson's disease.

4. C   The strongly positive family history suggesting dominant transmis-
         sion, the psychiatric abnormality, involuntary abnormal movements
         all are typical of chronic progressive (Huntington's) chorea.

         Sydenham's chorea is a disease of childhood, usually lasting 3-6
         weeks, and is generally considered to be a manifestation of rheumatic
         fever, with 3/4 of the cases showing, at some time in their lives,
         other forms of the disease, with carditis or arthritis. Alzheimer's
         disease is not associated with chorea. Seronegative neurosyphilis
         refers to cases of neurosyphilis in which nonspecific serological tests
         as the VDRL are negative whereas specific serological tests as the
         FTA or TPI are positive.

5. C   If H=dominant Huntington gene
         n=normal, then

	n	n
H	Hn	Hn
n	nn	nn

CASE STUDY #34

6. C

7. ABDE

8. BD

9. D

10. L

11. A. worsen   C. improve   E. improve   G. worsen
    B. improve   D. improve   F. improve   H. worsen

It has been proposed that a balance between neurotransmitters, especially dopamine and acetylcholine in the corpus striatum, is necessary for normal motor function. Klawans has suggested that the chorea of Huntington's disease may be associated with increased responsiveness of striatal cells to dopamine.

Worsening of chorea seems to be related to an increase in the ratio of dopamine to acetylcholine activity in the central nervous system. This can be due to an increase in dopamine concentration following administration of levodopa or amphetamine (which releases dopamine from presynaptic neurons in the striatum), or a decrease in acetylcholine due to anticholinergic agents such as benztropine.

Improvement in chorea is associated with agents which lower the dopamine/acetylcholine ratio. This can be done by either lowering dopamine effect, as with reserpine (which depletes CNS dopamine), alpha methyl para tyrosine (which blocks dopamine synthesis), or haloperidol and the phenothiazines (which block dopamine receptor sites), or by increasing CNS acetylcholine concentration with physostigmine (a centrally active inhibitor of cholinesterase).

The choreic movements seen in some patients on chronic treatment with phenothiazines or reserpine (the tardive dyskinesias) have been explained as due to hypersensitivity of dopamine receptors following drug induced chemical "denervation."

12. A   Since the mode of hereditary transmission indicates an autosomal dominant gene with complete penetrance, couples with a family history of this disease should be counselled to avoid having children. It is important to recall that the onset of symptoms of this disease may be delayed until the fourth or fifth decade, so that the asymptomatic young person of childbearing age may still develop the disease years or decades later.

Thalamotomy has not been useful in the treatment of this disease. Some drugs of the phenothiazine and butyrophenone families have been helpful in decreasing the intensity of the chorea. Levodopa worsens the intensity of chorea, and has been used as a possible provocative test to predict the future development of Huntington's disease in those genetically susceptible.

REFERENCES

1. Bruyn, G.W., Huntington's Chorea, Handbook of Clinical Neurology, Vol. 6, P.J. Vinken, and G.W. Bruyn, Ed., North Holland Publishing Co. 1968.

2. Fidler, S., R. O'Rourke, and H. Buchsbaum, Choreoathetosis as a Manifestation of Thyrotoxicosis, Neurology 21:55, 1971.

CASE STUDY #34

3. Sciarra, D., and B. Sprofkin, Symptoms and Signs Referable to the Basal Ganglia in Brain Tumor, AMA Arch Neur and Psych 69:450, 1953.

4. Huntington, G., On Chorea, Med and Surg Reporter, Philadelphia, 26:317, 1872.

5. Gamboa, E., et al., Chorea Associated with Oral Contraceptive Therapy, Arch Neurol 25:112, 1971.

6. Christiansen, N., and P. Hansen, Choreiform Movements in Hypoparathyroidism, New Eng J Med 287:569, 1972.

7. Klawans, H., et al., Use of L-DOPA in the Detection of Presymptomatic Huntington's Chorea, New Eng J Med 286:1332, 1972.

8. Editorial, Presymptomatic Detection of Huntington's Chorea, Brit Med J Sept. 2, 1972.

9. Fermaglich, J., et al., Chorea Associated with Systemic Lupus Erythematosus, Arch Neurol 28:276, 1973.

10. Candelise, L., Treatment of Huntington's Chorea, New Eng J Med 289:1201, 1973.

11. Klawans, H., The Pharmacology of Extrapyramidal Movement Disorders, S. Karger, 1973.

12. Tarsy, D., et al., Physostigmine in Choreiform Movement Disorders, Neurology 24:28, 1974.

13. Klawans, H., and W. Weiner, The Effect of D-Amphetamine on Choreiform Movement Disorders, Neurology 24:312, 1974.

14. Kooiker, J., and S. Sumi, Movement Disorder as a Manifestation of Diphenylhydantoin Intoxication, Neurology 24:68, 1974.

CASE STUDY #35

Headache and Double Vision Following Head Trauma

HISTORY: A 63 year-old housewife developed a headache while at work. The headache was mild, dull, steady, and located in the right parietal area. Two hours later she experienced vertical diplopia.

QUESTION:

1.   OTHER RECENT HISTORY OF IMPORTANCE WOULD BE:
     A. Subjective abnormal sounds in her head
     B. Weakness of any extremity
     C. Nasal speech

None of these complaints were present initially.

QUESTIONS:

2.   ADDITIONAL INFORMATION OF IMPORTANCE WOULD INCLUDE:
     A. History of diabetes mellitus   C. Previous similar episodes
     B. History of head trauma   D. History of alcoholism

3.   IF SHE HAD A HISTORY OF ALCOHOLISM, THE DIPLOPIA MIGHT BE DUE TO:
     A. Wernicke's syndrome
     B. Methyl alcohol poisoning
     C. "Boozer's Eye"
     D. Tobacco-alcohol amblyopia (nutritional amblyopia)

Two weeks earlier, while shopping at a market she slipped on a grape, falling backwards and striking her occiput. She did not lose consciousness. There were no immediate sequelae.

CASE STUDY #35

QUESTIONS:

4. HEAD TRAUMA MAY PRODUCE DIPLOPIA BY:
    A. Trapping of the inferior rectus muscle in a fractured orbital floor
    B. Injury to the fibers of the III, IV, and VI cranial nerve
    C. Injury to the nuclei of the III, IV, and VI cranial nerve
    D. Injury to the medial lemniscus

5. HEAD TRAUMA MUST BE SEVERE TO PRODUCE DIPLOPIA, WHATEVER
    THE CAUSE:
    A. True
    B. False

EXAMINATION: The physical examination was negative. Blood pressure was
120/70. The neurological examination was normal except for the ocular findings.
When she looked up and to the left, she complained of vertical diplopia. When
the right eye was covered, the higher image disappeared.

QUESTION:

6. WHAT SIMPLE TEST MAY HELP IDENTIFY THE WEAK MUSCLE(S)
    RESPONSIBLE FOR THE DIPLOPIA?:
    A. Rotating drum
    B. Red glass
    C. Caloric testing
    D. Orbital X-rays

This test revealed right inferior oblique weakness. The visual acuity was normal.
The pupils were 3 mm in diameter, round and regular, and reacted well to light
and in convergence. The fundi were normal. There were no bruits.

QUESTIONS:

7. APPROPRIATE TESTS TO BE ORDERED AT THIS TIME SHOULD
    INCLUDE:
    A. Two hour post prandial blood sugar
    B. Skull series
    C. Sedimentation rate
    D. Pneumoencephalogram
    E. Serology

8. THE FOLLOWING SIMPLE TESTS SHOULD BE DONE IN THE OFFICE ON
    PATIENTS PRESENTING WITH DIPLOPIA:
    A. Tensilon test
    B. Angio-Conray test
    C. Queckenstedt test

9. IN PERFORMING THE TENSILON TEST, AFTER AN INTRAMUSCULAR
    INJECTION, THE EXAMINER WAITS THIRTY TO FORTY-FIVE MINUTES
    FOR RESULTS:
    A. True
    B. False

Blood sugar, sedimentation rate, VDRL, Tensilon test and skull series were all
normal. During the next several weeks, she continued to complain of head pain,
but the diplopia disappeared. She did not return for two months. At that time she
reported that her headaches had subsided. However, for the past three weeks she
had heard a constant swishing sound in both ears, louder in the right. She also

CASE STUDY #35

had begun to note horizontal diplopia. A systolic bruit was heard over the right eye and temple. It could be obliterated by pressure on the right carotid artery. She had horizontal diplopia when she looked to the right, and there was weakness of abduction of the right eye. There was no exopthalmos. The patient was admitted to the hospital for further evaluation.

QUESTIONS:

10. BRUITS MAY BE HEARD BY EITHER THE PATIENT OR EXAMINER IN:
   A. Arteriovenous malformations
   B. Non chromaffin paragangliomas
   C. Carotid cavernous sinus fistulas
   D. Venous sinus thrombosis

11. IN CHILDREN, OCULAR BRUITS ALWAYS INDICATE DISEASE:
   A. True
   B. False

12. IN CAROTID-CAVERNOUS FISTULAS, IPSILATERAL CAROTID ARTERY COMPRESSION CAUSES:
   A. Cessation of the bruit
   B. Increase in the degree of exopthalmos
   C. Loss of vision

13. WITH THE HISTORY GIVEN, THE TEST MOST LIKELY TO PROVIDE A DEFINITE DIAGNOSIS IS:
   A. Right carotid angiogram
   B. Left carotid angiogram
   C. Left vertebral angiogram
   D. Pneumoencephalogram

Selective right internal and external carotid angiograms were performed. The internal carotid angiogram was normal. An external carotid angiogram showed an abnormal fistula (Fig. 37) between the external carotid artery and the cavernous sinus.

QUESTIONS:

14. MOST CAROTID-CAVERNOUS FISTULAS ARE DUE TO HEAD INJURY:
   A. True
   B. False

15. SUCH FISTULAS USUALLY OCCUR AS ABNORMAL CONNECTIONS BETWEEN THE CAVERNOUS SINUS AND:
   A. The internal carotid artery
   B. The external carotid artery

16. MOST SPONTANEOUSLY OCCURRING CAROTID CAVERNOUS SINUS FISTULAS DEVELOP WHEN PRE-EXISTING ANEURYSMS RUPTURE:
   A. True
   B. False

17. EXOPHTHALMOS OCCURRING IN UNILATERAL CAROTID CAVERNOUS FISTULA MAY BE:
   A. Unilateral
   B. Contralateral
   C. Bilateral
   D. All of the above

CASE STUDY #35

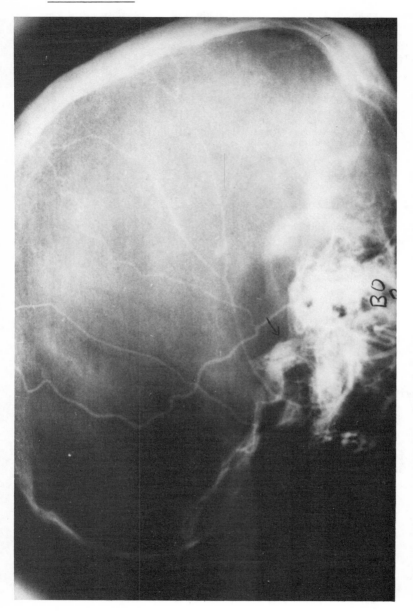

Fig. 37A - EXTERNAL CAROTID ANGIOGRAMS. There is abnormal early filling of the cavernous sinus in the arterial phase by branches of the internal maxillary artery. In the AP view there is early filling of the cavernous sinus as well as retrograde filling of the superior orbital veins.

CASE STUDY #35

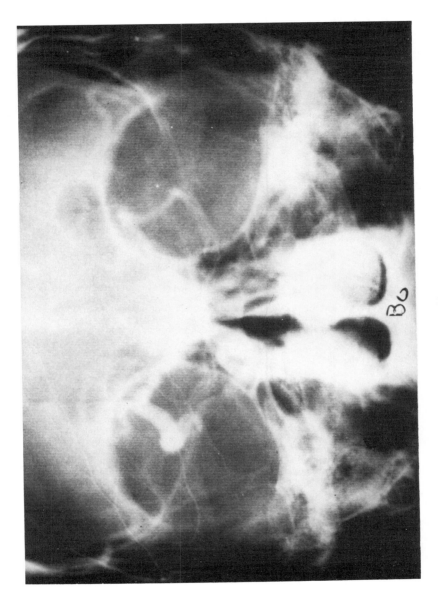

Figure 37B

CASE STUDY #35

18. WHICH OF THE FOLLOWING MECHANISMS MAY BE RESPONSIBLE FOR
VISUAL IMPAIRMENT IN PATIENTS WITH CAROTID CAVERNOUS SINUS
FISTULAS?:
   A. Compression of the optic nerve by an intracavernous aneurysm
   B. Compression of the optic nerve by distended venous channels within
      the orbital fissure
   C. Stretching of the optic nerve with increasing exophthalmos
   D. Retinal damage as retinal veins engorge
   E. Poor arterial perfusion due to "steal" from the ophthalmic artery

COURSE: The right external carotid artery was ligated. In the early post
operative period, there was a faint residual bruit. This disappeared gradually,
as did the diplopia.

ANSWERS AND DISCUSSION:

1. ABC   Patients with a variety of intracranial vascular malformations
             may hear abnormal sounds. Constant or fluctuating weakness of
             one or more extremities suggests nervous system dysfunction.
             Nasal speech suggests dysfunction of the lower brain stem, or of
             the cranial nerves, myoneural junctions or muscles involved in
             speech.

2. ABCD

3. A   Wernicke's syndrome is due to deficiency of thiamine and
             includes extraocular muscle palsies, nystagmus and clouding of
             consciousness. Tobacco-alcohol amblyopia affects the optic
             nerves rather than the nerves to the extraocular muscles. Methyl
             alcohol poisoning produces visual loss. "Boozer's eye" is a col-
             loquialism for the conjunctivitis seen in many active alcoholics.

4. ABC   Trapping of the inferior rectus muscle in a traumatic bony defect
             in the orbital floor is called a "blow out fracture."

5. B

6. B   In performing the red glass test, the patient is asked to look at a
             light. A red glass is placed before one eye. Two images are pro-
             duced, a red light seen by one eye, a white light seen by the other.
             The patient describes the degree of separation between these two
             images in each of the cardinal directions of gaze. Maximum sep-
             aration occurs in the field of action of the paretic muscle. By
             considering the relative positions of the two images at the point
             of maximum separation,the paretic muscle can be readily
             identified. (See also questions and discussion in Case #1).

7. ABCE   Ocular muscle palsies may occur as the initial clinical manifesta-
             tion of diabetes. Therefore the two hour postprandial blood sugar
             estimation is important in patients complaining of diplopia. A
             skull series might reveal abnormal intracranial calcifications, or
             other abnormalities. The sedimentation rate may be elevated
             markedly in cavernous sinus inflammation and in temporal
             arteritis. Diplopia may be a symptom in either of these con-
             ditions. Since syphillitic arteritis may produce palsies of the
             extraocular muscles, a VDRL and FTA are indicated. A
             pneumoencephalogram has significant risk and is not an appropriate
             "initial" test.

CASE STUDY #35

8. A   Myasthenia gravis is an important cause of weakness of the extraocular muscles. Thus the tensilon or negostigmine tests are indicated. Angio-Conray is the name of a contrast medium used to perform
angiograms. The Queckenstedt test is sometimes performed to de-
tect spinal block and is obviously inappropriate in this case.

9. B   Edrophonium (Tensilon) is given intravenously. Its effect begins in
thirty seconds, reaches its maximum in forty-five seconds and is
often completed after one minute.

10. ABCD

11. B   Bruits may be heard frequently over the eyes of children in the absence of underlying disease.

12. A

13. A   The presence of the bruit indicates a vascular lesion. Since the bruit
is obliterated with compression of the right common carotid artery,
the lesion would be located in the anterior circulation on the right side.

14. A

15. A

16. A

17. D   The fistula between the carotid artery and the cavernous sinus shunts
blood under arterial pressure to a venous channel. The sinus dilates.
The ophthalmic veins become dilated and tortuous in most instances.
Exophthalmos,which is frequently pulsating, results. There are venous branches between the right and left cavernous sinuses and therefore the pressure may rise bilaterally.

18. ABCDE

COMMENTS: The patient described in the case report demonstrates some of the
symptoms and signs seen with a carotid-cavernous fistula. One unusual feature
was the abnormal connection between the external carotid artery and the cavernous
sinus. More frequently this abnormal connection occurs between the internal carotid artery and the cavernous sinus. Interesting also was the mildness of the head
trauma which preceded and precipitated the development of the fistula. Several
authors have published strong evidence that hemodynamic disorders, produced by
trauma or other factors, change congenital arteriovenous dural shunts into clinically significant carotid-cavernous fistulas.

Some patients with carotid-cavernous fistulas have been followed without surgery.
Indications for operation include progressive exophthalmos and chemosis which may
cause deterioration of vision, as well as patient intolerance of the bruit. The pur-
pose of any type of operative procedure is to obliterate the abnormal communication between the artery, either internal or external carotid, and the cavernous sinus. There are differences of opinion as to the best surgical procedure. The
most direct approach of course, would be to expose the cavernous sinus, open the
dural covering, and directly ligate the abnormal communication. This is a form-
idable procedure but has been carried out in some instances, particularly by Parkinson.

The more standard approach is aimed at trapping the carotid supply to the fistula,
if the patient can tolerate occlusion of one carotid artery. The usual sequence is
a craniotomy, in order to ligate the carotid artery above the level of the cavernous sinus. Then the carotid artery is exposed in the neck and mechanical emboli

CASE STUDY #35

are introduced to occlude the communication between artery and sinus from within. After this the artery is ligated in the neck. In external carotid-cavernous sinus fistulas, some have exposed the external carotid artery in the neck and introduced emboli without intracranial ligation of the artery. In most cases, simple arterial ligation is inadequate because of collateral flow through other arterial channels which would keep the fistula open.

REFERENCES

1. Hamby, W., Carotid-Cavernous Fistula, Charles C Thomas, Springfield, 1966.

2. Isamat, E., V. Salleras, and A.M. Miranda, Artificial Embolization of Carotid-Cavernous Fistulas with Post-Operative Patency of Internal Carotid Activity, J Neurol Neurosurg and Psychiat 33:674, 1970.

3. Kosary, I.Z., M.A. Learner, M. Mozes, and M. Lazar, Artificial Embolic Oculsion of the Terminal Internal Carotid Artery in the Treatment of Carotid-Cavernous Fistulas, Technical Note, J Neurosurg 28:605, 1968.

4. Krayenbuhl, H., Article in Microvascular Surgery, Ed., R.M.P. Donaghy and M.G. Yasargil, C.V. Mosby Co., St. Louis, 1967.

5. Madsen, P.H., Carotid-Cavernous Fistulas, A Study of 18 Cases; Acta Ophth 48:731, 1970.

6. Parkinson, D., Transcavernous Repair of Carotid-Cavernous Fistula, Case Report, J Neurosurg 26:420, 1967.

7. Pool, J.L., and G. Potts, Aneurysms and Arterial Venous Anomalies of the Brain, Hoeber Medical Division, Harper and Row, 1965.

8. Sedzimir, C.B., and J.V. Occleshaw, Treatment of Carotid-Cavernous Fistulas by Muscle Embolization and Jalger's Maneuver, J Neurosurg 27:309, 1967.

9. Stern, W.E., et al., Surgical Challenge of Carotid-Cavernous Fistula, Critical Role of Intracranial Circulatory Dynamics, J Neurosurg 27:298 (Oct.) 1967.

10. Parkinson, D., Carotid Cavernous Fistula: Direct Repair with Preservation of the Carotid Artery, J Neurosurg 38:99, 1973.

11. Mahalley, M., and S. Boone, External Carotid-Cavernous Fistula Treated by Arterial Embolization, J Neurosurgery 40:110, 1974.

CASE STUDY #36

Headache and Amenorrhea

HISTORY: An 18 year-old girl had been seen in gynecology clinic at age sixteen because of amenorrhea of five months duration. Her periods had been previously normal since menarche at age twelve. She was otherwise in excellent health. Gynecological examination revealed sparse pubic hair, but was otherwise normal. A pregnancy test was negative. She was placed on enovid, with menses subsequently occurring, but, eight months later, when she discontinued the drug, her periods again stopped. She began to experience hot flashes. At about this time she also began to complain of headaches, bifrontal, severe, and aching. These gradually increased in frequency and severity and would occasionally awaken her from sleep.

CASE STUDY #36

QUESTIONS:

1. AT THIS POINT, WITH A HISTORY OF HEADACHE AND AMENORRHEA, YOU MIGHT SUSPECT THE PROBLEM TO BE:
   A. Multiple sclerosis
   B. Anorexia nervosa
   C. A tumor in the vicinity of the pituitary gland
   D. None of the above

2. YOU MIGHT NOW WISH FURTHER INFORMATION ABOUT:
   A. Visual function
   B. Endocrine function
   C. Urine output
   D. Thirst
   E. All of the above

A year after the onset of the amenorrhea, vision in her left eye began to deteriorate. When looking at objects she said that she saw a circular outline, but missed central portions of the object. She preferred hot to cool weather and frequently felt chilly when other members of her family did not. She did not drink or urinate excessively.

EXAMINATION: She was a well nourished pleasant young girl, with normal vital signs. Her breasts were well developed, but axillary and pubic hair were extremely sparse. Visual acuity was 20/300 in the left eye and was normal in the right. The left optic disc was pale. Visual fields were full peripherally, but there was a paracentral scotoma on the left.

Pupillary reactions, the extraocular movements, and the corneal reflexes were normal, as was the remainder of the neurological examination.

QUESTIONS:

3. OF THE FOLLOWING, THE MOST USEFUL LABORATORY TESTS WOULD INCLUDE:
   A. Urine specific gravity
   B. Spinal fluid gamma globulin
   C. Urine 17-ketogenic steroids
   D. PBI
   E. B and C

4. USEFUL RADIOLOGICAL PROCEDURES WOULD INCLUDE:
   A. Skull films
   B. Views of the optic foramina
   C. Pantopaque myelography of the posterior fossa
   D. Carotid angiography
   E. Pneumoencephalography

LABORATORY DATA: Protein bound iodine was 3.6mcg%. Radioiodine uptake was 8%. Urine 17 ketogenic and 17 ketosteroids were subnormal. Cerebrospinal fluid was normal. Urine specific gravity was normal.

Skull films showed the sella turcica expanded in all dimensions, with thinning of the posterior clinoids (Fig. 38).

CASE STUDY #36

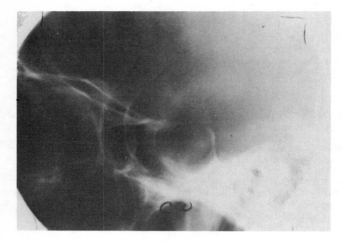

Figure 38

QUESTION:

5.   AT THIS POINT, DIAGNOSTIC POSSIBILITIES MIGHT INCLUDE:
      A. Craniopharyngioma
      B. Pituitary adenoma
      C. Aneurysm
      D. Optic glioma
      E. All of the above

X-rays of the optic foramina were normal.

Pneumoencephalogram showed an intrasellar mass with suprasellar extension (Fig. 39).

Carotid angiography showed elevation of the left internal carotid bifurcation and "opening" of the carotid siphon. No aneurysm was seen (Fig. 40).

COURSE: A craniotomy was performed. The left optic nerve was compressed by a large mass beneath it. The tumor proved to be a chromophobe adenoma (Fig. 41).

Following removal of the tumor, her vision gradually became normal. The scotoma disappeared, but the pallor of the left optic disc remained. She did well on endocrine replacement therapy for three years, when she began again to complain of headaches and diminishing vision of the left eye. The visual field of the left eye showed an inferior temporal quadrantic defect (Fig. 42).

A course of radiotherapy was given, the visual fields became normal, and she has since remained well.

CASE STUDY #36

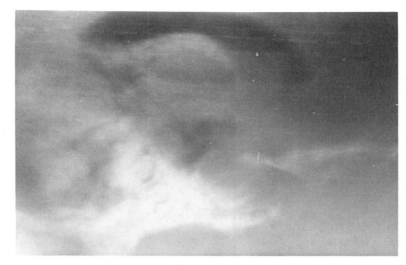

Figure 39

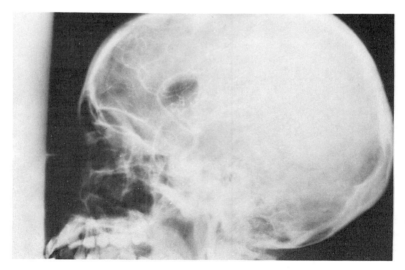

Figure 40

CASE STUDY #36

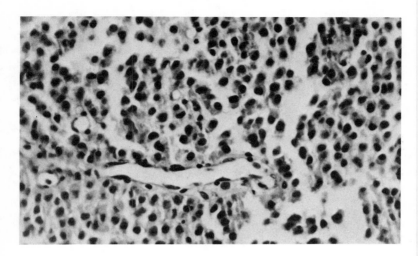

Figure 41

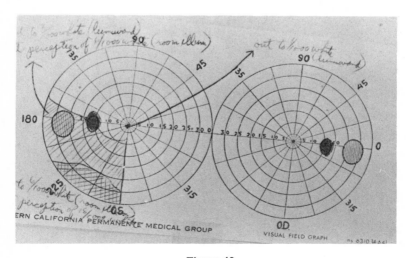

Figure 42

CASE STUDY #36

QUESTIONS:

TRUE OR FALSE:

6. This case is unusual since pituitary adenomas, although a common brain tumor of adult life, are relatively rare in childhood and adolescence.

7. Under age 20, craniopharyngioma is a much more common parasellar tumor than pituitary adenoma.

8. The absence of diabetes insipidus does not prove that the hypothalamic-posterior pituitary andidiuretic hormone pathway is intact, since anterior pituitary insufficiency may mask diabetes insipidus.

9. WHICH OF THE VISUAL FIELD ABNORMALITIES SCHEMATICALLY DIAGRAMMED BELOW IS THE MOST COMMON ONE IN PITUITARY ADENOMAS?:

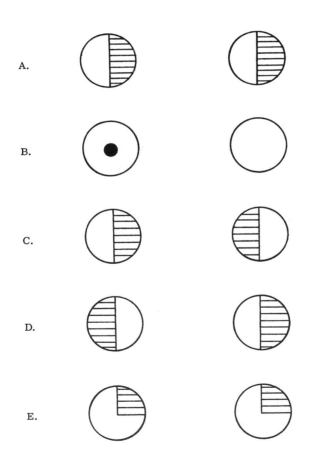

A.

B.

C.

D.

E.

CASE STUDY #36

MATCH THE POSSIBLE DIRECTION OF GROWTH OF A PITUITARY
TUMOR WITH THE NEUROLOGICAL COMPLICATION WHICH MIGHT
THEN BE SEEN:

10. ___ Upward, into the third ventricle
11. ___ Laterally to the temporal lobe
12. ___ Downward into the sphenoid sinus
13. ___ Laterally, involving cranial nerves
14. ___ Backwards to the cerebral
peduncles

A. Spinal fluid rhinorrhea
B. Spasticity, weakness, Babinski signs
C. Psychomotor seizures
D. Increased intracranial pressure with hydrocephalus
E. Diplopia

15. IF YOU WERE CALLED TO THE HOSPITAL EMERGENCY AREA BECAUSE
THIS PATIENT HAD BEEN ADMITTED WITH THE SUDDEN ONSET OF
HEADACHE, OBTUNDATION, AND IMPAIRED MOVEMENTS OF BOTH
EYES, THE MOST LIKELY DIAGNOSIS WOULD BE:
A. Meningitis
B. Drug abuse
C. Acute cranial polyneuritis
D. Pituitary apoplexy
E. Intracranial aneurysm

ANSWERS AND DISCUSSION:

1. C   The combination of severe headache with evidence of endocrine deficiency should suggest the possibility of a lesion in the pituitary-
hypothalamic area.

2. E   Disease in the vicinity of the pituitary gland frequently is associated
with visual disturbance due to involvement of the closely adjacent
optic nerves and chiasm.

Information about fluid intake, thirst and urine output is important to
evaluate the function of the hypothalamic-posterior pituitary pathway
which controls antidiuretic hormone synthesis, storage, and release.

3. ACD   The specific gravity of the urine, tested after a period of withholding
fluid for 12 hours, is a measure of the ability to conserve water and
concentrate the urine, which depends on the integrity of the antidiuretic hormone secretory pathway.

Urine ketogenic steroid measurement and blood protein bound iodide
are tests of adrenal and thyroid function which may be secondarily
impaired with pituitary hypofunction.

The spinal fluid gamma globulin content is elevated in many cases of
multiple sclerosis and occasionally in a variety of other neurological
conditions. A clinical picture of progressive headaches, visual impairment and endocrine hypofunction does not suggest the diagnostic
possibility of multiple sclerosis.

4. ABDE Skull films would give very significant information about possible enlargement or erosion of the sella turcica. The optic nerve foramen
is typically enlarged in cases of gliomata of the optic nerve, but occasionally with other tumors, as meningiomas or neurofibromas.

Both pneumoencephalography and carotid angiography can give important information about a mass in the parasellar area. An additional reason for the angiogram is to delineate a possible aneurysm.

5. E

CASE STUDY #36

6. True

7. True

8. T   "Following extensive neurohypophysial injury, the development of
adenohypophysial, adrenal cortical, or thyroid insufficiency may
cause severe diabetes insipidus to become mild or even latent. The
administration of anterior pituitary or target gland hormones can con-
vert latent diabetes insipidus to an overt state or make mild diabetes
insipidus more severe."[1]

9. D   The bitemporal field cut results from compression by the tumor of
fibers from the nasal retina and optic nerve of one side, crossing
medially in the optic chiasm to the other side (see figure p. 194). The
nasal retina receives light impulses from the temporal visual fields
because of light refraction by the lens of the eye.

The result of the pattern of crossing of fibers from the nasal retina in
the optic chiasm, while fibers from the temporal retina do not cross,
is that vision from the left half of the visual field travels in the right
optic tract to reach the right occipital lobe and vice versa.

The diagram (A) is that of a homonymous hemianopsia which results
from a lesion damaging the entire optic tract or optic radiations opposite the side of the hemianopsia.
(B) portrays a left central scotoma, often seen with optic nerve disease.
(C) is a binasal hemianopsia, which is uncommonly seen. Can you
visualize where the lesions would be to produce this pattern?
(E) is a right superior quadrantanopsia, resulting from a lesion in
the left temporal lobe, involving the lower half of the optic radiations.
Lesions of the parietal lobe, involving the upper half of the visual
radiations, result in a contralateral inferior quadrantanopsia.

10. D

11. C

12. A

13. E

14. B

15. D   The major clinical features of acute pituitary apoplexy are sudden
headache, depressed consciousness, ophthalmoplegia, and signs of
optic nerve or chiasmal compression. Signs of meningeal irritation
may be present. The cause is acute infarction and/or hemorrhage
in a pituitary neoplasm. CSF may be clear or bloody. Although some
patients with mild neurological deficits have been treated medically,
neurosurgical decompression (with cortisol administration) is required if vision or level of consciousness is deteriorating.

CASE STUDY #36

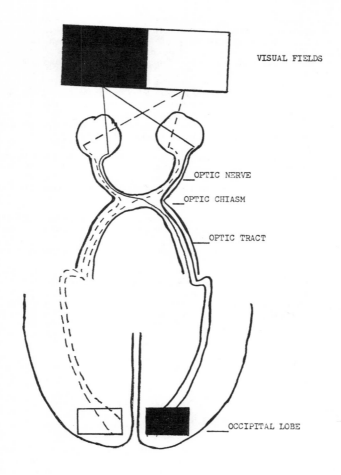

VISUAL FIELDS

OPTIC NERVE

OPTIC CHIASM

OPTIC TRACT

OCCIPITAL LOBE

CASE STUDY #36

COMMENTS: Surgery was performed in this patient because of the seriousness of visual loss and her age, at which pituitary adenomas are uncommon, whereas relatively radioresistant tumors such as craniopharyngiomas are more frequent. Many neurologists will treat adult patients with a typical clinical and radiological (including pneumography and angiography) picture of a chromophobe pituitary adenoma with radiotherapy initially. Indications for surgery vary among clinicians, and include rapid or profound visual loss, increased intracranial pressure, and lack of response to radiotherapy.

REFERENCES

1. Timmons, R.L., and G.S. Dugger, Water and Salt Metabolism Following Pituitary Stalk Section, Neurology 19:790, 1969.

2. Walsh, F.B., and W.B. Hoyt, Clinical Neuro-ophthalmology, Williams and Wilkins, Baltimore, 1969.

3. Heuser, G. (moderator), UCLA Interdepartmental Conf. Trends in Clinical Neuroendocrinology, Ann Int Med 73:783, 1970.

4. Wilson, P., M. Falconer, Patterns of Visual Failure with Pituitary Tumors, Brit J Ophth 52:94, 1968.

5. Svien, H., et al., Status of Vision Following Surgical Treatment for Pituitary Adenomas, J Neurosurg 22:47, 1965.

6. Elkington, S., Pituitary Adenoma, Preoperative Symptomatology in a Series of 260 Patients, Brit J Ophth 52:322, 1968.

7. Schlezinger, N., and R. Thompson, Pituitary Tumors with Central Scotomas Stimulating Retrobulbar Optic Neuritis, Neurol 17:782, 1967.

8. Reichlin, S., Function of the Hypothalamus, Am J Med 43:477, 1967.

9. Dawson, B., and P. Kothandaram, Acute Massive Infarction of Pituitary Adenomas, J Neurosurg 37:275, 1972.

10. Rovit, R., and J. Fein, Pituitary Apoplexy: A Review and Reappraisal, J Neurosurg 37:280, 1972.

11. Robert, C., et al., Ocular Palsy Occurring with Pituitary Tumors, J Neurosurg 38:17, 1973.

12. Jenkins, J., Pituitary Tumors, Appleton-Century-Crofts, 1973.

13. Samaan, N., Pituitary Tumors: Recent Advances in Diagnosis and Treatment, Texas Med 70:55, 1974.

14. Wirth, F., et al., Pituitary Adenomas: Factors in Treatment, pp. 8-25 in Clinical Neurosurgery, Wilkins, R.H. editor, Williams and Wilkins Co., 1974.

15. Pearson, O., et al., Endocrine Evaluation and Indications for Surgery of Functional Pituitary Adenomas, pp. 26-38, in Clinical Neurosurgery, Wilkins, R.H. editor, Williams and Wilkins Co., 1974.

16. Williams, R.H., Textbook of Endocrinology, W.B. Saunders Co., Philadelphia, 1974.

CASE STUDY #37

A Floppy Baby

HISTORY: This child was the first-born of normal parents. A grandmother was diagnosed as having myasthenia gravis. During the last trimester of the pregnancy fetal movements were thought to be weak. Delivery was normal but shortly thereafter he was noted to be hypoactive with only feeble movements of the extremities.

EXAMINATION (age 2 weeks): The infant lay alert but almost motionless, with hips externally rotated and knees flexed in a froglike posture (fig. 43).

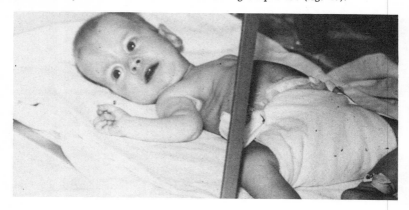

Figure 43

His head was of normal size and shape. The extremities were flaccid and moved only minimally in response to pinching. The Moro reflex was absent. In dorsal suspension (fig. 44) his head and legs hung limply. The deep tendon reflexes were absent. His cry was very weak and bilateral facial weakness was present. The optic fundi, pupillary reactions and extraocular movements were normal. Scattered rhonchi were heard in both lungs.

QUESTIONS:

1. WHICH OF THE FOLLOWING STATEMENTS APPLIES TO THE MORO REFLEX?
   A. When absent, a central nervous system lesion may be present
   B. It may be depressed or absent with dysfunction of the peripheral nervous system, neuromuscular junction or muscle fiber
   C. An asymmetrical response is usually pathological
   D. The reflex can be elicited by any sudden, uncomfortable sensory input
   E. All of above

CASE STUDY #37

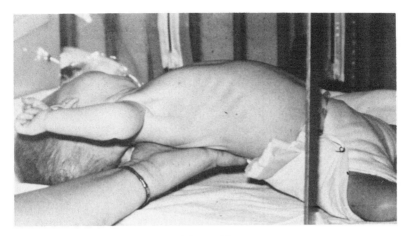

Figure 44

2. HYPOTONIA IS BEST EVALUATED BY:
   A. Careful observation of the patient at rest and during voluntary motor activity
   B. Careful palpation of muscle bellies while the patient is relaxed or sleeping
   C. Passive movement of a relaxed limb
   D. Observation of limb movements in response to startle
   E. Testing the deep tendon reflexes while the infant sleeps

3. WHAT ARE SOME OF THE MORE COMMON NEUROLOGIC CAUSES OF HYPOTONIA AND WEAKNESS AT BIRTH?
   A. Marfan's syndrome
   B. Infantile spinal muscular atrophy (Werdnig-Hoffman)
   C. Cerebral anoxia
   D. Phenylketonuria
   E. Polymyositis

4. WHAT STUDIES WOULD BE INDICATED?
   A. Bilateral carotid angiography   D. Nerve conduction velocities
   B. Electromyography   E. Brain biopsy
   C. Tensilon test   F. Muscle biopsy

LABORATORY STUDIES: Routine blood and urine studies were normal. 1 mg of edrophonium (Tensilon) I.V. and 0.1 mg of neostigmine (Prostigmin) I.M. resulted in no significant improvement in weakness. Nerve conduction velocities were within normal limits. Electromyography revealed evidence of diffuse fibrillatory activity in all four limbs. X-rays of the skull and cervical spine, protein bound iodine, serum potassium, cerebrospinal fluid examination and serum enzymes were all normal. The muscle biopsy was felt to be normal.

CASE STUDY #37

QUESTIONS:

5. WHAT IS THE MOST LIKELY DIAGNOSIS IN THIS CHILD?
   A. Myasthenia gravis
   B. Guillain-Barré syndrome
   C. Infantile spinal muscular atrophy (Werdnig-Hoffman)
   D. Benign congenital hypotonia
   E. Oppenheim's disease (amyotonia congenita)
   F. Myotonia congenita

COURSE: At age four months, he was noted to be an alert baby who could follow a light with his eyes, smiled at and recognized his mother. He had no head control or Moro response, and he remained areflexic and hypotonic. At about this time he began to have increasing difficulty with respiration and feeding, and was admitted to the hospital at age five months with pneumonia and atelectasis of the right lung. In spite of treatment, the child died several days later. Autopsy showed pneumonia and a denervation pattern of atrophy in most of the skeletal muscle. The spinal cord showed decreased numbers of anterior horn cells at all levels, with degenerative changes in the remaining neurons. Increased numbers of astrocytes were also seen in the anterior horns.

6. INFANTILE SPINAL MUSCULAR ATROPHY MAY BE CHARACTERIZED BY THE FOLLOWING:
   A. Degeneration of anterior horn cells of the brain stem and spinal cord
   B. Autosomal dominant in inheritance
   C. Atrophy and fasciculation of the tongue
   D. Increased cerebrospinal fluid protein
   E. Recurrent seizures

7. MYASTHENIA GRAVIS OF INFANCY:
   A. Occurs as a congenital form in which the mother is not myasthenic. The weakness may remit and exacerbate, as in adult myasthenia
   B. Is seen also in the neonatal form in infants of myasthenic mothers. The weakness disappears permanently after weeks to months
   C. Is important to diagnose since it is treatable
   D. Produces impairment of crying, sucking, swallowing, as well as generalized muscular weakness and limpness

8. IN THE REGULATION OF MUSCLE TONE:
   A. The sensory arc of the muscle stretch reflex consists of fibers from the muscle spindle; the motor arc of fibers from the alpha motoneurons in the spinal cord
   B. The gamma efferent system consists of fibers from the gamma motoneurons of the spinal cord to the muscle fibers of the muscle spindle; activity of this system alters the sensitivity of the muscle spindles to stretch
   C. The gamma efferent system is itself influenced by higher centers in the brain
   D. The gamma efferent system is unimportant in the regulation of muscle tone

9. WHICH OF THE FOLLOWING NEUROMUSCULAR DISORDERS COMMONLY ARE SYMPTOMATIC AT BIRTH?
   A. Duchenne muscular dystrophy
   B. Polymyositis
   C. Charcot-Marie-Tooth disease
   D. All of above
   E. None of above

CASE STUDY #37

10.   TRUE OR FALSE:

    A. Fibrillations are commonly seen in myasthenia gravis.

    B. Central core disease refers to a congenital lesion of the central portions of the brain, such as corpus callosum.

    C. The congenital form of myotonic muscular dystrophy frequently presents with facial weakness, sucking problems and dysphagia.

    D. Electromyography in the neonatal period is difficult to evaluate and often unreliable.

ANSWERS AND DISCUSSION:

1. E

2. C   Hypotonia refers to an alteration in tone which by definition is the resistance offered to passive limb movement. Tone cannot be observed or palpated. Evaluation of tone in an infant is difficult but can be achieved with persistence. Hypotonia must be differentiated from weakness which is more suggestive of damage to the motor unit.

3. BC

4. BCDF

5. C   Infantile spinal muscular atrophy is one of a group of clinical disorders which have in common a genetic tendency and pathology fairly well limited to motoneurons in spinal cord and brain stem. Related conditions include Kugelberg-Welander Disease, which begins later in life and has a slower and more benign course, and neurogenic forms of the facioscapulohumeral and limb-girdle syndromes. Although the muscle biopsy was negative the clinical and laboratory features were quite typical, and the post-mortem (see below) clearly established the nature of this child's illness. There is continuing debate as to whether the benign and more malignant forms are identical or separate in etiopathogenesis. Treatment is supportive and symptomatic, including genetic counselling.

6. AC

7. ABCD

8. ABC

9. E   See Case No. 21 for additional discussion of childhood weakness.

10.   A. False
      B. False
      C. True
      D. True
      The congenital form of myotonic dystrophy should be differentiated from myotonia congenita (Thompsen's disease). The former presents at birth with facial weakness, intellectual retardation and only

CASE STUDY #37

> modest myotonia. The latter rarely is symptomatic in infancy and usually presents in late childhood with the symptoms of myotonia alone.

REFERENCES

1. Kugelberg, E. and L. Welander, Familial Neurogenic (Spinal?) Muscular Atrophy Simulating Ordinary Proximal Dystrophy, Acta Psych et Neurol Scand 29:42, 1954.

2. Smith, J.B., and A. Patel, The Wohlfahrt-Kugelberg-Welander Disease, Neurology 15:469, 1965.

3. Munsat, T.L., et al., Neurogenic Muscular Atrophy of Infancy with Prolonged Survival, Brain 92:9, 1969.

4. Dubowitz, V., The Floppy Infant. Clinics in Developmental Medicine No. 31, William Heinemann Medical Books Ltd., Lavenham, 1969.

5. Emery, A.E., Electromyographic Studies in Parents of Children with Spinal Muscular Atrophy, J Med Genet 10:8, 1973.

6. Pearn, J.H., Fetal Movements and Werdnig-Hoffman Disease, J Neurol Sci 18:373, 1973.

7. Diagnosis of Childhood Spinal Muscular Atrophy, Editorial, British Med J Oct. 6, 1973.

8. Munsat, T., Congenital Myopathies, in The Striated Muscle, Chapt. 21, Williams and Wilkins Co., Baltimore, 1973.

9. Saper, J., Benign Congenital Myopathy, Am J Med 57:157, 1974.

CASE STUDY #38

Lancinating Facial Pain

HISTORY: A 59 year-old woman was seen because of severe facial pain. The pain radiated from the corner of the mouth to just below the lateral corner of the eye. She described it as knifelike, excruciating, lancinating, lasting only a second, occurring in bursts, and triggered by speaking, chewing or tooth brushing.

QUESTIONS:

1. THE PAIN IS LOCATED IN THE DISTRIBUTION OF THE:
    A. Great auricular nerve
    B. Mandibular branch of the trigeminal nerve
    C. Maxillary branch of the trigeminal nerve
    D. Glossopharyngeal nerve

2. THE MOST LIKELY DIAGNOSIS IS:
    A. Cluster headache
    B. Maxillary sinusitis
    C. Common migraine
    D. Trigeminal neuralgia
    E. Glossopharyngeal neuralgia

CASE STUDY #38

3. IN THIS CONDITION, THE NEUROLOGICAL EXAMINATION SHOWS:
   A. A hyperactive jaw jerk
   B. Nothing abnormal
   C. Facial weakness
   D. A Babinski sign
   E. A, C, and D

EXAMINATION: The neurological examination was entirely normal.

QUESTION:

4. AT THIS POINT, YOU MIGHT NOW REQUEST:
   A. Carotid angiograms
   B. A myelogram
   C. Skull films
   D. A spinal tap
   E. Dental evaluation
   F. All of the above

LABORATORY DATA: Blood count, urinalysis, skull films, electroencephalogram, dental examination, blood sugar were all normal.

COURSE: She was begun on Dilantin, which even at high doses brought little relief. Carbamazepine (Tegretol) was then begun, initially at 200 mgm daily, gradually increasing to one gram daily. At this dosage, she experienced only moderate relief, but was very unhappy about the nausea, lethargy and vertigo produced by the drug.

QUESTIONS:

5. OTHER SIDE EFFECTS OF CARBAMAZEPINE INCLUDE:
   A. Skin rash
   B. Agranulocytosis
   C. Liver damage
   D. All of the above

6. CARBAMAZEPINE IS SIMILAR TO DILANTIN IN THAT:
   A. Both have anticonvulsant activity
   B. Both can cause blood dyscrasias
   C. Both can inhibit synaptic transmission
   D. All of the above

7. THE PERCENTAGE OF PATIENTS WITH THIS CONDITION WHO WILL SHOW CONSIDERABLE BENEFIT FROM TEGRETOL IS:
   A. 10%
   B. 25%
   C. 70%
   D. 98%

COURSE: Because of the partial and unsatisfactory response to carbamazepine, she was referred for a surgical procedure.

QUESTION:

8. THE PLANNED SURGERY MIGHT BE:
   A. Prefrontal lobotomy
   B. Cordotomy
   C. Thalamotomy
   D. Pallidectomy
   E. Alcohol block of the trigeminal nerve

CASE STUDY #38

After this procedure, the pain disappeared.

QUESTIONS:

9.   IN THE GREAT MAJORITY OF CASES OF THIS SYNDROME, THERE IS
     NO DEMONSTRABLE PATHOLOGY. OCCASIONALLY, THIS PAIN PAT-
     TERN CAN BE SEEN WITH:
     A. Multiple sclerosis
     B. Meningiomas
     C. Aneurysm
     D. Neurofibromas
     E. All of the above

10. CLUES TO THE PRESENCE OF UNDERLYING STRUCTURAL DISEASE
     ARE:
     A. Abnormalities in the neurological examination, such as numbness over
         the face
     B. Abnormalities of the skull films, spinal fluid
     C. Both A and B

11. THE NERVE INVOLVED IN THIS CONDITION SUPPLIES MUSCLES
     INVOLVED IN:
     A. Visual accomodation
     B. Chewing
     C. Protruding the tongue
     D. Closing the eyes
     E. B and D

ANSWERS AND DISCUSSION:

1. C

2. D   The description is classically that of trigeminal neuralgia, with
               lightning-like jabs of pain in the distribution of one or more
               branches of the 5th cranial nerve. As with this patient,
               characteristically there is a trigger zone, which when touched
               sets off the paroxysms of pain. This trigger zone may be
               stimulated by chewing, tooth brushing, or facial movement. The
               pain of migraine, cluster headache, and sinusitis typically per-
               sists for hours, and does not consist of a succession of knifelike
               momentary jabs of pain. The pain of glossopharyngeal neuralgia
               is similar to trigeminal neuralgia in its quality, but occurs in the
               region of the tonsils, posterior pharynx, back of the tongue and
               middle ear.

3. B   Objective neurological abnormality on examination should initiate
               a search for an underlying lesion (see also questions 9 and 10).

4. CE   Skull and sinus films and a dental evaluation should be obtained to
               rule out other causes of facial pain. A spinal tap is not ordinarily
               done where the clinical picture is typical. It should be performed,
               however, where there is a suspicion of secondary trigeminal
               neuralgia, as when abnormalities are found on the neurological
               examination or where the onset of symptoms occurs at an unusual
               age, as prior to 40. This is illustrated by case #3 of Abbott and
               Killeffer[2], of a 29 year-old man who had developed the typical
               pain pattern of tic doloreux five years earlier. The neurological
               examination and skull films were normal, but lumbar puncture
               showed an increase of protein and subsequently a tumor of the

CASE STUDY #38

posterior fossa was discovered. Neither myelography nor carotid angiography are appropriate studies in cases of typical trigeminal neuralgia.

5. D

6. D

7. C

8. E

9. E   Additionally, acoustic tumors, cerebellopontine angle dermoids, vascular lesions of the posterior fossa may also cause secondary trigeminal neuralgia. Kerr[3] in arguing for a peripheral site of pathogenesis in trigeminal neuralgia points out that the only central type of lesion known to produce trigeminal neuralgia is multiple sclerosis, but in cases where the brain was examined, a plaque was invariably found at the point of entrance of the posterior root into the pons on the affected side, producing in fact a peripheral or root lesion.

10. C

11. B   The fifth cranial nerve supplies motor fibers to the temporal and masseter muscles which elevate the mandible and close the jaw.

REFERENCES

1. Killian, J. M., and G. H. Fromm, Carbamazepine in the Treatment of Neuralgia, Arch Neuro 19:129, 1968.

2. Abbott, M., and F. Killeffer, Symptomatic Trigeminal Neuralgia, Bull LA Neurol Soc 35:1, 1970.

3. Kerr, F., The Etiology of Trigeminal Neuralgia, Arch Neur 8:31, 1963.

4. Miller, H., Pain in the Face, Brit Med J 2:577, 1968.

5. Procacci, P., A Survey of Modern Concepts of Pain, Handbook of Clinical Neurology, P. J. Vinken, and G. W. Bruyn, Ed., North Holland Publishing Co., 1969.

6. White, J., and W. Sweet, Pain and the Neurosurgeon; A Forty Year Experience, Charles C Thomas, 1969.

7. Stookey, B., and J. Ransohoff, Trigeminal Neuralgia; History and Treatment, Charles C Thomas, 1959.

8. Yoshimasu, F., et al., Tic Douloureux in Rochester, Minnesota 1945-1969, Neurology 22:952, 1972.

9. Wepsic, J., Tic Douloureux, New Eng J Med 288:680, 1973.

10. Amols, W., Medical Treatment of Tic Douloureux, New Eng J Med 289:159, 1973.

11. Jannetta, P., Pain Problems of Significance in the Head and Face, Some of which Often are Misdiagnosed, Current Problems in Surgery Feb. 1973.

12. Crill, W., Carbamazepine, Ann Int Med 79:844-847, 1973.

13. Nugent, G. R., and B. Berry, Trigeminal Neuralgia Treated by Differential Percutaneous Radiofrequency Coagulation of the Gasserian Ganglion, J Neurosurg 40:517, 1974.

CASE STUDY #39

Baldness, Muscle Weakness and Cataracts

HISTORY: A 45 year-old male was seen because of weakness. As a child and youth he was quite athletic, but, during the past ten years, he had noted progressive weakness and wasting of both arms and legs.

QUESTION:

1.   THE HISTORY SO FAR SUGGESTS:
    A. Myelopathy
    B. Neuropathy
    C. Myopathy
    D. Any of the above

During this time he had also noted that when he clenched his hands tightly, he was unable to open them rapidly. This did not worsen in cold weather.

QUESTION:

2.   THIS PHENOMENON IS CALLED:
    A. Myasthenia
    B. Myokymia
    C. Myotonia
    D. None of the above

Ocular cataracts had been diagnosed several years ago.

QUESTION:

3.   THE MOST LIKELY DIAGNOSIS OF THIS PATIENT'S ILLNESS IS:
    A. Paramyotonia
    B. Myotonic muscular dystrophy
    C. Myotonia congenita
    D. None of the above

He was the father of four children, all of whom were said to be well. There was no history of familial neuromuscular disease or cataracts, but information about many members of his family could not be obtained.

EXAMINATION: He was bald, and showed atrophy of the temporal and masseter muscles (Fig. 45). There was also muscle atrophy in all extremities, most marked distally. Weakness was present in the facial muscles and in all extremities, worse distally. The deep tendon reflexes were hypoactive.

When asked to clench his fists forcibly and then rapidly open his hands, he could only open the hands partially (Fig. 46).

Percussion of the tongue produced dimpling, and percussion of the thenar eminence (Fig. 47) produced opposition of the thumb with very slow relaxation.

QUESTION:

4.   THIS IS NOT ONLY A NEUROMUSCULAR, BUT A MULTISYSTEM DISEASE, WITH ABNORMALITIES OFTEN NOTED IN EXAMINING THE:
    A. Eyes, scalp, and liver
    B. Liver, spleen and skin
    C. Eyes, lungs and scalp
    D. Eyes, testes, and scalp

CASE STUDY #39

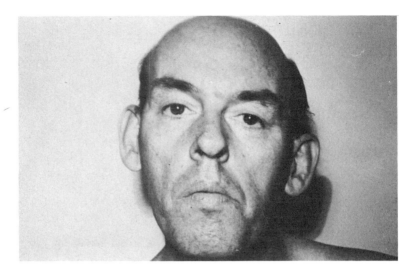

Figure 45

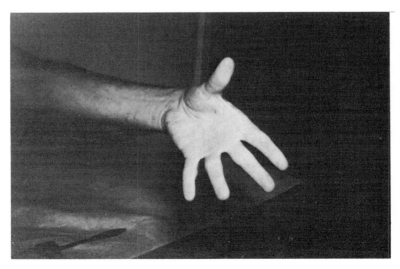

Figure 46

CASE STUDY #39

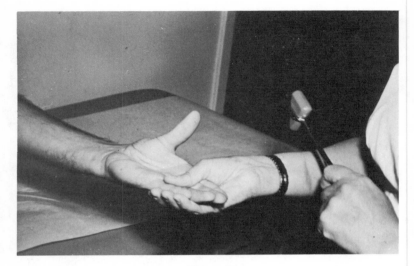

Figure 47

Bilateral cataracts were present, and the testes were atrophic.

QUESTIONS:

5.　　PARTICULARLY USEFUL IN CONFIRMING THE DIAGNOSIS WOULD BE:
　　　A. Electromyography
　　　B. Tensilon test
　　　C. Myelography
　　　D. All of the above

6.　　THE DISTINCTIVE PATTERN OF MUSCLE ACTIVITY HEARD WITH THE
　　　ELECTROMYOGRAM IN THIS CONDITION HAS BEEN COMPARED TO
　　　THE SOUND OF:
　　　A. Raindrops
　　　B. Static electricity
　　　C. A dive bomber
　　　D. A machine gun

7.　　IN THIS CONDITION, ABNORMALITIES HAVE BEEN NOTED IN:
　　　A. Basal metabolism rate
　　　B. Urine 17 ketosteroids
　　　C. Serum immunoglobulin
　　　D. Cardiac function
　　　E. Pneumoencephalogram
　　　F. None of the above

LABORATORY DATA: The electromyogram showed the classical bursts of
myotonia in all muscles tested. Serum creatine phosphokinase and lactic
dehydrogenase were both significantly elevated. The electrocardiogram showed

CASE STUDY #39

a left bundle branch block. Biopsy of the deltoid muscle showed considerable variation in fiber size, with long chains of centrally placed nuclei. Urine 17 ketosteroids were decreased; 17 ketogenic steroids were normal. Blood sugar was normal.

QUESTIONS:

8. THE WEAKNESS AND WASTING OF THIS DISEASE ARE IMPROVED BY:
   A. L Dopa
   B. Quinine
   C. Mestinon
   D. Vitamin E
   E. No drug presently known

9. THE MYOTONIA CAN BE DECREASED WITH:
   A. Dilantin
   B. Quinine
   C. Procaineamide
   D. All of the above

Myotonia and myasthenia gravis are in some ways pharmacological opposites.

MATCH THE FOLLOWING:

10. ___ Myotonia is improved by   A. Curare
                                          B. Potassium
11. ___ Myotonia is worsened by   C. Quinine
                                          D. Neostigmine
12. ___ Myasthenia is helped by   E. Mestinon

13. ___ Myasthenia is worsened by

14. MYOTONIA CAN BE EXPERIMENTALLY PRODUCED BY:
    A. Extracts of thymus gland
    B. Antibodies to muscle
    C. Slow virus infection
    D. Certain drugs which inhibit the synthesis of cholesterol from desmosterol
    E. Metapyrone

15. THE SYNDROME OF MYOTONIA AND RECURRENT ATTACKS OF FLACCID PARALYSIS OF THE EXTREMITIES IS USUALLY ASSOCIATED WITH INTERMITTENT:
    A. Hypercalcemia
    B. Hypermagnesemia
    C. Hyperkalemia
    D. Hypernatremia

16. THE FUNDAMENTAL DEFECT IN MYOTONIA:
    A. Is at the neuromuscular junction
    B. Is associated with a delay in relaxation of muscle
    C. Is probably in the muscle membrane
    D. Has been proven to be an abnormality of the sodium pump mechanism

CASE STUDY #39

17. OTHER CAUSES OF PROLONGED MUSCLE CONTRACTION WHICH ARE
     TO BE DIFFERENTIATED FROM MYOTONIA INCLUDE:
     A. Tetanus
     B. Tetany
     C. Rigidity
     D. Spasticity
     E. Phosphorylase deficiency
     F. All of the above

ANSWERS AND DISCUSSION:

1. D

2. C

3. B   The combination of myotonia, muscle weakness, and cataract
             most strongly suggests the diagnosis of myotonic muscular
             dystrophy.

4. D   Cataracts, testicular atrophy and baldness are typical of
             myotonic dystrophy.

5. A

6. C

7. ABCDE   The decrease in serum immunoglobulin G in myotonic dystrophy
             is due to an accelerated rate of degradation of this protein.
             Ventricular enlargement seen on pneumoencephalography has
             been reported in some patients with myotonic dystrophy. Low
             urinary 17 ketosteroids in patients with myotonic dystrophy are
             unassociated with other evidence of adrenal hypofunction.
             Similarly, a low basal metabolic rate frequently found in this
             condition is unassociated with other evidence of thyroid
             hypofunction.

             About 80% of these patients have involvement of cardiac muscle,
             and diabetes mellitus occurs in about 25% of cases. Myotonic
             dystrophy is a multisystem disease affecting many organs.

8. E

9. D

10. C

11. BDE

12. BDE

13. AC   Most compounds which have depolarizing activity intensify
              clinical and electrical myotonia. This includes acetylcholine,
              neostigmine and potassium. On the other hand, agents which
              stabilize (prevent depolarization) or hyperpolarize (raise the
              transmembrane potential) show an improvement in the myotonic
              state. Pharmacological agents which fall into the category of
              "stabilizers" and relieve myotonia would include quinine, calcium,
              and procaine. Curare, which has no significant effect on the
              muscle membrane per se or the transmembrane potential, does
              not alter the myotonic phenomenon.

14. D

CASE STUDY #39

15. C   This is the syndrome of hyperkalemic periodic paralysis
              associated with myotonia.

16. BC   Current theory suggests that myotonia is caused by altered
              muscle membrane physiology resulting in a muscle fiber that is
              hypersensitive to mechanical, electrical and biochemical stimuli.
              Electromyography demonstrates abnormal repetitive discharge
              of single or groups of muscle fibers in response to a variety of
              stimuli.

17. F

REFERENCES

1. Myotonia, A Review of Its Clinical Implications, Neurological Grand
    Rounds of the Sacramento Medical Center, Calif Med 114:16, 1971.

2. Engel, W. K., Myotonia - A Different Point of View, Calif Med 114:32,
    1971

3. Munsat, T. L., Therapy of Myotonia, Neurology 17:359, 1967.

4. Kilburn, K., J. Eagan, H. Sieker, and A. Heyman, Cardiopulmonary
    Insufficiency in Myotonic and Progressive Muscular Dystrophy, New Eng
    J Med 261:1089, 1959.

5. Marshall, J., Observations on Endocrine Function in Dystrophic Myotonia,
    Brain 82:221, 1959.

6. Jensen, H., K. Jensen, and S. Jarnum, Turnover of IgG and IgM in
    Myotonic Dystrophy, Neurology 21:68, 1971.

7. Refsum, S., A. Lonnum, O. Sjaastad, and A. Engeset, Dystrophica
    Myotonica, Neurology 17:345, 1967.

8. Caughey, J., and N. Myrianthopoulos, Dystrophica Myotonica and Related
    Disorders, Charles C Thomas, Springfield, 1963.

9. Bundey, S., C. Carter, and J. Soothill, Early Recognition of Hetero-
    zygotes for the Gene for Dystrophica Myotonica, J Neurol Neurosurg
    Psych 33:279, 1970.

10. Rosman, N., and B. Kakulas, Mental Deficiency Associated with
    Muscular Dystrophy, Brain 89:769, 1966.

11. UCLA Interdepartmental Conference: Skeletal Muscle; Basic and Clinical
    Aspects and Illustrative New Diseases, C. Pearson, moderator, Ann Int
    Med 67:614, 1967.

12. Wochner, R., et al., Accelerated Breakdown of Immunoglobulin G in
    Myotonic Dystrophy, J Clin Invest 45:321, 1966.

13. Rosman, N., and J. Rebeiz, The Cerebral Defect and Myopathy in
    Myotonia, Neurology 17:1106, 1967.

14. Zellweger, H., V. Ionasescu, Myotonic Dystrophy and its Differential
    Diagnosis, Acta Neurologica Scandinavica, Supp 55 v. 49:5, 1973.

CASE STUDY #40

Progressive Tremor

HISTORY: A 54 year-old man was referred because of a tremor of the left arm of several months duration. He held that arm in a flexed position at the elbow and there was, at rest, a rapid, regular, "pill-rolling" tremor. As the hand was flexed and extended at the wrist, cogwheeling rigidity was apparent. The neurological examination was otherwise normal. When seen two years later, the tremor was worse, involving both arms. The posture was stooped, he blinked infrequently, and showed little emotional affect (Figs. 48A, B).

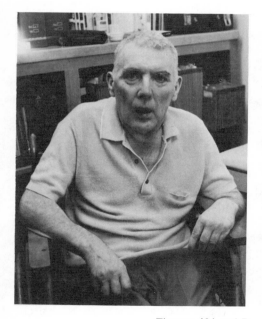
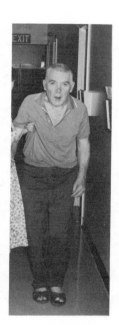

Figures 48A and B

QUESTIONS:

1.   THE PATIENT HAS:
      A. Chorea
      B. Athetosis
      C. Parkinsonism
      D. Ballism

CASE STUDY #40

2.   THIS IS A SYNDROME OF VARIABLE CAUSE. MOST OFTEN THE
     ETIOLOGY IS UNKNOWN. IT MAY FOLLOW A RARE FORM OF
     ENCEPHALITIS. SOMETIMES THE CAUSE CAN BE DIRECTLY
     TREATED, AND THE PATIENT CURED IF THE ETIOLOGY IS:
     A. Reserpine toxicity
     B. Phenothiazine toxicity
     C. Hypocalcemia
     D. Any of the above

There was no history of drug ingestion or encephalitis. Skull films,
electroencephalogram, serology, ceruloplasmin, calcium were all normal. He
was begun on artane,but developed urinary retention which disappeared when the
drug was stopped. A urologist found moderate prostatic hypertrophy.

QUESTION:

3.   URINARY RETENTION IS A SIDE EFFECT OF ARTANE; SO IS BLURRED
     VISION AND DRY MOUTH. THIS IS BECAUSE ARTANE IS:
     A. Sympathomimetic
     B. Cholinergic
     C. Anticholinergic
     D. Muscarinic
     E. None of the above

His condition deteriorated, with rigidity and tremor becoming worse. He fell
frequently, once fracturing the right hip. He gradually became unable to walk by
himself. In 1969 he showed modest improvement after receiving amantadine.
Later L-Dopa was begun, with impressive and dramatic benefit. He became able
to walk unaided, and his speech, which had been almost unintelligible became
almost normal. At eight grams of L-Dopa per day, nausea and vomiting became
persistent and severe. The dosage was decreased to 7 gm, the vomiting stopped,
but he then became badly depressed and despondent. Further lowering of the dose
of L-Dopa resulted in improvement of the depression while maintaining most of
the benefit noted in the tremor, rigidity, and speech.

QUESTIONS:

4.   CLINICAL FEATURES OF THIS DISEASE INCLUDE:
     A. Masked facies
     B. Akinesia
     C. Retropulsion
     D. Athetosis
     E. Dysarthria

5.   STEREOTACTIC NEUROSURGICAL PROCEDURES HAVE PRODUCED
     CONSIDERABLE BENEFIT IN PATIENTS WITH THIS DISEASE. THE
     LESION IS MADE IN THE:
     A. Substantia nigra
     B. Nucleus ruber
     C. Caudate nucleus
     D. Putamen
     E. Thalamus

6.   THE CARDINAL FEATURES OF MEDICAL TREATMENT ARE:
     A. Drug therapy
     B. Increasing copper excretion
     C. Exercise therapy
     D. Psychotherapy
     E. Genetic counselling

CASE STUDY #40

7. THE MOST EFFECTIVE ANTIPARKINSON DRUG IS:
   A. Parsidol   D. Benadryl
   B. Artane   E. Cogentin
   C. L-Dopa

8. USING THIS DRUG THE PERCENTAGE OF PATIENTS WHO WILL ACHIEVE
   SIGNIFICANT IMPROVEMENT IS ABOUT:
   A. 50%   C. 30%
   B. 10%   D. 65%

9. SIDE EFFECTS OF THIS DRUG INCLUDE:
   A. Sialorrhea   D. Agitation
   B. Cardiac arrhythmia   E. Hallucinations
   C. Hypotension

10. CHOREIFORM MOVEMENTS ALSO OCCUR AS A SIDE EFFECT OF THIS
    DRUG. THESE MAY BE HELPED BY DECREASING THE DRUG DOSAGE,
    OR BY ADMINISTERING:
    A. Thiamine   D. Pyridoxine
    B. Niacin   E. Tocopherol
    C. Riboflavin

11. COMMONLY SEEN IN THE BRAINS OF PATIENTS DYING WITH THIS DIS-
    EASE IS DEPIGMENTATION OF THE:
    A. Cerebral cortex   C. Substantia nigra
    B. Area postrema   D. Caudate nucleus

12. THIS AREA IS ALSO FOUND TO CONTAIN IN THIS SYNDROME:
    A. An increased amount of dopamine
    B. A decreased amount of dopamine
    C. An increased amount of homovanillic acid
    D. Both A and C

13. DOPAMINE:
    A. Is formed from the decarboxylation of Dopa
    B. Is not given directly for the therapy of this patient's condition since it does
       not cross the blood-brain barrier
    C. Is decreased both in the substantia nigra and in the caudate nucleus in
       this condition
    D. Will be lower in concentration in the brain when L-Dopa and a peripheral-
       ly acting dopa decarboxylase inhibitor are given than when L-Dopa is given
       alone
    E. All of the above

14. THE DRUGS WHICH ARE BENEFICIAL IN THIS CONDITION FALL INTO TWO
    MAIN GROUPS:
    A. Those which supply both serotonin and acetylcholine
    B. Those which supply both acetylcholine and dopamine
    C. Those which supply acetylcholine and block dopamine
    D. Those which supply dopamine and block acetylcholine

15. THE RIGIDITY SEEN IN THIS CONDITION DIFFERS FROM SPASTICITY IN
    THAT:
    A. There is no "clasp-knife" phenomena
    B. The deep tendon reflexes are normal
    C. There is no Babinski sign
    D. Cogwheeling is present
    E. All of the above

CASE STUDY #40

ANSWERS AND DISCUSSION:

1. C

2. D

3. C   Anticholinergic drugs are one of the major classes of useful anti-parkinson medications.

4. ABCE

5. E   Lesions in the ventrolateral nucleus of the thalamus have been found to produce significant benefit in many cases of parkinsonism.

6. ACD

7. C

8. D   Although the parkinsonism continues to progress despite L-Dopa treatment, life expectancy is increased, and the quality of survival, both medically and socially, is significantly improved.

9. BCDE

10. D   Pyridoxine is thought to reverse the action of levodopa by increasing its decarboxylation to dopamine which does not readily cross the blood-brain barrier.

11. C

12. B   Homovanillic acid is one of the metabolites of dopamine and is also decreased in this area of the brain.

13. ABC   The administration of a dopa decarboxylase inhibitor plus levodopa results in impairment of the decarboxylation of levodopa to dopamine. Therefore the blood concentration of levodopa rises. This increased amount of l-dopa can cross the blood-brain barrier, and so the brain concentration increases. Since the decarboxylase inhibitor does not cross the blood-brain barrier, brain dopamine concentration also increases. Clinically, the addition of a dopa decarboxylase inhibitor to a levodopa regimen markedly reduces dopa-induced nausea and vomiting, but may produce an increase in chorea.

14. D   One (admittedly oversimplified) way of looking at parkinsonism is that there is an abnormal decrease in the ratio of dopaminergic to cholinergic activity in the basal ganglia. This concept is suggested by pharmacological evidence as follows: Parkinsonism is produced or worsened by drugs which either block CNS dopamine receptors as the phenothiazines, or deplete dopamine storage as reserpine, or which increase central cholinergic activity as physostigmine. Parkinsonism is improved by drugs which block cholinergic transmission as atropine, artane, etc., or which supply dopamine, as L-Dopa.

15. E   Spasticity is a specific pattern of steadily increasing muscular resistance to continuous passive stretch, up to the point of a relatively sudden decreased resistance, the classical clasp-knife reaction.[2] It is associated clinically with increased deep tendon reflexes, diminished or absent superficial reflexes, and pathological reflexes, such as the Babinski response. The spasticity and hyperreflexia may represent an exaggeration of reactivity of the alpha motor neuron at the spinal segmental level.[2]

CASE STUDY #40

In contrast to the normal and spastic muscle, in which, at rest, muscle is quiet and inactive, the muscles in parkinsonian rigidity show a continuously increased level of muscle contraction, even when the patient is at rest and relaxed. The rigidity which one notes in flexing and extending an affected limb is regularly interrupted, producing a "cogwheeling" effect. The normal level of the deep tendon reflexes in parkinsonism suggests that there is not an abnormal hyperreactivity of the alpha motor neurons, but that there is abnormal stimulation of these motor neurons, via suprasegmental pathways due to lesions in motor control centers at a forebrain level. Put another way, this is a "busy-line"[2] hypothesis, in which the descending motor pathways are "cluttered" with abnormal messages, and so the lines are not available for normal motor activity without the "static" of the tremor and rigidity.

REFERENCES

1. Yahr, M.D., R.C. Duvoisin, M.J. Schear, R.E. Barrett, and M.M. Hoehn, Treatment of Parkinsonism with Levodopa, Arch Neurol 21:343, 1969.

2. Landau, W.M., Spasticity and Rigidity, Recent Advances in Neurology, F. Plum, Ed., F.A. Davis Co., 1969.

3. Cotzias, G., P. Papavasiliou, and R. Gellene, Modification of Parkinsonism-Chronic Treatment with L-Dopa, New Eng J Med 280:337, 1969.

4. Waltz, J., M. Riklan, S. Stellar, and I. Cooper, Cryothalamectomy for Parkinson's Disease, Neurology 16:994, 1966.

5. Recent Advances in Parkinson's Disease, F.H. McDowell, and C.H. Markham, Ed., F.A. Davis, Co., 1971.

6. Goodwin, F., Psychiatric Side Effects of Levodopa in Man, JAMA 218:1915, 1971.

7. Sourkes, T., Actions of Levodopa and Dopamine in the Central Nervous System, JAMA 218:1909, 1971.

8. Klawans, H., The Pharmacology of Extrapyramidal Movement Disorders, S. Karger AG, 1973.

9. Markham, C., et al., Carbidopa in Parkinson Disease and in Nausea and Vomiting, Arch Neurol 31:128, 1974.

10. Barbeau, A., High Level Levodopa Therapy in Parkinson Disease: Five Years Later, Arch Neurol 30:422, 1974.

11. Miller, E., and L. Wiener, RO 4602 and Levodopa in Treatment of Parkinsonism, Neurology 24:482, 1974.

12. Birdsong, J., and A. McKinney, Long Range Motor Performance Changes in Levodopa Treated Patients with Parkinson's Disease, Neurology 24:107, 1974.

13. Miller, E., L Tryptophan in the Treatment of Levodopa Induced Psychiatric Disorders, Diseases of the Nervous System 35:20-23, 1974.

14. Markham, C., et al., Parkinson's Disease and Levodopa, West J Med 121: 188, 1974.

CASE STUDY #41

Headache in an Elderly Woman

HISTORY: An 83 year-old woman began for the first time to complain of head-aches, nine weeks previously. These were dull, aching, severe, and bitemporal.

QUESTIONS:

1. THE MOST LIKELY DIAGNOSIS IS:
   A. Headache secondary to cerebral arteriosclerosis
   B. Migraine
   C. Muscle contraction headaches
   D. None of the above

2. IF SHE ALSO COMPLAINED OF SUDDEN LOSS OF VISION IN ONE EYE, THE MOST LIKELY DIAGNOSIS WOULD BE:
   A. Hemorrhage into a pituitary adenoma
   B. Glioblastoma
   C. Aneurysm
   D. None of the above

EXAMINATION: She was a pleasant, alert, cooperative elderly woman. The deep tendon reflexes were normal, and the plantar responses were flexor. Mentation, sensation, strength, and the cranial nerve examination were normal.

QUESTION:

3. THE MOST IMPORTANT FURTHER INFORMATION TO DETERMINE NOW WOULD BE:
   A. Whether there is a positive family history of migraine
   B. Whether there is a bruit over the carotid arteries
   C. The condition of the temporal arteries
   D. None of the above

The blood presure was 170/105. The temporal arteries were thickened, nodular and tender bilaterally (Fig. 49).

QUESTIONS:

4. THE MOST USEFUL TESTS TO OBTAIN WOULD BE:
   A. Electroencephalogram
   B. Spinal tap
   C. Sedimentation rate
   D. Pneumoencephalogram
   E. Temporal artery biopsy

5. IF THE SEDIMENTATION RATE WERE ELEVATED YOU WOULD THEN:
   A. Begin an intravenous infusion of mannitol, to reduce the intracranial pressure
   B. Administer intravenous magnesium sulfate
   C. Begin a course of adrenal corticosteroids
   D. Obtain an immediate neurosurgical consultation

6. YOU MIGHT EXPECT A BIOPSY OF THE TEMPORAL ARTERY TO MOST LIKELY SHOW:
   A. No abnormalities
   B. Severe arteriosclerosis
   C. Giant cells
   D. Complete or partial obstruction of the vessel lumen by connective tissue and round cells

CASE STUDY #41

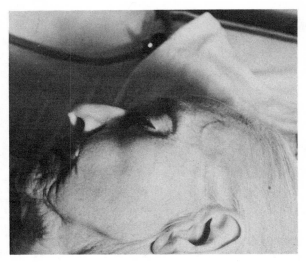

Figure 49

The diagnosis of temporal arteritis was made and she was begun on a course of prednisone, 50 mgm daily. The erythrocyte sedimentation rate was 34mm/hour. Biopsy of the right temporal artery showed a granulomatous arteritis with giant cells. Hemoglobin was 10.9 gm%. The headaches disappeared, and the sedimentation rate became normal. The steroids were discontinued after a three week course. Two months later she developed an organic mental syndrome. The neurological examination was otherwise normal. Sedimentation rate was 32 mm/hour. Steroids were again begun, but with only slight improvement in her confusion. An electroencephalogram showed bitemporal slowing. Normal tests included complete blood count, urinalysis, skull films, lumbar puncture, diagnex blue, PBI, electrolytes.

QUESTIONS:

7. THE SYNDROME OF TEMPORAL ARTERITIS MAY INCLUDE:
   A. Headache
   B. Jaw pain
   C. Dementia
   D. Fever
   E. Anemia
   F. Weight loss
   G. All of the above

CASE STUDY #41

8. 40% OF PATIENTS WITH CLASSICAL TEMPORAL ARTERITIS DEVELOP SOME TYPE OF VISUAL SYMPTOMS, HENCE THE URGENCY OF INITIATING STEROID TREATMENT. THE MOST COMMON TYPE OF VISUAL IMPAIRMENT IS:
    A. Visual loss
    B. Ptosis
    C. Diplopia
    D. Internuclear ophthalmoplegia

9. THE PATHOLOGICAL ARTERIAL CHANGES ARE NOT LIMITED TO THE TEMPORAL ARTERY BUT MAY BE SEEN IN THE:
    A. Intracranial arteries
    B. Subclavian arteries
    C. Coronary arteries
    D. Renal arteries
    E. All of the above

10. THE MOST COMMON CAUSES OF DEATH IN PATIENTS WITH TEMPORAL ARTERITIS ARE:
    A. Cerebral vascular thrombosis
    B. Pulmonary emboli
    C. Opportunistic infections such as cryptococcosis
    D. Myocardial infarction

    TRUE OR FALSE:

11. An elderly patient who complains of acute onset of pain and stiffness of the muscles of limbs and neck should be initially referred for physiotherapy.

12. A normal temporal artery biopsy rules out the diagnosis of temporal arteritis.

13. The sedimentation rate is important both in the diagnosis of temporal arteritis as well as a guide to the duration of steroid treatment.

14. The usual onset of temporal arteritis is between the ages of 55 to 85.

ANSWERS AND DISCUSSION:

1. D

2. D

3. C

4. CE

5. C

6. CD

7. G

8. A

9. E

10. AD

CASE STUDY #41

11. False   The symptoms of muscle pain and joint stiffness in this age group have been termed polymyalgia rheumatica. The importance of recognition of this syndrome is that there is often associated temporal arteritis in these patients.

12. False   As with any biopsy, an area may be sampled which does not show the typical pathology. Occasional patients are seen with normal biopsies, but with typical clinical features, increased sedimentation rate, and dramatic relief from corticosteroids.

13. True

14. True   When a person over 50 begins for the first time to suffer from headaches, a serious illness must be suspected, since the two most common causes of headaches - migraine and muscle contraction (tension) - produce symptoms at a younger age. Indeed, migraine which has been lifelong often disappears in the 60's. It is particularly important to suspect temporal arteritis when the onset of headache is over 50, first, because some type of visual symptoms, usually blindness, but also ptosis or diplopia, occurs in 40% of these patients, and secondly because the visual impairment which is due to retinal artery thrombosis may be preventable. Visual loss is usually severe and sudden, and the second eye may be involved after several days or weeks. Classically one finds a pulseless, firm, enlarged tender temporal artery, but occasionally the artery may feel quite normal.

    The single most reliable test is the sedimentation rate which is almost invariably elevated.

    Biopsy changes include round cell infiltration, primarily in the media, with multinucleated giant cells, intimal thickening, and luminal narrowing.

    Some clinicians, in otherwise classical cases, do not even biopsy the artery, and a normal biopsy does not rule out this disease.

    Neither the cause of nor the relationship between temporal arteritis and other forms of vasculitis is known.

    The only known treatment is the adrenal corticosteroids, and the improvement, in sense of well being and in relief of headache, is often dramatic.

REFERENCES

1. Beasley, H., Cranial Arteritis, Headache 9:119, 1969.

2. Andrews, J.M., Giant-Cell ("Temporal") Arteritis, Neurology 16:963, 1966.

3. Hauser, W., R. Fergusen, K. Holley, and L. Kurland, Temporal Arteritis in Rochester, Minnesota, 1951 to 1967, Mayo Clin Proc 45:597, 1971.

4. Gutrecht, J., Occult Temporal Arteritis, JAMA 213:1188, 1970.

5. Harrison, M.J.G., and A.T. Bevan, Early Symptoms of Temporal Arteritis, Lancet 2:638, 1967.

6. Hamilton, C.R., Jr., et al., Giant Cell Arteritis: Including Temporal Arteritis and Polymyalgia Rheumatica, Medicine 50:1, 1971.

7. Ostberg, G., Temporal Arteritis in a Large Necropsy Series, Ann Rheumat Dis 30:224, 1971.

CASE STUDY #41

8. Healey, L. A., et al., Polymyalgia Rheumatica and Giant Cell Arteritis, Arthritis & Rheumat 14:138, 1971.

9. Fauchald, P., et al., Temporal Arteritis and Polymyalgia Rheumatica. Clinical and Biopsy Findings, Ann Int Med 77:845, 1972.

10. Anderson, L. G., and T. B. Bayles, Polymyalgia Rheumatica and Giant Cell Arteritis, Disease-a-Month, Jan. 1974.

CASE STUDY #42

Back Pain and Paraparesis

HISTORY: A 45 year-old man claimed that three months previously, while he was bending over at work, he felt something "give" in his back. Since then he experienced pain in the mid to low dorsal spine area, radiating around to either side, and increased in severity with coughing or sneezing. Four days before, he had become constipated, and felt that his lower abdomen and both legs were numb. On the day of admission his legs became weak and he could barely walk. He also noted increasing difficulty with urination. Past medical history was unremarkable.

QUESTION:

1.   THE HISTORY TO THIS POINT SUGGESTS:
      A. A stroke
      B. Guillain-Barré syndrome
      C. Acute polymyositis
      D. None of the above

EXAMINATION: The superior border of the bladder was palpable at the level of the umbilicus. Rectal sphincter tone was poor. There was considerable tenderness over the mid dorsal spine. Pin sensation was impaired from the costal margin downward. The deep tendon reflexes were normal in the arms, hyperactive in the legs. Bilateral Babinski responses were present. Abdominal reflexes were absent. He was unable to move his legs, except for feeble contractions of the quadriceps. Strength in the upper extremities was normal.

QUESTIONS:

2.   THE EXAMINATION CONFIRMS THE IMPRESSION OF:
      A. Myopathy
      B. Neuropathy
      C. Myelopathy
      D. None of the above

3.   THE ABNORMALITIES SEEN ON EXAMINATION CAN BEST BE EXPLAINED BY LESIONS INVOLVING THE:
      A. Rubrospinal and corticospinal tracts
      B. Spinothalamic and reticulospinal tracts
      C. Corticospinal and spinothalamic tracts
      D. Spinothalamic tract and fasciculus gracilis

CASE STUDY #42

4. CONSIDERING THE HIGHEST LEVELS OF MOTOR, SENSORY, AND
   REFLEX ABNORMALITY, THE LEVEL OF THE SPINAL CORD LESION
   IS:
   A. Cervical
   B. Thoracic
   C. Lumbar
   D. Sacral

5. CAN ALL OF THE NEUROLOGICAL ABNORMALITIES BE EXPLAINED
   BY ONE LESION?:
   A. Yes
   B. No
   C. There is insufficient evidence to reach a decision

6. ALL OF THE FOLLOWING CAN CAUSE THE CLINICAL PICTURE OF
   PARAPLEGIA WITH A THORACIC SENSORY LEVEL, EXCEPT:
   A. Acute transverse myelitis
   B. Spinal epidural abscess
   C. Cord compression from thoracic disc herniation
   D. Amyotrophic lateral sclerosis
   E. Syphillis
   F. Cord compression from metastatic carcinoma

7. THE MOST IMPORTANT PROCEDURE TO DO FIRST WOULD BE:
   A. Spinal tap
   B. X-rays of the thoracic spine
   C. Myelogram
   D. Electromyogram

LABORATORY DATA: Hemoglobin was 10. X-rays of the thoracic spine
(Fig. 50) were taken.

QUESTIONS:

8. THESE FILMS SHOW:
   A. Severe arthritic changes
   B. Spina bifida occulta
   C. Pathological collapse of the 9th thoracic vertebra
   D. None of the above

9. A SPINAL TAP AND QUECKENSTEDT TEST:
   A. Would be most important to perform quickly now to see if there were a
      block to spinal fluid flow
   B. Would be important to perform now mainly to see if there were an
      increase in spinal fluid protein ("chemical" block)
   C. Should not be done, since there is some risk of worsening the signs of
      cord compression, and the spinal fluid can be examined at the time of
      myelography
   D. Should be done, but only with a #22 needle

COURSE: An emergency myelogram was performed. This revealed a complete
extradural block to the cephalad flow of pantopaque at the T9-10 interspace
(Fig. 51).

10. THE MAIN DIAGNOSTIC POSSIBILITIES WOULD INCLUDE:
    A. Metastatic carcinoma
    B. Lymphoma
    C. Meningioma
    D. All of the above

CASE STUDY #42

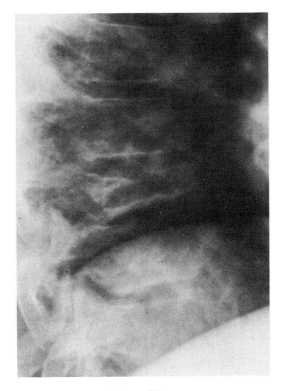

Figure 50

At surgery, a vascular, greyish-red tumor was seen surrounding the cord substance and invading the adjacent vertebrae. The spinal cord was decompressed. The tumor microscopically was composed almost exclusively of plasma cells, some of which were moderately pleomorphic. Occasional mitotic figures were seen. The pathological diagnosis was a plasma cell myeloma. Postoperatively the patient showed improvement in strength and sensation. A bone marrow specimen showed infiltration of plasma cells. Serum immunoelectrophoresis showed a gamma A immunoglobulin paraprotein. The urine was negative for Bence-Jones protein. Following the surgery and a course of radiotherapy to the lower thoracic spine, he made an excellent improvement, and became able to ambulate with the aid of a walker.

Skull films taken several months later showed multiple areas of bone destruction (Fig. 52).

CASE STUDY #42

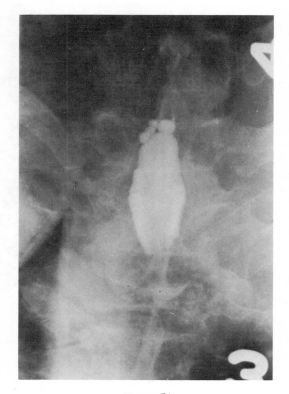

Figure 51

TRUE OR FALSE:

11. Myeloma is a relatively radioresistant tumor.

12. Little benefit is obtained in myeloma with chemotherapy.

13. The most common presenting abnormalities in multiple myeloma are
     anemia, bone pain, bone lesions and abnormal serum proteins.

14. A short history, a total flaccid paraplegia, paraplegia of sudden onset are
     all indications of a poor surgical outcome in cord compressions due to
     malignant tumors.

15. Complications of multiple myeloma include amyloidosis and impaired
     capacity for antibody formation.

CASE STUDY #42

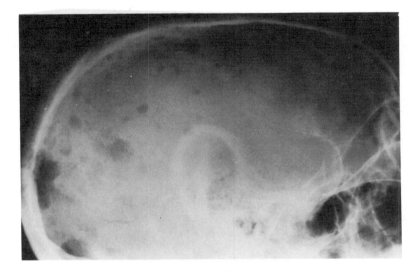

Figure 52

ANSWERS AND DISCUSSION:

1. D   The history is a progressive one of back and radicular pain, numbness and weakness of the legs, and impaired urination. This story strongly suggests an advancing spinal cord lesion. Myopathy is unassociated with sensory abnormality unless it is due to some etiology which also affects peripheral nerves or the central nervous system (sarcoid or collagen disease for example). The back pain and bladder involvement are against the possibility of infectious polyneuritis. Bowel and bladder impairment do occur, but quite rarely in the Guillain-Barré syndrome, whereas this is a common feature of myelopathy of diverse etiology.

2. C   The Babinski signs, hyperactive deep tendon reflexes, sensory level, sphincter impairment are all consistent with a myelopathy. Myopathy produces proximal limb weakness without pathological reflexes or sensory impairment. In neuropathic disease the weakness is distal, the deep tendon reflexes are decreased or absent, and pathological reflexes are not present.

3. C   The hyperactive deep tendon reflexes and Babinski signs occur with lesions of the corticospinal tracts, and the impairment of pain sensation with involvement of the spinothalamic tracts.

4. B   The upper level of segmental involvement is as follows: (1) motor: the paralyzed ilio-psoas muscles which flex the leg at the hip are innervated primarily from the 1st and 2nd lumbar segments. (2) sensory: pin sensation is impaired below the ninth thoracic

CASE STUDY #42

dermatomal level. (3) reflex: the hyperactive deep tendon reflexes in the legs and absent abdominal reflexes indicate a lesion at or above the lower thoracic cord levels.

Since reflexes, sensation, and strength are normal in the arms which are innervated from the cervical spinal cord, and since the motor, sensory and reflex levels indicate a lesion above the lowest thoracic segments, the disease process must lie in the upper 3/4 of the thoracic spinal cord. The site of the radicular pain and the tenderness over the mid dorsal spine are further localizing clues.

5. A

6. D   Amyotrophic lateral sclerosis is purely a motor system disease causing signs of lower motor neuron and corticospinal tract dysfunction.

7. B

8. C

9. C

10. AB

11. False

12. False

13. True

14. True

15. True

REFERENCES

1.   Garrett, M., Spinal Myeloma and Cord Compression, Clin Radiol 21:42, 1970.

2.   Alexanian, R. et al., Treatment for Multiple Myeloma, JAMA 208:1680, 1969.

3.   Millburn, L., G. Hibbs, and F. Hendrickson, Treatment of Spinal Cord Compression from Metastatic Carcinoma, Cancer 21:447, 1968.

4.   Smith, R., An Evaluation of Surgical Treatment for Spinal Cord Compression due to Metastatic Carcinoma, J Neurol Neurosurg Psych 28:152, 1965.

5.   Greenwald, E.S., Cancer Chemotherapy, Medical Examination Publishing Co., New York, 1967.

6.   Williams, W., et al., Hematology, McGraw-Hill, 1972.

CASE STUDY #43

An Unwashed, Confused and Euphoric Alcoholic

HISTORY: A 39 year-old woman was referred because of poor memory and decreasing vision. She had a history of heavy alcoholic intake. When seen in the office, she looked and smelled as if she hadn't taken a bath in months. She joked and was inappropriately euphoric. There was a strongly positive snout reflex.

QUESTION:

1. INAPPROPRIATE JOCULARITY CAN BE SEEN WITH:
    A. Pseudobulbar palsy
    B. Frontal lobe disease
    C. Schizophrenia
    D. All of the above

Vision was 20/80 in the right eye and 20/30 in the left. Bilateral papilledema was present. The neurological examination was otherwise normal except for some impairment of memory and calculating ability. Examination of the visual fields revealed enlarged blind spots.

QUESTIONS:

2. THE CRITERIA FOR THE DIAGNOSIS OF PAPILLEDEMA INCLUDE:
    A. Blurred optic disc margins
    B. A whiter color of the disc
    C. An increase in the ratio of the diameters of retinal veins/arteries which is usually about 3/2
    D. All of the above

3. YOU MIGHT CONSIDER IN THE DIFFERENTIAL DIAGNOSIS:
    A. Brain tumor
    B. Hydrocephalus
    C. Chronic subdural hematoma
    D. Brain abscess
    E. All of the above

4. ALL OF THE FOLLOWING TESTS MIGHT GIVE USEFUL INFORMATION, EXCEPT:
    A. Electromyography
    B. Skull films
    C. Electroencephalography
    D. Brain scan

5. A SPINAL TAP, IN THE PRESENCE OF PAPILLEDEMA:
    A. Is always contraindicated
    B. Should be done only if there is an urgent need to examine the spinal fluid, as to rule out meningitis
    C. Should be done, if necessary, with caution, using a small gauge needle
    D. Requires the Queckenstedt maneuver to be done with care

6. THE ENLARGED BLIND SPOTS SEEN IN THE VISUAL FIELDS ARE DUE TO:
    A. Edema of the optic discs
    B. Damage to the maculae
    C. Lesions of the papillo-macular bundles
    D. None of the above

CASE STUDY #43

LABORATORY DATA: Skull films showed some demineralization of the dorsum sellae. The optic foramina were normal. A huge focus of increased isotope uptake was seen on the brain scan (Figs. 53A, B)

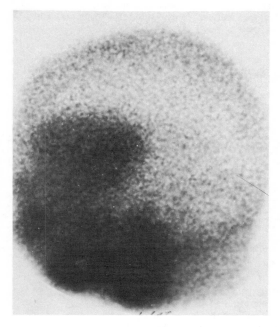

Figure 53 A

Carotid angiograms disclosed a large left subfrontal mass supplied by branches of the opthalmic artery, suggesting a subfrontal meningioma. There was a large shift of the anterior cerebral artery across the midline(Figs. 54A, B)

At craniotomy there was a 7 cm tumor arising from the medial aspect of the olfactory groove, which was resected, and proved to be a meningioma. Postoperatively she did well, with marked improvement in visual and mental function.

QUESTIONS:

7. MENINGIOMAS DAMAGE THE CENTRAL NERVOUS SYSTEM PRIMARILY BY:
   A. Compression
   B. Infiltration
   C. Metastasis

   TRUE OR FALSE:

8. Meningiomas are a common tumor of childhood

9. A brain tumor is more likely than a spinal tumor to be a meningioma.

CASE STUDY #43

10.   Most meningiomas are extremely radiosensitive.

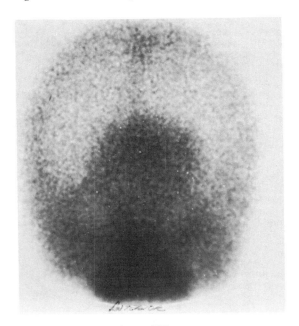

Figure 53B

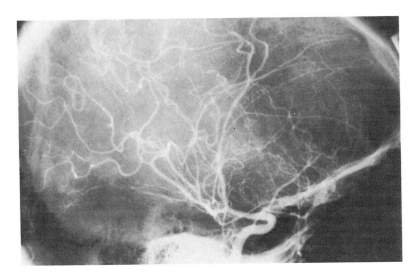

Figure 54A

CASE STUDY #43

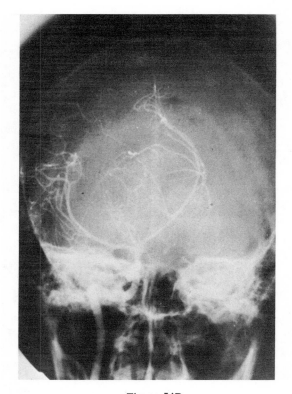

Figure 54B

ANSWERS AND DISCUSSION:

1. D   Pseudobulbar palsy refers to the syndrome of weakness of the
        bulbar muscles of speech, swallowing, etc., due to a bilateral
        lesion of the corticobulbar tracts innervating bulbar lower motor
        nuclei. Emotional incontinence, i. e. laughing or crying without
        appropriate cause commonly accompanies this syndrome.

2. AC   In papilledema the color of the optic disc becomes more
        erythematous.

3. E

4. A   Electromyography is primarily useful in differential diagnosis of
        disease of the motor unit and would not be appropriate here.

        A positive brain scan is present in approximately 85% of cases
        of brain tumor, and the scan may also outline a brain abscess
        and subdural hematomas. It is further useful in being able to
        indicate multiple lesions. A negative brain scan does not rule

CASE STUDY #43

out neoplasm or any of the other diagnostic possibilities mentioned.

The importance of skull films and the electroencephalogram in the localization of cerebral lesions has been discussed previously.

5. BC   The Queckenstedt maneuver of jugular compression, which produces a rise in spinal fluid pressure which then can be measured with a needle in the lumbar sac is used only in the diagnosis of a lesion blocking spinal fluid flow at the spinal level, or in the diagnosis of lateral sinus thrombosis. It is otherwise useless, and, in cerebral disease, particularly with increased intracranial pressure, absolutely contraindicated, as it may precipitate cerebral herniation and death.

6. A

7. A

8. False

9. False   Meningiomas comprise 15% of brain tumors and 29% of spinal tumors.

10. False   Meningiomas are in general poorly responsive to radiotherapy.

COMMENT: A frontal lobe meningioma is one of the curable causes of chronic dementia and this case illustrates the importance of not passing off the demented alcoholic as suffering from chronic degenerative brain disease, since papilledema may not be present at all, or may be a late sign in intracranial tumors. Chronic subdural hematomas, lues, electrolyte abnormalities, hypoglycemia, hepatic encephalopathy and vitamin deficiency are some other treatable causes of dementia to be ruled out in the chronic alcoholic patient.

Meningiomas are common intracranial tumors which may cause increased intracranial pressure and a variety of focal neurological abnormalities, depending on the location of the tumor. The most common locations include the parasagittal area, over the convexity of the cerebral hemispheres or, as in this case, on the floor of the anterior fossa. Some less common sites include the peritorcular area and the posterior fossa. Merritt divides the meningiomas of the floor of the anterior fossa into two groups. The first arising from the tuberculum sellae compresses the optic chiasm and produces a syndrome similar to that of a pituitary adenoma. The second group arises from the olfactory groove. Unilateral anosmia from compression of the olfactory nerve may be an early finding. Headache, mental deterioration, and visual failure ensue as the tumor grows, from pressure of the frontal lobes and optic nerves, or visual failure can be a result of optic atrophy due to chronic papilledema.

REFERENCES

1.   Merritt, H.H., A Textbook of Neurology, 5th Ed.,Lea and Febiger, Philadelphia, 1973.

2.   Cushing, H., and L. Eisenhardt, Meningiomas, Charles C Thomas, Springfield, 1938.

3.   Jane, J., and W. McKissock, Importance of Failing Vision in Early Diagnosis of Suprasellar Meningiomas, Brit Med J (July 7,) 1962.

CASE STUDY #44

Headaches, Nuchal Rigidity and Cerebrospinal Fluid

HISTORY: A 32 year-old woman was in good health until two months before admission, when she began to experience severe headaches which were steady, aching, and usually centered around the right temple.

QUESTION:

1.   IT WOULD BE IMPORTANT TO INQUIRE, IN THIS HISTORY, ABOUT:
     A.   Use of oral contraceptives
     B.   Familial history of migraine
     C.   Hypertension
     D.   Visual abnormalities
     E.   All of above

The headaches did not awaken her from sleep, were relieved by codeine, and were not associated with nausea, vomiting or visual symptoms. There was no history of trauma, oral contraceptive use, hypertension or familial headaches. Her headaches were not benefited by Caffergot, Fiorinal or Valium.

General physical and neurological examinations were normal, and a psychiatric consultant felt that the headaches were a psychophysiologic reaction.

QUESTION:

2.   AT THIS POINT YOU MIGHT ORDER:
     A.   Carotid angiography
     B.   Isotope cisternography
     C.   Vertebral angiography
     D.   Cervical myelography
     E.   None of the above

She complained that the headaches were becoming more frequent and more severe. Examination now showed mild nuchal rigidity, but was otherwise normal. She was afebrile.

LABORATORY DATA: Blood count, urinalysis, skull films, chest films, cervical spine X-rays, echoencephalogram, serology were all normal. Electro-encephalogram was mildly abnormal with small amounts of slowing noted bitemporally. Lumbar puncture showed clear fluid, with a protein of 68 mgm%, sugar of 50 mgm% and normal cell count and serology. For several weeks her condition remained unchanged except for increasing neck stiffness.

QUESTION:

3.   THE CAUSES OF NUCHAL RIGIDITY INCLUDE:
     A.   Meningitis
     B.   Subarachnoid hemorrhage
     C.   Cervical osteoarthritis
     D.   Cerebellar herniation through the foramen magnum
     E.   All of the above

She began to have episodes of confusion and excitement, and a left Babinski response was seen. Examination of the visual fields revealed a left homonymous hemianopsia (Fig. 55).

A brain scan was negative. The lumbar puncture was repeated and the spinal fluid contained 150 mgm% of protein, 28 mgm% sugar, and 20 wbc/cu mm of which 90% were mononuclear, 10% polymorphonuclear.

CASE STUDY #44

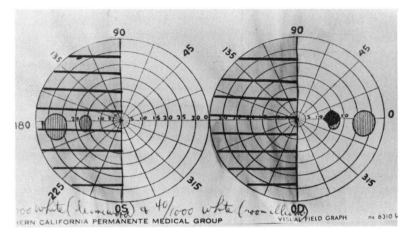

Figure 55

QUESTION:

4. THIS SPINAL FLUID FORMULA SUGGESTS ANY OF THE FOLLOWING, EXCEPT:
   A. Cryptococcal meningitis
   B. Meningococcal meningitis
   C. Tuberculous meningitis
   D. Coccidioidal meningitis
   E. Viral meningitis

COURSE: Skin tests with ppd, histoplasmin, coccidioidin were all negative. There was no history of travel through the San Joaquin Valley. Spinal fluid cultures for pyogens and fungi were negative.

QUESTIONS:

5. THE SAN JOAQUIN VALLEY OF CALIFORNIA IS NOTED FOR BOTH ITS AGRICULTURE AND ITS INCREASED PREVALENCE OF:
   A. Cryptococcosis
   B. Blastomycosis
   C. Mucormycosis
   D. Salmonellosis
   E. Coccidioidomycosis

CASE STUDY #44

6. MOST LIKELY, IN ADDITION TO MENINGITIS, THIS PATIENT HAS A
    LESION OF THE:
    A. Cervical spinal cord
    B. Left mesencephalon
    C. Right cerebral hemisphere
    D. Left cerebral hemisphere
    E. Pons

7. BECAUSE OF THE EVIDENCE OF THIS FOCAL LESION, AN
    APPROPRIATE DIAGNOSTIC STUDY WOULD BE:
    A. A cervical myelogram
    B. A carotid angiogram
    C. An electromyogram
    D. None of the above

8. THE PRESENCE OF AN ORGANIC MENTAL SYNDROME WITH AN
    APPARENT UNILATERAL CEREBRAL LESION MIGHT SUGGEST:
    A. Actual bilateral cerebral disease
    B. Possible hydrocephalus
    C. Possible increased intracranial pressure
    D. All or any of the above

COURSE: Electroencephalogram showed a right anterior temporal slow wave
focus. Brain scan was normal. Bilateral carotid angiography showed generalized narrowing of the arterial tree, suggesting diffuse spasm. There was no shift
and the ventricles were of normal size. Vertebral angiography also showed
generalized narrowing of the posterior circulation. Another spinal tap showed a
protein of 116 mgm%, sugar of 15 mgm%, and 29 white cells/cu mm, 70% of
which were mononuclear. Numerous india ink preparations, acid fast, pyogen,
and fungal cultures were negative. Examination of the spinal fluid for tumor cells
was negative.

She was given a therapeutic trial on antituberculous therapy without benefit.
Gradually, she became more lethargic, but complained of very severe headaches.
A pneumoencephalogram was normal. Occasionally she was found to be incontinent of urine. A course of amphotericin B was given, again without benefit.
Bilateral plantar extensor responses were found, and the right pupil was noted to
react more sluggishly to light than the left. A repeat right carotid angiogram
again showed generalized vessel spasm. A cardiac arrest occurred; she was
resuscitated, but remained comatose, with pupils fixed and dilated, requiring a
respirator. She died several days later, following another cardiac arrest.

QUESTIONS:

9. THE COURSE OF THIS PATIENT'S ILLNESS MIGHT BEST BE
    DESCRIBED AS:
    A. Progressive
    B. Remitting and exacerbating
    C. Apoplectic
    D. None of the above

10. THIS ILLNESS IS COMPATIBLE WITH:
    A. Infectious disease
    B. Demyelinating disease
    C. Vascular disease
    D. Disease due to toxins
    E. Neoplastic disease

WHAT DO YOU THINK IS THE MOST LIKELY DIAGNOSIS?:

CASE STUDY #44

Autopsy revealed a diffuse infiltration of the meninges, as well as nodules of cells within the substance of the central nervous system which appeared reticuloendothelial in origin. The neuropathological diagnosis was reticulum cell sarcoma involving the cerebral hemispheres, brain stem, and meninges, sparing other organs in the body.

ANSWERS AND DISCUSSION:

1. F   Birth control pills may worsen or precipitate migraine headaches.

Migraine is often familial and may be associated with a variety of visual symptoms which precede the headache, such as scotomata, hemianopsia etc. and which are due to transient local constriction of retinal or cerebral arteries.

The pattern of visual symptoms may be a most important clue to localization of a neurological lesion. Episodes of flashing lights in the right visual fields would suggest the possibility of an irritative lesion in the left occipital cortex, for example.

Plum[5] notes that about 10% of persons with arterial hypertension may experience severe, even disabling headaches, which are principally of the vascular and muscle contraction type.

2. F   Simpler and safer tests are in order, such as skull films, electroencephalogram, brain scan, and lumbar puncture.

3. F

4. BF   This spinal fluid composition--of a lymphocytic pleocytosis, low sugar and elevated protein--is typical of the granulomatous meningitides such as those caused by fungi or the tubercle bacillus. Cysticercosis and sarcoid meningitis may show a similar spinal fluid formula, as also carcinomatous and gliomatous invasion of the meninges. In untreated pyogenic meningitis, the pleocytosis is typically polymorphonuclear. Although there have been a few reported cases of viral meningitis in which the spinal fluid sugar has been low, it is almost always normal.

5. F

6. C   Because of the left Babinski sign and left hemianopsia.

7. B

8. D

9. A

10. AF

CASE STUDY #44

REFERENCES

1. Case Records of the Massachusetts General Hospital (Case 88-1961) New Eng J Med 265:1205, 1961.

2. Gonzalez-Angulo, A., M. Rabiela, and L. Lombardo, Reticuloendothelial Sarcoma of the Brain, J Neurosurg 28:560, 1968.

3. Craig, D., T. Cobb, and H. Huntington, Reticulum Cell Sarcoma of the Septum Pellucidum, J Neurosurg 29:183, 1968.

4. Burstein, S.D., J.W. Kernohan, and A. Uihlein, Neoplasms of the Reticulo-endothelial System of the Brain, Cancer 16:289, 1963.

5. Plum, F., Headache, in Cecil-Loeb Textbook of Medicine, 13th Ed., P.B. Beeson, and W. McDermott, Ed., W.B. Saunders Co., Philadelphia, 1971.

6. Schaumberg, H., et al., The Reticulum Cell Sarcoma-Microglioma Group of Brain Tumors, Brain 95:199, 1972.

7. Gregory, M., and J. Hughes, Intracranial Reticulum Cell Sarcoma Associated with Immunoglobulin A Deficiency, J Neurol Neurosurg Psych 36:769, 1973.

8. Lambert, C., and P. Trewby, Microglioma with Paraproteinaemia, J Neurol Neurosurg Psychiat 37:835-840, 1974.

9. Wechsler, A., and U. Tomiyasu, An Unusual Radiographical-Brain Scan Dissociation Pattern with Reticulum Cell Sarcoma of the Brain, Bull LA Neuro Soc 39:1, 1974.

CASE STUDY #45

An Elderly Woman with Intermittent Numbness

HISTORY: A 77 year-old widow, over a six week period, noted five episodes of numbness in the right hand and forearm. There were no other sensory phenomena. She had moderate weakness of the right hand and wrist with the two most recent episodes of numbness so that she could not hold a cup of tea. All of the symptoms resolved spontaneously after approximately fifteen minutes total duration.

QUESTIONS:

1. WITH THIS HISTORY, THE EXAMINER WOULD BE INTERESTED PARTIC-ULARLY IN:
   A. Visual symptoms
   B. Speech difficulty
   C. Loss of awareness or consciousness
   D. All of the above

She had none of the above symptoms, either concomitant with the attacks or at any other time.

2. IF SHE IS RIGHT HANDED, WITH THE ABOVE SYMPTOMS YOU WOULD NOT EXPECT ANY DIFFICULTY UNDERSTANDING OR EXPRESSING WORDS:
   A. True
   B. False

3. IN A YOUNGER WOMAN WITH THESE SYMPTOMS, YOU WOULD WANT TO CONSIDER IN THE DIFFERENTIAL DIAGNOSIS:
   A. Migraine
   B. Migraine or vascular insufficiency related to birth control pills
   C. Focal epileptic seizures
   D. The aortic arch syndrome (Takayasu's syndrome)
   E. All of the above

CASE STUDY #45

She had noted occasional brief "light headed feelings" over the past month without any other concurrent symptoms. She was unaware of any past neurological problems of any kind. Arteriosclerotic heart disease had been diagnosed fifteen years ago. She had an acute myocardial infarction eight years ago. She had episodes of premature ventricular contractions for many years, treated periodically with procaine amide.

QUESTIONS:

4. CARDIAC DISEASES THAT MAY CAUSE CEREBRAL SYMPTOMS INCLUDE:
   A. Myocardial infarction
   B. Myxoma of the heart
   C. Subacute bacterial endocarditis
   D. Aortic valvular disease
   E. Heart block
   F. All of the above

5. CHANGES OF CARDIAC RATE OR RHYTHM MAY CAUSE CEREBRAL SYMPTOMS:
   A. True
   B. False

6. DRUGS USED TO RETURN THE CARDIAC RATE OR RHYTHM TO WITHIN NORMAL LIMITS MAY BE ASSOCIATED WITH CEREBRAL SYMPTOMS:
   A. True
   B. False

7. OTHER DRUGS THAT MAY CAUSE CARDIAC RATE OR RHYTHM CHANGES INCLUDE:
   A. Aspirin
   B. Tri-cyclic anti-depressants
   C. Diphenylhydantoin (Sodium Dilantin)
   D. Phenobarbital
   E. B and C
   F. A and D

Over the past year she had taken none of the drugs mentioned, and had stopped the procaine amide. Premature contractions apparently had been rare. She had many years of mild hypertension. Her blood pressure had been in the normal range for the last five years, taking hydrochlorthiazide and potassium supplements.

QUESTION:

8. LOW SERUM POTASSIUM MAY CAUSE SYMPTOMS OF:
   A. Malaise and generalized fatigue
   B. Convulsions
   C. Weakness
   D. Migraine headaches

She reported no symptoms suggesting hypokalemia, congestive heart failure, coronary insufficiency, or bleeding from any part of the body. Serologic tests for syphilis were always negative. Nine months prior to her present symptoms, an abdominal aortic aneurysm was resected with insertion of a graft below the renal arteries.

CASE STUDY #45

EXAMINATION: An alert, cooperative elderly woman who appeared to be healthy and younger than her chronological age. Pulse: 80, normal sinus rhythm. Blood pressure: 180/100 mm. Hg. Her neck was supple. The carotid arteries had equal pulse strength by palpation, but there was a high pitched systolic bruit on auscultation over the left carotid artery that was maximal just below the mandible.

QUESTIONS:

9. CAROTID BRUITS IN ADULTS ARE USUALLY OF NO SIGNIFICANCE:
   A. True
   B. False

10. UNILATERAL CAROTID BRUITS ARE SIGNIFICANT, BILATERAL BRUITS ARE NOT:
    A. True
    B. False

11. WITH UNILATERAL CAROTID BRUITS:
    A. The bruit is always on the side of the pathological vessel
    B. May be on the side of the clinically uninvolved vessel, especially over the eye-ball
    C. If particularly severe, is called "bruit de diable"

12. SUPRACLAVICULAR BRUITS ARE:
    A. Never significant
    B. Sometimes of no definite significance
    C. Of significance when coupled with cerebral symptoms when the upper extremity on that side is exercised
    D. B and C

There were no other bruits and no cardiac murmurs. The remainder of her physical examination was within normal limits. The neurological examination was completely normal.

QUESTIONS:

13. THE NORMAL NEUROLOGICAL EXAMINATION EFFECTIVELY RULES OUT ANY SIGNIFICANCE TO THE HISTORY:
    A. True
    B. False

14. THE MOST LIKELY DIAGNOSIS IS:
    A. Brain tumour   C. Cerebral lacunar infarct
    B. Transient cerebral ischemia   D. Multiple sclerosis

15. THE SYMPTOMS AND FINDINGS SUGGEST THE OFFENDING VESSEL IS:
    A. The right vertebral artery
    B. The left vertebral artery
    C. The right carotid artery
    D. The left carotid artery

LABORATORY DATA: hemoglobin: 14; Hematocrit: 37; White blood count: 6,300, with a normal differential count; urinalysis: normal; sedimentation rate: 6mm/hour. Serum sodium: 142; potassium: 3.5; Chloride: 100. (All in milliequivalents per liter). Two hour postprandial sugar: 95 mg% (normal). Blood urea nitrogen: 7 mg%. Chest X-ray: clear lung fields with normal cardiac configuration. Skull X-rays: normal. Electroencephalogram: Normal. Electrocardiogram: Frequent premature atrial contractions. Minimal S-T-T wave changes with U-waves, compatible with hypokalemia. Ophthalmodynanometry: Pressure significantly lower on the left than the right. (She was treated with oral potassium supplements, and the serum potassium rose to 4.0 mEq/liter and the EKG became normal.)

CASE STUDY #45

16. WITH THESE LABORATORY VALUES THE MOST LIKELY DIAGNOSIS NOW
    IS:
    A. Brain tumour   C. Cerebral lacunar infarct
    B. Transient cerebral ischemia   D. Multiple sclerosis

17. OPHTHALMODYNANOMETRY IS:
    A. A contrast dye test
    B. A measurement of retinal artery systolic/diastolic pressure
    C. A radioactive scan technique
    D. Of no use

Because of her excellent physical condition, despite her age, it was elected to perform an aortic arch angiogram through a femoral artery catheter. This was followed by selective catheterization of the carotid and vertebral vessels, via the
same route to evaluate the intracerebral circulation. The aortic arch study is below. The arrow indicates the major lesion (Fig. 56).

One of the vessels has been catheterized and the dye injected into it.

QUESTIONS:

18. IT IS:
    A. A carotid artery   D. The left vertebral artery
    B. The innominate artery   E. The basilar artery
    C. The right vertebral artery

19. THE ARTERY OR ITS BRANCHES IS:
    A. Normal   C. Stenotic
    B. Occluded   D. Congenitally absent

20. THE BRANCH WITH THE MAJOR ABNORMALITY IS:
    A. The internal carotid artery
    B. The external carotid artery
    C. The posterior inferior cerebellar artery
    D. No branch is abnormal

The intracerebral circulation was completely within normal limits. She tolerated
the procedure well.

QUESTION:

21. THERE IS ONLY ONE WAY TO TREAT EXTRACRANIAL INSUFFICIENCY
    SYNDROMES:
    A. True
    B. False

A left carotid thromboendarterectomy was performed. The electroencephalogram
was monitored and did not change during the operation. A large hard clot was
found at the bifurcation of the common carotid artery extending into the internal
carotid artery and almost completely occluding it. The clot also extended into the
external carotid artery. The surgeon noted that: "Within the obstructing arterial
plaque, there was an ulcerative area measuring approximately 1/2 cm. in diameter with loose debris within it." The pathological microscopic interpretation
was: "blood vessel with moderate to marked arteriosclerotic changes. An organized thrombus is also noted."

Post operatively, she did well without significant complications. She subsequently
has had no return of her admitting symptoms.

CASE STUDY #45

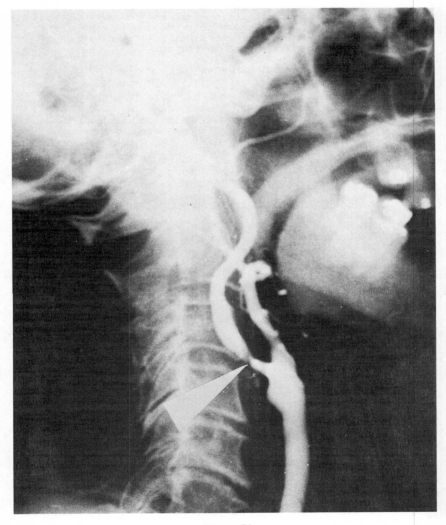

Figure 56

CASE STUDY #45

ANSWERS AND DISCUSSION:

1. D   The patient should be asked about any transient or permanent changes in her visual acuity and fields of vision. A scotoma is an area of partial or absolute loss of vision inside a field of vision that is otherwise normal. It is most commonly associated with retinal or optic nerve pathology but may be seen with occipital lobe lesions also. Scotomas with occipital lobe lesions would be bilateral. With optic nerve or retinal lesions, the scotoma is unilateral. Dysarthria - difficulty articulating words clearly, causing thick or slurred speech - is found secondary to disease in several locations in the nervous system. It may be due to disease of muscle, the neuromuscular junction (as in myasthenia gravis) the lower motor neurone, as in poliomyelitis and lower brain stem tumours and vascular insults. Bilateral lesions of the cortico-bulbar tracts cause dysarthria of the pseudo-bulbar type. Extrapyramidal lesions may cause poor articulation. This is typified by Parkinson's syndrome. There may be combinations of pyramidal and extra-pyramidal disturbances. Finally, cerebellar lesions may cause dysarthria. Dysphasia - difficulty expressing or understanding words - is seen when the speech areas of the dominant hemisphere are involved. There are different types of dysphasia depending on the area of the brain affected. Dysphasia varies from total inability to express any words, to jargon, to minor and occasional errors in speech. Loss of awareness or consciousness is experienced in a number of conditions that could have significance in this case. These conditions include cardiac arrhythmias, transient cerebral ischemia, and seizures secondary to focal brain disease.

2. B   The patient's symptoms are in the territory of the left middle cerebral artery. This vessel also goes to the speech areas of the brain in the dominant hemisphere. In right-handed persons, the left hemisphere is dominant.

3. E   Migraine can cause similar focal neurological symptoms. The apparent relationship of migraine and vascular insufficiency syndromes to estrogenic hormones is discussed elsewhere in the book. Focal epileptic seizures could cause these symptoms. A patient with these symptoms, on the basis of focal seizures, should be thoroughly evaluated regarding the possibility of a structural lesion of the central nervous system. The aortic arch syndrome is an unusual syndrome of granulomatous arteritis, first described in young women in Japan but since reported from other parts of the world.

4. F   Myocardial infarction may be associated with systemic hypotension and cerebral symptoms, arterial embolism to the brain vessels, arrhythmias and heart block producing syncope (Adams-Stokes syndrome) etc. Myxoma is an endocardial lesion which may produce episodes of syncope with change of position, or may embolize to the cerebral circulation. Subacute bacterial endocarditis may lead to cerebral embolism with symptoms. Syncope is one of the cardinal symptoms of aortic valvular stenosis.

5. A   Both bradycardia and tachycardia may cause cerebral symptoms.

6. A   Drugs used in the treatment of cardiac arrhythmias include atropine, isoproterenol, digitalis, phenylephrine, diphenylhydantoin, quinidine, procainamide, propanolol, and lidocaine. Which of the drugs is used depends on the type of arrhythmia. The side effects that affect the nervous system vary among these drugs. Side effects include headaches, con-

CASE STUDY #45

        vulsions, and syncope. Successful treatment itself of an arrhythmia may produce cerebral symptoms. An example of this is conversion of atrial fibrillation to normal sinus rhythm. This occasionally dislodges an atrial clot into the vascular tree, including to the brain.

7. E   Diphenylhydantoin has been used for both supraventricular and ventricular arrhythmias, and with lesser success for atrial tachycardia. Side effects following IV administration with these problems have included asystole and ventricular fibrillation, AV block and apnea. The tri-cyclic anti-depressants including desipramine HCl, imipramine HCl and amitriptylin HCl, may cause conduction defects, arrhythmias and tachycardia.

8. AC

9. B

10. B   Bilateral bruits should be evaluated with equal concern as a unilateral bruit. In many cases they are significant and there is stenosis in both carotid arteries.

11. B   This particularly occurs with occlusion of one carotid artery producing increased flow and a bruit in the opposite side carotid artery. Bruit de diable is an unusual humming sound auscultated over the neck in patients with very severe anemia.

12. D   Some supraclavicular bruits are benign and positional and do not indicate significant vascular disease and usually lessen or disappear with hyperextension of the extremity behind the back of the patient. "C" is a description of the subclavian steal syndrome, wherein the proximal subclavian artery is occluded and blood is shunted into the arm by retrograde flow from the vertebral artery on that side.

13. B

14. B   The history is not the inexorable progression of most brain tumors. A patient with cerebral lacunar infarction would be expected to have symptoms for several days at least and possibly abnormal findings on neurological examination. This is also true for multiple sclerosis, and this would be a very late and unlikely time of onset for multiple sclerosis.

15. D   The patient had no vertigo, diplopia, dysphagia, dysarthria, tinnitus or other symptoms of brain stem dysfunction.

16. B   Regarding her cerebral problem, the only specifically helpful findings are those of ophthalmodynanometry as explained in the answer to #17.

17. B   Both pupils are dilated with a mydriatic drug and the corneas anesthetized topically. A pressure gauge instrument is applied to the temporal sclera while the disc is observed with an ophthalmoscope. As the pressure is increased slowly, a notable arterial pulse in the papilla is seen. The reading at this point is the diastolic pressure. Further pressure produces collapse of the arteries. Pressure is slowly decreased until the arteries suddenly fill. This is the systolic pressure. 80/40 is an average reading, but the greater value comes with comparison of the systolic/diastolic pressure between each eye. A difference of more than 20% is significant. The test is of use in carotid artery stenotic and occlusive disease. However, the pressures are not altered invariably in the presence of significant pathology.

CASE STUDY #45

18. A

19. C

20. A

21.   (See Comments.)

COMMENTS: The present concept of the pathogenesis of transient ischemic attacks is that emboli are intermittently released from arteriosclerotic plaques in the walls of the great vessels that leave the aorta and go to the brain.

In evaluating a patient who may have TIA's, other conditions which produce transient neurological symptoms as epilepsy, hypoglycemia, conversion reaction, hyperventilation, labyrinthine disorders and migraine should be ruled out. Cardiac arrhythmia, systemic hypotension, polycythemia, anemia, birth control pill use, and carotid sinus hypersensitivity should be searched for and treated. Hypertension, hyperlipidemia and diabetes should be treated.

After careful history and examination, including auscultation of the neck vessels and bilateral brachial blood pressure readings, further evaluation should include blood count, urinalysis, serologic test for syphilis, glucose tolerance test, serum lipid profile, electrocardiogram and ophthalmodynanometry. Skull X-rays, lumbar puncture, EEG, brain scan, EMI scan (Computerized Axial Tomography), are useful in ruling out infarction or an unusually presenting brain tumor. Radioisotope flow studies as part of the brain scan may give additional information. Because of the occasional serious complications of angiography, most neurologists do not consider this a routine test in the patient with transient ischemic attacks, but reserve its use for patients who are good risks for both the test and subsequent surgery, if a remediable lesion is found, or in patients whose diagnosis is uncertain. The patient in this case report was felt to meet these criteria despite her age.

Transient ischemic attacks can be precursors of ischemic stroke, since about 35% of affected patients are likely to have a cerebral infarct within the next five years. However, the natural history is variable, and some patients who are untreated continue to have TIA's without apparent permanent residua, others progress to a completed stroke, and others spontaneously stop having the episodes. Controversy continues regarding the comparative benefit and risk, in the patient with TIA's of endarterectomy, anticoagulation, and drugs such as aspirin and sulfinpyrazone which inhibit platelet aggregation. Recent evidence suggests that in patients without neurological deficit, surgery has the greatest probability of success in stopping the attacks and avoiding progression to a major stroke. It cannot be stressed enough that each patient with this problem must be evaluated individually as to which course of action will be taken. Most neurologists agree that a patient with a stroke in progress, who shows increasing evidence of progressively infarcting brain secondary to thrombosis, should be treated with immediate anticoagulation. Most physicians feel that a completed stroke due to an occlusion of an extracranial vessel should neither be operated to remove the thrombus, nor anticoagulated.

CASE STUDY #45

In summary, the realization that a large number of strokes stem from disease
extracranially, and that many of these strokes may be prevented, has made
considerable difference in the evaluation, diagnosis, and treatment of cerebrovascular disease which now ranks third among the leading causes of death in the
United States.

REFERENCES

1.   Browne, T.R., and D.C. Poskanzer, Treatment of Strokes, New Eng J
        Med 281:594-602; 650-657, 1969.

2.   Fields, W.S., et al., Joint Study of Extracranial Arterial Occlusion,
        JAMA 211:1993-2003, 1970.

3.   Fisher, C.M., Occlusion of the Internal Carotid Artery, Arch Neurol
        65:346-377, 1951.

4.   Hass, W.K., et al., Joint Study of Extracranial Arterial Occlusion, II.
        Arteriography Techniques, Sites, and Complications, JAMA 203:961-968,
        1968.

5.   Marshall, J., The Natural History of Transient Ischemic Cerebrovascular
        Attacks, Quart J Med 33:309-324, 1964.

6.   Marshall, J., The Management of Stroke, Little Brown Co., Boston, 1970.

7.   Whisnant, J., et al., Clinical Prevention of Stroke, Stroke 3:806, 1972.

8.   Shaw, D., Investigation of Stroke, Brit Med J 1:91, 1972.

9.   Hass, W., Occlusive Cerebrovascular Disease, Med Clin N Am 56:1281,
        1972.

10.   Ziegler, D., et al., Prognosis in Patients with Transient Ischemic At-
        tacks, Stroke 4:666, 1973.

11.   Van Horn, G., Cerebrovascular Disease, Disease-a-Month, June 1973.

12.   Stroke: Diagnosis and Management. Fields, W., Moossy, J., Editors,
        Warren H. Green Co., 1973.

13.   Medical and Surgical Management of Stroke, Report of the Joint Committee
        for Stroke Facilities, Stroke 4:269, 1973.

14.   Editorial; Carotid Endarterectomy and TIA's, Lancet Jan.12, 1974.

CASE STUDY #45

15. Transient Ischaemic Attacks, Editorial, Brit Med J, Feb. 15, 1975.

16. Toole, J. F., et al., Transient Ischemic Attacks Due to Atherosclerosis,
     Arch Neurol 32:5, 1975.

CASE STUDY #46

Tremor in a Young Woman

HISTORY: A 22 year-old woman was admitted to the hospital for evaluation of
tremor of both arms of four years duration. The tremor was present at rest, but
worsened with movements of the arms.

QUESTIONS:

1. TREMOR AND RIGIDITY ARE COMMONLY SEEN WITH LONG-TERM
    INTAKE OF:
    A. Marijuana
    B. LSD
    C. Trifluperazine
    D. Meprobamate
    E. Mescaline

2. IN THE DIFFERENTIAL DIAGNOSIS OF TREMOR, YOU WOULD CON-
    SIDER:
    A. Familial tremor
    B. Thyrotoxic tremor
    C. Cerebellar tremor
    D. Parkinsonian tremor
    E. All of the above

3. IN COMPARING TREMOR DUE TO CEREBELLAR DISEASE WITH
    TREMOR SEEN IN PARKINSONISM:
    A. The cerebellar tremor is present primarily on movement of the limbs
       -so called "intention" tremor
    B. The parkinson tremor is present at rest
    C. The parkinson tremor always disappears with movements of the
       affected limbs
    D. Both types of tremor may be abolished by a lesion in the ventrolateral
       nucleus of the thalamus

There was no history of drug ingestion. Past medical history was negative except for an episode of jaundice at age 7. One sister had died at age 28 from
hematemesis and another had been admitted to a mental hospital at age 38. Five
other siblings were normal.

CASE STUDY #46

EXAMINATION: A young cheerful woman with a pronounced resting tremor of the head, both arms, and the left leg. The tremor persisted, though with decreased amplitude with movement. There was no rigidity, drooling, or dysarthria. The liver and spleen were both moderately enlarged. A ring of golden brown pigmentation encircled the rim of both corneas (Fig. 57).

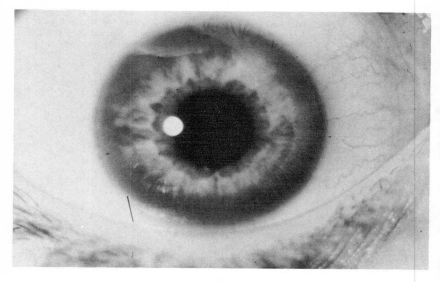

Figure 57

QUESTIONS:

4. THIS PATIENT SUFFERS FROM A DISTURBANCE IN THE METABOLISM OF:
   A. Serotonin
   B. Iron
   C. Lead
   D. None of the above

5. ONE WOULD PREDICT THAT:
   A. 25% of her siblings of either sex would neither have this disease nor be carriers of it
   B. 50% of her female siblings would have liver but not central nervous system disease
   C. 50% of her siblings of either sex would be heterozygous carriers of the disease
   D. 75% of her siblings of either sex would have the same corneal pigmented ring

CASE STUDY #46

6. THE EPONYM FOR THE PIGMENTED PERICORNEAL RING IN THIS
   DISEASE IS:
   A. Jacob-Creutzfeldt
   B. Erb-Duchenne
   C. Hallevorden-Spatz
   D. Kayser-Fleischer
   E. None of the above

7. LABORATORY ABNORMALITIES IN THIS DISEASE INCLUDE:
   A. Increased urine delta aminolevulinic acid
   B. Aminoaciduria
   C. Decreased serum ceruloplasmin
   D. Decreased hepatic copper
   E. Increased serum albumin bound copper

LABORATORY DATA: Serum ceruloplasmin was markedly decreased. Liver
function tests were mildly abnormal. There was one-plus proteinuria. Liver
biopsy showed a greatly increased copper level. The electroencephalogram
showed a triphasic wave pattern often associated with liver disease. The
platelet count was reduced.

QUESTIONS:

8. TYPICAL PATHOLOGIC FINDINGS IN THIS DISEASE INCLUDE:
   A. Hepatic cirrhosis
   B. Atrophy of the basal ganglia
   C. Depigmentation of the substantia nigra
   D. Lewy bodies

   TRUE OR FALSE:

9. When neurological abnormalities are due to Wilson's disease, Kayser-
   Fleischer rings are always present.

10. Mental disturbance may occur but is extremely rare.

11. The disease may present as parkinsonism, chorea, dystonia or ballism.

12. There is no effective treatment for this disease.

13. This disease is ruled out by a normal level of serum ceruloplasmin.

14. Cure is achieved by the intravenous administration of ceruloplasmin.

15. Kayser-Fleischer rings are seen in this disease, in Hallevorden-Spatz
    disease and in other degenerative and metabolic central nervous system
    diseases.

ANSWERS AND DISCUSSION:

1. C   A parkinsonian syndrome is seen frequently with long-term
            administration of phenothiazine drugs, such as trifluperazine.

2. E

3. ABD   A curious feature of parkinson tremor is that, although often
            worse with movements of the limbs, so that the patient's chief
            complaints may be impaired ability to write, or spilling and
            dropping the glass while drinking, yet the tremor can totally
            disappear if the limb is rapidly moved under conditions which
            are unexpected or a surprise to the patient. It is quite striking
            to see a parkinson patient, severely disabled by tremor, stop
            shaking entirely when a ball is tossed at him, catch the ball,
            and then resume the shaking.

CASE STUDY #46

4. D   Abnormal movements, liver disease and a brownish ring around
           the cornea are diagnostic features of hepatolenticular degen-
           eration or Wilson's disease, characterized by disturbances in
           the metabolism of copper.

5. AC   Since Wilson's disease is a heredofamilial disorder with an
           autosomal recessive inheritance pattern, one would predict that
           25% of the siblings of a patient's family would be homozygous
           and have the disease, 50% would be heterozygous carriers, and
           25% would not carry the gene.

6. D   The Kayser-Fleischer ring is best identified with slit lamp
           examination.

7. BCE   The evidences of disturbed copper metabolism in Wilson's
           disease include decreased serum ceruloplasmin, increased
           "free" or nonceruloplasmin copper in serum, increased
           absorption of copper from the GI tract, increased urinary out-
           put of copper, increased copper in brain, liver, cornea and
           kidney, delayed incorporation of copper into ceruloplasmin.

8. AB   Spongy necrosis, neuronal loss and sometimes cavitation are
           seen in the basal ganglia. There is a nodular cirrhosis of the
           liver.

           Depigmentation of the substantia nigra and Lewy bodies are
           pathologic features of idiopathic parkinsonism.

9. True

10. False   Mental disturbance is not uncommon in this disorder.

11. True

12. False   The most commonly used and effective regimen includes
           penicillamine, a copper-chelating agent, low copper diet, and
           potassium sulfide to bind copper in the GI tract and prevent its
           absorption.

13. False   A number of patients have been reported with normal or near
           normal levels of serum ceruloplasmin at some stage in the
           course of the disease.

14. False   This has not been helpful.[1]

15. False   The Kayser-Fleischer rings are not found in other than Wilson's
           disease.

REFERENCES

1.   O'Reilly, S., Problems in Wilson's Disease, Neurology 17:137, 1967.

2.   Richardson, J.C., Treatment of Wilson's Disease, Modern Treatment
      5:321, 1968.

3.   O'Reilly, S., M. Pollycove, M. Tono, and L. Herradora, Abnormalities
      of the Physiology of Copper in Wilson's Disease, Arch Neurology 24:481,
      1971.

4.   Wilson, S.A.K., Progressive Lenticular Degeneration: A Familial
      Nervous Disease Associated with Cirrhosis of the Liver, Brain 34:295,
      1911.

CASE STUDY #46

5. Scheinberg, I., Copper Metabolism; A review, Wilson's Disease; Some Current Concepts, J. Walshe, and J. Cumings, Ed., Oxford: Blackwell, 1961.

6. Deiss, A., R. Lynch, R. Lee, and G. Cartwright, Long Term Therapy of Wilson's Disease, Ann Int Med 75:57, 1971.

7. Symposium on Copper Metabolism and Wilson's Disease, Mayo Clinic Proceedings, June 1974, pp. 363-411.

8. Scheinberg, I., Letter to the Editor, Arch Neurol 29:449, 1974.

CASE STUDY #47

Sudden Loss of Speech

HISTORY: A 55 year-old right handed woman, a diabetic receiving insulin, was seen as an emergency because of a possible acute "stroke." She was said to have been well until the morning of admission when she was found by her husband to be unable to move the left side of her body, to speak, or to make any sound.

QUESTION:

1. WHAT IS UNUSUAL ABOUT THE HISTORY SO FAR?
   A. If she had a cerebral lesion, then acute expressive aphasia should occur in a right handed person with a left or dominant hemisphere injury; one would therefore expect a right, not a left hemiplegia; most left handed people have the speech center in the left cerebrum also
   B. One might suspect that she was originally left handed, with the right hemisphere dominant, but forced to use her right hand in childhood
   C. If the lesion were unilateral in the brain stem, one would not expect anarthria
   D. All of the above

Her last injection of NPH insulin was at 8:00 AM that morning. She apparently fell down a short staircase and was found by her husband at the foot of the stairs, fully alert, but mute.

EXAMINATION: She was able to walk, although with great difficulty, staggering and dragging her left leg, and supported by her husband. There was no evidence of head trauma. Blood pressure was 168/100. There was no respiratory difficulty or stridor. The right carotid pulsation was slightly weaker than the left. She was alert and able to follow commands, both verbal and written. She could write her name and sentences with her right hand. She could also, upon request, imitate such actions as lighting a match. She was able to silently form words with her lips, and to respond appropriately in this way, although she could make no sound. She was oriented and could name objects appropriately. She could cough normally.

QUESTIONS:

2. AT THIS POINT, IN CONSIDERING THE DIFFERENTIAL DIAGNOSIS:
   A. She is not aphasic as she can understand and communicate well, though soundlessly
   B. The lack of respiratory difficulty or stridor rules out bilateral abductor paralysis of the vocal cords
   C. Her ability to cough vigorously proves that she can adduct the vocal cords
   D. All of the above

CASE STUDY #47

3. THE MOST PROBABLE DIAGNOSIS IS:
   A. Cerebrovascular accident involving the right side of the medulla
   B. Right cerebral infarct in a person whose right hemisphere is the dominant one
   C. Brain stem neoplasm invading medullary structures bilaterally
   D. Conversion hysteria

The deep tendon reflexes were normal, with no pathological responses. She claimed to be unable to move the left arm and leg more than feebly, but showed a left Hoover sign. (To elicit this, the examiner places his hands under the heels of the supine patient, who is then asked to lift one leg. Counter pressure downward is exerted by the other leg, which can be felt by the examiner. This contralateral counterpressure downward is preserved as the patient attempts to lift an organically but not a hysterically "paralyzed" leg.) Pin and touch were claimed to be decreased on the left side of the body, but the point of change to normal sensation was exactly at the midline. (Organic sensory loss due to nerve, root or tract disease does not sharply change at the midline of the body.)

She claimed that vibratory perception was less on the left than the right side of the sternum (also a sign of hysterical illness since there is overlapping innervation over the sternum by the left and right intercostal nerves). The cranial nerves were normal, and indirect laryngoscopy showed that the cords moved inward normally on coughing and then returned to physiological position. Skull films and an electroencephalogram were normal.

Subsequently, the husband related that early that morning he and his wife had an intense argument. The patient then locked herself in the bathroom and loudly threatened that she was going to slash her wrists. He kicked down the door, took a razor blade out of her hands, and told her harshly to "cut out the nonsense." Half an hour later, when he found her mute, he became upset, guilty, repentant and worried.

The patient was referred to a psychiatrist, and, with reassurance and encouragement, she was able to speak and walk normally in a few hours. When seen a week afterwards, she was able to express her anger at her husband, and also complained that for the past few months, she had been depressed and had experienced frequent severe anxiety, particularly in crowds. She was also disturbed by impulses to strike visitors who came to her house. She had no delusions or hallucinations. She is currently receiving psychotherapy for what is considered to be a neurosis with depressive, phobic and hysterical features.

QUESTIONS:

4. FINDINGS ON THE NEUROLOGICAL EXAMINATION ASSOCIATED WITH HYSTERIA INCLUDE:
   A. Sensory loss in the arm ending abruptly at the shoulder or in the leg at the inguinal ligament
   B. Apparent indifference to the severity of the symptoms
   C. Visual loss in one eye and weakness of the opposite arm and leg
   D. All of the above

TRUE OR FALSE:

5. A conversion reaction means that a psychic conflict is converted to symptoms of dysfunction of the autonomic nervous system.

CASE STUDY #47

6. The symptoms often seem to symbolize the unconscious psychic conflict, i. e., the soldier afraid to charge up the hill who develops "paralysis" of the legs.

7. The "primary gain" in hysteria refers to the relief of anxiety.

8. Secondary gain includes other reinforcements to the hysterical illness, as sympathy, domination over others, financial gain.

9. No abnormality of laryngeal function is seen with a unilateral cerebral lesion because the nucleus ambiguus in the brainstem, which supplies the nerve fibers to the larynx, receives innervation from the upper motor neuron fibers of both hemispheres.

MATCH COLUMNS A AND B:

A			B
Breathing	Voice	Cough	
10. Normal	Normal or slightly hoarse	Normal or slightly weak	A) Bilateral total vocal cord paralysis
11. Normal	Lost	Lost	B) Bilateral abductor paresis of the vocal cords
12. Normal	Lost	Normal	C) Unilateral total vocal cord paralysis
13. Stridor and Dyspnea	Normal	Normal	D) Hysteria

ANSWERS AND DISCUSSION:

1. D

2. D

3. D   A unilateral brainstem lesion might produce distorted, hoarse, slurred speech, i. e., dysarthria, but not aphonia. She does not have an aphasia-causing cerebral lesion since her ability to comprehend and use language is intact. She can understand spoken and written sentences and communicate in writing and with speech, though soundlessly. A bilateral medullary lesion affecting the vagal nuclei bilaterally would produce not only severe difficulty with speech but impairment of cough and swallowing. Conversion hysteria is the most likely diagnosis.

4. AB   C describes a typical pattern of neurological deficit in occlusive disease of the carotid artery, with retinal ischemia producing decreased visual acuity while inadequate blood flow to the cerebral hemisphere results in contralateral hemiparesis.

5. False

CASE STUDY #47

6. True

7. True

8. True

9. True

10. C

11. A

12. D

13. B

COMMENTS: The medical history of hysteria is most fascinating. The word hysteria comes from the Greek word for uterus, since the ancient Greeks believed that hysterical illness was a disease of women caused by a wandering or abnormally moving uterus. The study of hysterical phenomena was the bridge, for Sigmund Freud, which led from neurology to psychoanalysis. During his time there was a bitter debate between the followers of Charcot, who felt that although hysterical phenomena could be produced and cured by hypnosis, the susceptibility to both hypnosis and hysteria reflected an underlying hereditary degenerative central nervous system disease, and those of Bernheim who felt that the condition was solely psychological, a result of excessive suggestibility. Freud's first psychiatric paper was about hysteria, and his observations and analyses of the underlying psychodynamics of hysterical illness led both to his concepts of defense mechanisms and personality structure.

The differential diagnosis of organic neurological illness from hysteria is a frequent problem in neurological practice. The range of hysterical symptoms parallels the spectrum of neurological disease - including seizures, blindness, deafness, paralysis, and tremor. At times, particularly with pain problems, the differential diagnosis may be extremely difficult. Particularly is the physician likely to have diagnostic difficulty with the patient who has both organic illness and a hysterical "overlay." The diagnosis of conversion hysteria should be based on both the absence of organic neurologic disease and positive evidence of psychiatric illness, including a recent conflict situation in which the symptom represents a kind of solution.

REFERENCES

1. Brain, Sir Russell, Clinical Neurology, 3rd Ed., Oxford University Press, 1969.

2. Haymaker, W., Bing's Local Diagnosis in Neurological Diseases, 15th Ed., C.V. Mosby, St. Louis, 1969.

3. Zeigler, F., Hysterical Conversion Reactions, Postgrad Med 47:174, 1970.

4. Stevens, H., Conversion Hysteria - A Therapeutic Opportunity for the Neurologist, Trans Am Neurol Assoc 96:313, 1971.

5. Kolb, L.C., Noyes' Modern Clinical Psychiatry, 8th Ed., W.B. Saunders Co., Philadelphia, 1973.

CASE STUDY #48

Headaches, Vertigo and Nystagmus

HISTORY: A 34 year-old Mexican grocery clerk was well until several months before admission when he began to suffer from severe occipital headaches, together with episodes of vertigo and ringing in his ears. The vertigo was not related to head position.

QUESTION:

1. IN ANY PATIENT WITH VERTIGO ONE SHOULD INQUIRE ABOUT SYMP-TOMS OF BRAINSTEM DYSFUNCTION. THESE INCLUDE:
   A. Ability to speak only jargon
   B. Bitemporal visual field cut
   C. Dysarthria, dysphagia and diplopia
   D. Grand mal seizures

He denied dysphagia, speech difficulty or double vision.

EXAMINATION: General physical examination was normal. Neurological examination revealed horizontal nystagmus when looking to the right and an increased right ankle jerk.

QUESTIONS:

2. THE LOCATION OF THE HEADACHE AND THE NEUROLOGICAL SYMP-TOMS AND SIGNS WOULD PERMIT YOU AT THIS POINT TO POSTULATE A LESION IN:
   A. The anterior fossa
   B. The middle fossa
   C. The posterior fossa
   D. There is insufficient evidence to localize the disturbance

3. NYSTAGMUS CAN BE:
   A. Congenital
   B. Caused by various drugs
   C. Caused by a lesion of the vestibulo-cerebellar connections
   D. All of the above

4. IN THE DIFFERENTIAL DIAGNOSIS OF THIS CASE, YOU MIGHT CON-SIDER:
   A. Cerebellar tumor
   B. Meningovascular syphilis
   C. Fungal meningitis
   D. Any of the above

LABORATORY DATA: Blood count, urine, serology were all normal, as was the spinal fluid. Audiograms showed a mild bilateral high tone hearing loss. Caloric testing was normal. A pneumoencephalogram was performed which showed poor filling of the left cerebellopontine angle.

Because of neck pain, a myelogram was performed (Fig. 58).

From the appearance of this abnormal myelogram, with multiple spherical lucent filling defects, the neuroradiologist was able to suggest the correct diagnosis. Can you guess it? (see Fig. 58)

CASE STUDY #48

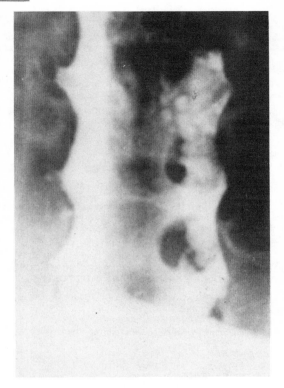

Figure 58

A suboccipital craniotomy was performed. About a dozen translucent cysts were found, measuring from 0.5 to 1.5 cm in size. These were located mainly in the cisterna magna, but also almost filled the left cerebellopontine angle cistern. Some of the cysts were gingerly removed. Pathologically, typical cysticerci were seen. Postoperatively the patient's symptoms were improved.

LABORATORY DATA: Blood complement fixation tests were positive for cysticercosis at a dilution of 1:800. Stool examinations showed no ova or parasites and at no time was there any peripheral eosinophilia.

QUESTIONS:

5. IN CEREBRAL CYSTICERCOSIS, ONE FINDS IN THE BRAIN THE:
    A. Adult worms
    B. Eggs
    C. Encysted larvae
    D. Any of the above

6. WHEN INFECTED AND UNDERCOOKED PORK IS EATEN, ONE INGESTS THE:
    A. Adult worms
    B. Eggs
    C. Encysted larvae
    D. A and C

CASE STUDY #48

7. THESE THEN DEVELOP, IN THE HUMAN INTESTINE, INTO:
   A. Cysts
   B. Adult worms
   C. Larvae
   D. Any of above

8. MAN, LIKE THE PIG, DEVELOPS DISSEMINATED SPREAD OF ENCYSTED LARVAE IN HIS TISSUES AFTER INGESTING:
   A. Eggs in fecally contaminated food
   B. Cysts in raw meat
   C. Segments of tapeworm
   D. None of the above

9. CYSTICERCOSIS IS RARE IN THE UNITED STATES; IN MEXICO, OF PATIENTS SUSPECTED OF HAVING A BRAIN TUMOR, CYSTICERCOSIS WILL BE FOUND IN:
   A. 1%
   B. 3%
   C. 5%
   D. 25%

10. CENTRAL NERVOUS SYSTEM CYSTICERCOSIS MAY BE ASSOCIATED WITH:
    A. Seizures
    B. Hydrocephalus
    C. Organic mental syndrome
    D. Headaches
    E. All of above

11. LABORATORY ABNORMALITIES WHICH MAY BE SEEN IN CYSTICERCOSIS OF THE CENTRAL NERVOUS SYSTEM INCLUDE:
    A. Cerebrospinal fluid pleocytosis
    B. Decreased sugar in the cerebrospinal fluid
    C. Peripheral eosinophilia
    D. Increased urinary delta amino levulinic acid

12. A TYPICAL RADIOLOGICAL ABNORMALITY IN CEREBRAL CYSTICERCOSIS IS:
    A. Hyperostosis frontalis
    B. Scattered intracranial calcifications
    C. Widening of the internal auditory canal
    D. None of the above

13. CURE OF CEREBRAL CYSTICERCOSIS CAN BE ACHIEVED WITH HIGH DOSES OF:
    A. Tetracycline
    B. Colchicine
    C. Atabrine
    D. No currently known drug
    E. Amphotericin B

ANSWERS AND DISCUSSION:

1. C   Dysarthria, an impairment in the quality, but not the content of speech, dysphagia, and diplopia all can result from brainstem disease. Grand mal seizures and jargon speech occur with cerebral lesions. A bi-temporal field cut is seen with lesions in the parasellar area involving the optic chiasm.

CASE STUDY #48

2. C   The symptoms of vertigo, tinnitus and occipital headache, and the finding of nystagmus, all suggest a posterior fossa lesion.

3. D   Dilantin and the barbiturates are two of the many drugs which may produce nystagmus.

4. D

5. C

6. C

7. B

8. A

9. D

10. E

11. ABC   An increase in urinary delta amino levulinic acid is seen in acute intermittent porphyria.

12. B   Multiple scattered small calcifications are frequently seen on the skull films of patients with cerebral cysticercosis.

13. D

REFERENCES

1. Olive, J., and P. Angulo-Rivero, Cysticercosis of the Nervous System - Introduction and General Aspects, J Neurosurg 19:632, 1962.

2. Cardenas, J., Cysticercosis of the Nervous System, Pathologic and Radiologic Findings, J Neurosurg 19:635, 1962.

3. Goni, P., Cysticercosis of the Nervous System, Clinical Findings and Treatment, J Neurosurg 19:641, 1962.

4. Ahlmen, J., A Case of Cysticercosis Cerebri, Acta Med Scand 184:177, 1968.

5. Greenspan, G., and L. Stevens, Infection with Cysticercus Cellulosae, New Eng J Med 264:751, 1961.

6. Kagan, I., Serologic Diagnosis of Parasitic Diseases, New Eng J Med 282: 685, 1970.

7. Clinical Neuropathological Conference, S. Aronson, and B. Aronson, Ed., Dis of Nervous System 28:757, 1967.

8. Bickerstaff, E., Cerebral Cysticercosis, Brit Med J p. 1055, April 30, 1955.

9. Dorfsman, J., The Radiologic Aspects of Cerebral Cysticercosis, Acta Radiol 1:836-842, 1963.

CASE STUDY #49

Depression and Confusion

HISTORY: A 57 year-old male was well until five years previously when, after an unsuccessful attempt at owning his own business, he seemed to become depressed and withdrawn. He slept much more than usual, refused to work, sat constantly in a dark room, and showed little interest in his surroundings. In the ensuing months he became confused and showed evidence of impaired memory. He also began to walk with a slow shuffling gait.

QUESTION:

1. AT THIS POINT IN THE STORY YOU MIGHT SUGGEST:
   A. Treatment with electroshock, because of the obvious severity of the depression
   B. Treatment with a tricyclic antidepressant drug
   C. Further evaluation, since memory loss and gait disturbance suggest organic central nervous system disease
   D. Referring the patient for analysis
   E. Referring the patient for behavior therapy

Two years ago, he was hospitalized elsewhere and carotid angiography was performed, after which his family was told that he suffered from Alzheimer's disease. Following the angiogram, he became transiently confused and paranoid.

QUESTION:

2. YOU MIGHT CONJECTURE THAT THOSE ANGIOGRAMS SHOWED:
   A. Failure of the intracranial circulation to fill
   B. Failure of the vertebral artery to fill
   C. A more rapid intracranial circulation time
   D. A widened sweep of the thalamostriate vein suggesting ventricular dilation

Six months ago he was placed in a psychiatric hospital. Electroshock was urged, but refused by the family.

During the week prior to admission he experienced increasing difficulty in walking.

There was no history of cough, weight loss, or serious medical illness. One sister had a history of depression treated with electroshock.

EXAMINATION: He was a well developed apathetic appearing male. The general physical examination was normal. He did not know where he was. He knew the month and year but not the day or date. He could give his own name, but was unable to subtract serial sevens. His affect seemed "flat" and he would frequently respond to questions by repeating the phrase "I am too nervous."

QUESTION:

3. THE MENTAL EXAMINATION DESCRIBED ABOVE BEST FITS:
   A. Paranoid schizophrenia
   B. Organic mental syndrome
   C. Hebephrenic schizophrenia
   D. Involutional depression
   E. Pseudoneurotic schizophrenia

CASE STUDY #49

His gait was unsteady with a tendency to fall backwards. The deep tendon reflexes were equal. Bilateral snout and Babinski responses were present. There was no nuchal rigidity and he was afebrile. Strength was normal.

QUESTIONS:

4. THE DIFFERENTIAL DIAGNOSIS OF THIS PATIENT'S CONDITION WOULD INCLUDE BOTH TREATABLE AND INCURABLE DISEASE. AMONG THE TREATABLE CONDITIONS TO BE RULED OUT IN THIS PATIENT WOULD BE:
   A. Chronic subdural hematoma
   B. Brain tumor
   C. Syphilitic encephalitis
   D. Pernicious anemia
   E. Chronic poisoning
   F. "Normal pressure" hydrocephalus
   G. All of the above

5. SOME OF THE POSSIBLE CAUSES OF HIS CONDITION FOR WHICH THERE IS NO DEFINITIVE TREATMENT ARE:
   A. Alzheimer's disease
   B. Huntington's chorea
   C. Dementia secondary to cerebrovascular arteriosclerosis with multiple cerebral infarcts
   D. All of the above

6. SOME INITIAL USEFUL TESTS MIGHT INCLUDE:
   A. Creatine phosphokinase
   B. Electromyography
   C. Lumbar puncture
   D. FTA-ABS
   E. All of the above

LABORATORY DATA: Blood count, urinalysis, blood sugar, serology were all normal. Bilateral carotid angiograms showed increased ventricular size. Pneumo-encephalography was attempted but the ventricles could not be filled. However, the spinal fluid obtained contained 500 mgm of protein, 147 white blood cells per cu mm, 78% of which were mononuclear, the remainder polymorphonuclear. The sugar was 30 mgm%. Gram stain, culture for pyogens, india ink stain, stain and culture for acid fast bacteria were normal.

QUESTION:

7. THE SPINAL FLUID FINDINGS RULE OUT THE DIAGNOSIS OF:
   A. Alzheimer's disease
   B. Huntington's chorea
   C. Dementia from multiple cerebral infarcts due to cerebrovascular arterio-sclerosis
   D. All of the above

Ventriculography was performed. (Fig. 59)

CASE STUDY #49

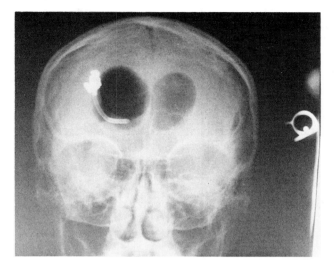

Figure 59

The ventricular system was hugely dilated without evidence of intraventricular obstruction.

8. SOME OF THE CAUSES OF CHRONIC PLEOCYTOSIS IN THE SPINAL FLUID
ASSOCIATED WITH A DECREASED SUGAR INCLUDE:
A. Tuberculous meningitis
B. Fungus meningitis
C. Sarcoidosis
D. Seeding of the meninges with malignant cells
E. Cysticercosis
F. All of above

9. HYDROCEPHALUS WHICH IS CAUSED BY OBLITERATION OF THE SUB-
ARACHNOID SPACES AROUND THE BRAIN, AS MAY OCCUR IN MENINGITIS,
IS CALLED:
A. Communicating
B. Noncommunicating
C. Hydrocephalus ex vacuo
D. None of the above

10. IN THIS TYPE OF HYDROCEPHALUS, THE INTRAVENTRICULAR PRESSURE
AND THE SPINAL FLUID PRESSURE AS MEASURED CONVENTIONALLY AT
THE LUMBAR AREA MAY BE:
A. Elevated
B. Normal
C. Either A or B

CASE STUDY #49

11. ISOTOPIC SERUM ALBUMIN, IF INJECTED INTO THE LUMBAR SAC, MIGHT LATER SHOW:
   A. A pathologic concentration within the ventricles
   B. A delay in disappearing from the cranial cavity
   C. More rapid filling of the superior longitudinal sinus
   D. All of above

COURSE: The ventricular fluid also showed a pleocytosis with a high protein and decreased sugar. This time the india ink test was positive, and cryptococci were grown in culture.

QUESTIONS:

12. THE DRUG OF CHOICE FOR CRYPTOCOCCAL MENINGITIS IS:
   A. Ampicillin
   B. Potassium iodide
   C. Griseofulvin
   D. Amphotericin
   E. Mycostatin

13. THE UNTOWARD EFFECTS OF THIS DRUG INCLUDE:
   A. Fever
   B. Thiamine deficiency
   C. Renal impairment
   D. Anemia
   E. Phlebitis

14. IF INJECTED INTRATHECALLY, THE DRUG CAN CAUSE:
   A. Chemical meningitis
   B. Neuritic pain
   C. Paresthesiae
   D. Headache
   E. All of the above

15. THE MAIN SOURCE OF CRYPTOCOCCI HAS BEEN FOUND TO BE:
   A. Rats
   B. Pigeon excreta
   C. The kissing bug
   D. Fleas

16. ANOTHER, MORE RECENTLY DESCRIBED, DRUG WHICH APPEARS USEFUL IN THE TREATMENT OF CRYPTOCOCCAL MENINGITIS IS:
   A. Gentamicin
   B. 5 fluorocytosine
   C. Chlorambucil
   D. Lincomycin

17. IN ADDITION TO THE ANTIFUNGAL DRUG, THE PATIENT MAY REQUIRE A SURGICAL PROCEDURE FOR RELIEF OF THE HYDROCEPHALUS. THIS PROCEDURE WOULD BE:
   A. Subtemporal decompression
   B. A shunt from a cerebral ventricle to the cisterna magna
   C. A shunt from a cerebral ventricle to an extracranial site such as the cardiac atrium
   D. Hemispherectomy

CASE STUDY #49

ANSWERS AND DISCUSSION:

1. C

2. D   Ventricular dilation or hydrocephalus has many causes, which can be divided into three main groups: that due to overproduction of cerebrospinal fluid as with a choroid plexus papilloma; that due to obstruction of cerebrospinal fluid flow either within the ventricular system or outside it, as in the subarachnoid spaces around the brain; and the ex vacuo type, due to atrophy of cerebral tissue, as might be seen in Alzheimer's disease.

3. B   He shows a severe organic mental syndrome. This term describes a set of criteria including impairment of memory, orientation, learning, problem solving, and calculating ability, which have been found useful in identifying and distinguishing mental disturbance of demonstrable organic etiology (of diverse causes as toxic, neoplastic, infectious, degenerative etc.) from that of unknown etiology as the schizophrenias and affective psychoses. In any organic mental syndrome, "psychiatric" abnormalities of thought and affect, such as paranoia, depression and anxiety are often interwoven with the "organic" features.

4. G   Many treatable diseases can cause chronic dementia and it is most important that they be ruled out before a diagnosis of an incurable illness is made. Some of these treatable conditions include chronic subdural hematomas, luetic encephalitis, "normal pressure" hydrocephalus, intoxications, as with heavy metals or various drugs (atropine, L-DOPA, dilantin, barbiturates especially in the elderly, amphetamines, bromides, etc., hypo- and hyperthyroidism, hypo- and hyperadrenalism, hyper- and hypocalcemia, hypo- and hypernatremia, pulmonary, cardiac, renal and hepatic decompensation, hyperlipidemia, recurrent hypoglycemia, colloid ventricular cysts, Wilson's disease, deficiency of vitamins B1, B2 and B12.

5. D   Chronic dementia due to cerebrovascualr arteriosclerosis is diagnosed frequently but is actually an uncommon cause of dementia.

           Huntington's chorea may present initially with either the choreic movements or the mental disturbance.

6. CD   Creatine phosphokinase determination is useful in the diagnosis of myopathic disease, and the electromyogram too is primarily important in the differential diagnosis of diseases of the motor unit.

7. D   In the presenile dementias such as Alzheimer's disease the spinal fluid is usually normal, with occasional cases showing a slight increase in protein concentration. In Huntington's chorea the spinal fluid is also normal. In cerebrovascular disease with multiple infarcts the spinal fluid may be normal or may show a moderate increase in protein and/or cells, but not the gross protein elevation, pleocytosis and decreased sugar as in this case.

8. F

9. A   Communicating hydrocephalus is due to extraventricular obstruction in the subarachnoid spaces surrounding the brain, through which the cerebrospinal fluid passes on its way to the arachnoid villi, to empty into the superior longitudinal sinus. The term communicating is used because a dye placed in the ventricles can later be detected in the

CASE STUDY #49

lumbar subarachnoid space. Noncommunicating hydrocephalus is due to intraventricular obstruction of cerebrospinal fluid flow so that the ventricular system and the lumbar subarachnoid space are not in open communication.

10. C

11. AB

12. D

13. ACDE

14. E

15. B

16. B   Because treatment failure is common using 5 fluorocytosine alone for cryptococcal meningitis, this drug is best used in combination with Amphotericin B. Leukopenia and thrombocytopenia may result from fluorocytosine, especially in azotemic patients.

17. C   A shunting procedure would be required, but one from the lateral cerebral ventricle to the cisterna magna would be useless since the site of obstruction of flow of the spinal fluid would not be bypassed. Shunting from the ventricle to an extracranial site such as the cardiac atrium would be the operation of choice.

COMMENTS:

This case is an excellent example of the risk of premature diagnosis of a degenerative disease without adequate testing to rule out the treatable causes of dementia.

Extraventricular obstruction, causing hydrocephalus and dementia, can occur with normal ventricular and lumbar pressures and, although the mechanism has not been fully elucidated, Adams et al.[4] suggest that ventricular enlargement can be maintained by less pressure elevation than needed to produce it, since, according to the formula, force=pressure X area, the greater the ventricular area, the less the given pressure necessary to maintain the distending force. Others have postulated that the intraventricular pressure must be intermittently elevated. This syndrome of "normal" pressure hydrocephalus includes primarily dementia, unsteady gait and incontinence. Other symptoms, as parkinsonism, seizures, and combativeness have also been described. The traditional laboratory criteria for the diagnosis of this syndrome and treatment with shunting procedures have been:

1. Pneumoencephalogram: (a) there is absence or a decreased amount of air over the cerebral convexity
(b) the callosal angle is less than 120 degrees

2. Isotope cisternography: There is an abnormal intraventricular accumulation as well as a slow disappearance of the isotope from the cranium.

3. CSF infusion test: Infusion into the lumbar subarachnoid space of saline or artificial spinal fluid results in a greater rise of spinal fluid pressure per amount infused than in the normal.

CASE STUDY #49

Although some patients with clinical and laboratory features of this syndrome show dramatic and remarkable improvement following shunting, many patients do not. Often the criteria above correlate only poorly with each other and with the clinical response to shunting. The shunting procedure itself has significant morbidity and mortality. The search continues for ways to identify those patients who will benefit from surgery.

REFERENCES

1. Goodman, J., L. Kaufman, and M. Koenig, Diagnosis of Cryptococcal Meningitis, New Eng J Med 285:434, 1971.

2. Vijayan, N., J. Cuanang, and P. Dreyfus, Dementia, Current Concepts, Calif Med 111:208, 1969.

3. Raskin, N., Dementia, Calif Med 111:227, 1969.

4. Adams, R., C.M. Fisher, S. Hakim, R. Ojemann, and W. Sweet, Symptomatic Occult Hydrocephalus with "Normal" Cerebrospinal Fluid Pressure, New Eng J Med 273:117, 1965.

5. Geschwind, N., The Mechanism of Normal Pressure Hydrocephalus, J Neuro Sci 7:481, 1968.

6. Samuelson, S., et al., Subdural Hematoma as a Complication of Shunting Procedures for Normal Pressure Hydrocephalus, J Neurosurg 37;548, 1972.

7. Wolinsky, J., et al., Diagnostic Tests in Normal Pressure Hydrocephalus, Neurology 23:706, 1973.

8. Crowell, R., et al., Aggressive Dementia Associated with Normal Pressure Hydrocephalus, Neurology 23:461, 1973.

9. Gonyea, E., Cisternal Puncture and Cryptococcal Meningitis, Arch Neurol 28:200, 1973.

10. Chawla, J., et al., Intracranial Pressure in Patients with Dementia and Communicating Hydrocephalus, J Neurosurg 40:376, 1974.

11. Martin, W., and A. Smith, The Evaluation of Dementia, Diseases of the Nervous System 35:262, 1974.

12. Messert, B., and B. Wannamaker, Reappraisal of the Adult Occult Hydrocephalus Syndrome, Neurology 24:224, 1974.

13. Wood, J., et al., Normal Pressure Hydrocephalus: Diagnosis and Patient Selection for Shunt Surgery, Neurology 24:517, 1974.

14. Hoff, J., and R. Barber, Transcerebral Mantle Pressure in Normal Pressure Hydrocephalus, Arch Neurol 31:101, 1974.

15. Heilman, K., and W. Fisher, Hyperlipidemic Dementia, Arch Neurol 31:67, 1974.

16. Bennett, J., Chemotherapy of Systemic Mycoses, New Eng J Med 289:30, 1974 and 289:320, 1974.

17. Meyer, R., and J. Axelrod, Fatal Aplastic Anemia Resulting from Flucytosine, JAMA 228:1573, 1974.

18. Baum, G., and J. Schwarz, Diagnosis and Treatment of Systemic Mycoses, Med Clin N America 58:661, 1974.

CASE STUDY #49

18. Baum, G., and J. Schwarz, Diagnosis and Treatment of Systemic Mycoses, Med Clin N America 58:661, 1974.

19. Diamond, R., and J. Bennett, A Subcutaneous Reservoir for Intrathecal Therapy of Fungal Meningitis, New Eng J Med 288:186,1973.

20. Diamond, R., and J. Bennett, Prognostic Factors in Cryptococcal Meningitis, Ann Int Med 80:176, 1974.

21. Eraut, D., Idiopathic Hypoparathyroidism Presenting as Dementia, Brit Med J 1:429, 1974.

22. Harder, E., and P. Hermans, Treatment of Fungal Infections with Flucyto- sine, Arch Int Med 135:231, 1975.

23. Poser, C., The Presenile Dementias, JAMA 233:81, 1975.

CASE STUDY #50

Muscle Cramps in a Young Woman

HISTORY: A 29 year-old pregnant woman noted an increase of symptoms that had begun when she was fourteen. Leg cramps and difficulty typing because of cramps of her fingers were previously static, except that they worsened during the winter when she was exposed to cold. She noted that once movement was initiated and repeated several times, the cramps or tightness improved.

QUESTIONS:

1. INCREASE IN SYMPTOMS WHEN EXPOSED TO COLD IS SEEN IN:
   A. Duchenne muscular dystrophy
   B. Acute porphyria
   C. Infantile spinal muscular atrophy
   D. Myotonia congenita
   E. Myotonic muscular dystrophy

2. SYMPTOMS USUALLY OCCUR ONLY WHEN EXPOSED TO COLD IN:
   A. Paramyotonia congenita
   B. Paroxysmal myoglobinuria
   C. Myasthenia gravis
   D. Syringomyelia

3. THE EXAMINER WOULD BE PARTICULARLY INTERESTED IN ELICITING FINDINGS OR HISTORY OF:
   A. Early frontal baldness
   B. Weakness
   C. Atrophy of muscle
   D. Cataracts

All of the above were absent in this patient. Her biceps were prominent (Fig. 60), the calves were hypertrophied with a "hard, wooden feel" to palpation (Fig. 61). Percussion myotonia was notable in the trapezii, calves, thenar eminences, biceps, and to a lesser degree in the tongue.

The patient's thenar muscles have been percussed with a soft rubber hammer (Fig. 62). The muscle mounds-up in contraction. Relaxation of the muscle is delayed. Opening and closing of the hands and the initiation of other movements were severe- ly myotonic, but became normal with repetition of the movement. She had no atrophy or demonstrable weakness.

QUESTION:

4. DO YOU THINK SHE HAS MYOTONIC MUSCULAR DYSTROPHY?:
   A. Yes
   B. No

   WHY?

CASE STUDY #50

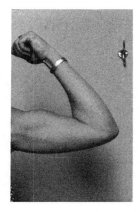

Figure 60

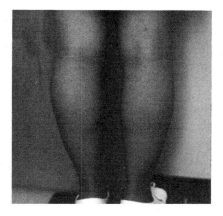

Figure 61

CASE STUDY #50

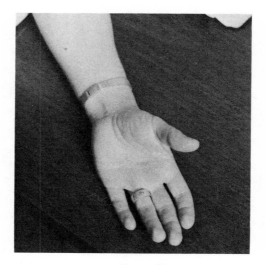

Figure 62

The patient's 27 year-old brother is considerably more symptomatic, and has marked muscle hypertrophy. He does not have cataracts, testicular atrophy or frontal alopicia. There is no family history of mental disease, or of cataracts, but much of the patient's family history on the father's side is unknown. The father died when the patient was 9 years old, of unknown causes.

QUESTIONS:

5.   IN MYOTONIC MUSCULAR DYSTROPHY, FAMILY HISTORY MAY REVEAL:
        A. Dominant mode of transmission
        B. Recessive mode of transmission
        C. Members with mental retardation
        D. Tendency to increased severity in succeeding generations
        E. Members with cataracts prematurely but no demonstrable muscle disease

6.   IN MYOTONIA CONGENITA, FAMILY HISTORY MAY REVEAL:
        A. Dominant mode of transmission
        B. Recessive mode of transmission
        C. Members with mental retardation
        D. Members with cataracts but no demonstrable muscle disease
        E. Tendency to increased severity in succeeding generations

7.   IN MYOTONIC MUSCULAR DYSTROPHY, MYOTONIA USUALLY BEGINS:
        A. In the calves
        B. In the trunk muscles
        C. In the tongue
        D. In the small hand muscles

CASE STUDY #50

The absence of signs of myotonic muscular dystrophy in addition to myotonia and the family history, made myotonia congenita the probable diagnosis.

QUESTIONS:

8. ANOTHER NAME FOR THIS DISEASE IS:
   A. Thomsen's disease
   B. Kugelberg-Welander syndrome
   C. Erb's disease
   D. Oppenheim's disease
   E. Walton's myotonia antarctica

9. SOME CASES OF MYOTONIA CONGENITA:
   A. May ultimately develop the features of myotonic dystrophy
   B. May remain as essentially "pure" myotonia without other features
   C. Have frequently associated endocrine abnormalities
   D. Have regression of the mytonia

10. IN MYOTONIA CONGENITA ONE WOULD EXPECT MUSCLE ENZYMES TO BE:
    A. Within normal limits in most cases
    B. Elevated in all cases
    C. Elevated in severe cases

11. MUSCLE BIOPSY IN MYOTONIA CONGENITA MAY:
    A. Be within normal limits
    B. Show some fibers that are hypertrophied
    C. Show central cores
    D. Reveal fiber necrosis

As the patient was having increasing functional difficulty with her myotonia, diphenylhydantoin 100 mg three daily was begun. There was striking subjective and objective improvement of the patient's myotonia.

QUESTION:

12. A LUPUS-LIKE SYNDROME HAS BEEN ASSOCIATED WITH THE TREAT-MENT OF MYOTONIA WITH:
    A. Procaine amide
    B. Quinine
    C. Dilantin

With a saddle-block anesthesia, the patient completed an uneventful pregnancy and delivered a healthy seven pound boy with no signs of myotonia. She has continued to do well with the administration of diphenylhydantoin.

ANSWERS AND DISCUSSION:

1. DE

2. A   Paramyotonia, also known as von Eulenburg's syndrome, is a non-progressive dominantly inherited syndrome with myotonia and attacks of flaccid weakness. Usually it is noted first in infancy or childhood. Patients with paramyotonia also may have their weakness provoked by potassium. It is probable that this condition is a form of hyperkalemic periodic paralysis. More basic knowledge of the pathophysiology of both conditions is needed to confirm this.

CASE STUDY #50

3. ABCD   All of these symptoms are prominent in myotonic muscular dystrophy.

4. B   She has a normal examination except for myotonia. None of the findings of myotonic muscular dystrophy are present. She has no atrophy or weakness of muscle, frontal baldness and "hatchet facies," or cataracts.

5. ACDE   Members of a family with myotonic muscular dystrophy may have symptoms or findings on examination of all or only part of the disease.

6. AB   Myotonia congenita is listed as a disease with a dominant pattern of inheritance, but autosomal recessive cases have been reported. See comments following.

7. D

8. A   Kugelberg-Welander syndrome or juvenile progressive spinal muscular atrophy is a neural disease that often mimics muscular dystrophy. Erb's disease is the eponym for facioscapulohumeral dystrophy. Oppenheim's disease is the eponym for amyotonia congenita, a category now thought to be invalid by most neurologists. "e" does not exist.

9. ABD   Answer "a" occurs, but is unusual. In most cases, it is due to miscalling myotonic muscular dystrophy rather than a patient with Thomsen's disease later developing myotonic dystrophy. Thomsen's disease usually remains as myotonia alone and tends to regress in severity as the patient grows older.

10. AC   Footnote #1

11. AB

12. AC

COMMENTS: Myotonia is found in several diseases. By definition, it is a delayed relaxation of voluntary muscle contraction. This is usually clinically detectable but, in some cases, only electromyography reveals the myotonia. The diseases in which it characteristically occurs are genetically determined. Several genetic lines of goats and horses also exhibit myotonia. It is of vital importance to the patient to distinguish between myotonia congenita with its usual benign course and myotonic muscular dystrophy (myotonia atrophica) with its associated physical findings, progressive course, and usually premature death. It recently has been suggested[5] that there are two forms of myotonia congenita. The classical dominant form begins shortly after birth with mild muscle hypertrophy and generalized myotonia. A recessive form begins between the 5th and 10th year, with the legs affected first in 50% of the cases, and with a greater degree of hypertrophy. Finally, although myotonia is presently felt by most authorities to be an abnormality of the excitable muscle membrane, Engel has recently theorized that myotonic dystrophy is a neuropathy rather than a myopathy. He bases this conclusion on the distal wasting, pathological features, the frequent lack of muscle enzyme elevation, and motor nerve ending abnormalities with methylene blue staining. Diphenylhydantoin is the treatment of choice because of low toxicity and usually good effect. Procaine amide or quinine have been used also.

CASE STUDY #50

REFERENCES

1. Becker, P.E., "Myopathies," Humangenetik, Georg Thieme Verlag, Stuttgart, 1964.

2. Bhatt, G.P., M. Vijayan, and P.M. Dreyfus, Myotonia: A Review of its Clinical Implications, Calif Med 114:16, (Feb.) 1971.

3. Engel, W. King, Myotonia: A Different Point of View, Calif Med 114:32, (Feb.) 1971.

4. Layzer, R.B., and L.P. Rowland, Cramps, New Eng J Med 285:31, 1971.

5. Caughey, J., Myrianthopolous, N., Dystrophica Myotonica and Related Disorders, Charles C Thomas, 1963.

6. Munsat, T.L., Therapy of Myotonia, A Double Blind Evaluation of Diphenylhydantoin, Procainamide and Placebo, Neurology 17:359, 1967.

7. Pennington, R.J., Chapter in Disorders of Voluntary Muscles, Ed., J.N. Walton, Little, Brown and Co., Boston, 1964.

8. Rowland, L.P., and R.B. Layzer, Ch. 37, Muscular Dystrophies, Atrophies, and Related Disorders, Clinical Neurology, Ed., Baker, A.B., Harper and Row, 1971.

9. "Skeletal Muscle Review", UCLA Conference, Ann Int Med 67:614, 1967.

10. Walton, J., Editor, Disorders of Voluntary Muscle, Little,Brown Co., 1969.

CASE STUDY #51

Paralysis Following an Upper Respiratory Infection

HISTORY: A 61 year-old man in previously good health developed a sore throat, low grade fever, and runny nose. Six days later, these symptoms were improving, but he began to ache in his neck, back, thighs and calves, and he noted numbness and tingling sensations in his fingers and toes. A day later, when he tried to get out of bed, he fell to the ground. He was able to stand and walk only with support. He tripped over his feet, because "his toes dragged."

QUESTION:

1. "TOE-DRAGGING" DUE TO WEAKNESS OF TOE AND FOOT DORSIFLEXION OCCURS IN:
   A. Posterior tibial nerve lesions
   B. First sacral root lesions
   C. Common peroneal nerve lesions
   D. Fifth lumbar root lesions
   E. Charcot-Marie-Tooth disease
   F. Distal myopathy

He denied any difficulty with swallowing, breathing, urination, or defecation. He had had no recent vaccinations or other injections. He had received no medication recently, except for ampicillin, taken orally when his upper respiratory symptoms began. He had no exposure to heavy metals, insecticides, or other known toxins, nor was there any history of diabetes or alcoholism.

PHYSICAL EXAMINATION: A well developed, tired appearing man, lying in bed complaining of back pain. Vital signs were normal. There was no skin rash. The general physical examination was normal.

CASE STUDY #51

NEUROLOGICAL EXAMINATION: He was unable to stand and was able to sit on
the edge of the bed only with difficulty due to weakness of the trunk muscles.
There was equal, and moderately severe, weakness distally and proximally of
all extremities.   The deep tendon reflexes were completely absent.
There was mild impairment of position and vibratory sensation in the feet.
There was hypalgesia in both legs from the mid-calf level distally.
Coordination, cranial nerve function, and mentation were normal.

QUESTION:

2.   GIVEN THE HISTORY AND PHYSICAL FINDINGS, THE MOST LIKELY
      SITE OF THIS PATIENT'S DISEASE IS:
      A. Muscle
      B. Neuromuscular junction
      C. Peripheral nerve
      D. Spinal cord
      E. Brainstem
      F. Basal ganglia
      G. Thalamus
      H. Cerebral cortex

LABORATORY DATA: Hematocrit: 36. WBC: 13,800, slight shift to left on
differential count; sedimentation rate: 56mm/hour corrected. Two hour post
prandial blood sugar: 94 mg.%. Serum potassium, sodium, chlorides, calcium,
phosphorus; blood urea nitrogen: All within normal limits. Urine for heavy
metals: normal. Serum protein electrophoresis: normal pattern. Antinuclear
antibody test and latex fixation: negative. Lumbar puncture: opening pressure
180 mm of water, 3 red blood cells, 1 lymphocyte/mm^3 sugar 67 mg.%., protein
124 mg.%. Immunoglobulin G (gamma globulin): 6% of the total protein. Urine
negative for porphobilinogen.

QUESTIONS:

3.   WHAT NEUROLOGICAL TESTS WOULD YOU WANT TO OBTAIN?:
      A. Carotid angiogram
      B. Pneumoencephalogram
      C. Nerve conduction times
      D. Electromyogram
      E. Isotope brain scan
      F. All of the above
      G. None of the above

4.   ACUTE AND SUBACUTE POLYNEUROPATHIES HAVE BEEN REPORTED
      ASSOCIATED WITH VARIOUS INFECTIONS:
      A. True
      B. False

5.   THESE INFECTIONS HAVE INCLUDED:
      A. Mumps
      B. Infectious mononucleosis
      C. Diphtheria
      D. Hepatitis
      E. All of the above
      G. None of the above

CASE STUDY #51

6. HEAVY METALS THAT MAY CAUSE POLYNEUROPATHY INCLUDE:
    A. Arsenic
    B. Lead
    C. Thallium
    D. Manganese
    E. Mercury

7. LEAD POISONING IN INFANTS USUALLY CAUSES A POLYNEUROPATHY:
    A. True
    B. False

As no underlying cause was found, this patient's illness was considered to be "infectious" polyneuritis.

8. CHARACTERISTIC, BUT NOT INVARIABLE,IN THIS SYNDROME ARE:
    A. Bilateral extensor plantar responses
    B. The objective motor loss more than sensory
    C. Loss of vision
    D. High spinal fluid protein, few cells
    E. All of the above
    F. None of the above
    G. A and C
    H. B and D

9. THE SPINAL FLUID FINDINGS OF HIGH PROTEIN AND FEW CELLS IS CALLED:
    A. The doppler effect
    B. Pancoast's syndrome
    C. The hyperviscosity syndrome
    D. Albumino-cytologic dissociation

10. HALLMARKS OF THE SYNDROME INCLUDE:
    A. Hyporeflexia or areflexia
    B. Paresthesiae of extremities,but sensory loss less then motor
    C. Progressive symmetrical motor loss, proximal or distal
    D. Acute or subacute course
    E. All of the above
    F. None of the above

11. THERE IS AN EXCELLENT CORRELATION BETWEEN SPINAL FLUID PROTEIN AND PROGNOSIS:
    A. True
    B. False

COURSE IN HOSPITAL: The patient's extremity weakness worsened over the next five days. He developed virtually complete quadriplegia and severe facial weakness. He had dysphagia and progressive difficulty handling his secretions. He could not abduct with either eye or adduct or elevate the right eye.

QUESTION:

12. THE CRANIAL NERVE MOST OFTEN AFFECTED IN THIS CONDITION IS:
    A. IX
    B. X
    C. III
    D. IV
    E. VII

CASE STUDY #51

Pupillary reflexes remained intact.

13.   THERAPY INCLUDES:
        A. Cortico-steroids
        B. Meticulous nursing care
        C. Respiratory assistance, including tracheostomy as needed
        D. All of the above
        E. None of the above

On the sixth hospital day, a tracheostomy was performed. His breathing was helped with a volume respirator.

QUESTION:

14.   VITAL IN EVALUATING AND TREATING RESPIRATORY INSUFFICIENCY ARE:
        A. Blood gases determinations
        B. Mechanical assistance in respiration as needed
        C. Tracheostomy as needed
        D. Prophylactic antibiotics

Intravenous steroids were begun in high doses. He began to show improving strength in the proximal extremities over the next several days.

QUESTIONS:

15.   IN RECENT YEARS, THE MORTALITY OF THIS ILLNESS HAS:
        A. Increased
        B. Decreased

16.   THE RECENT HIGHER SURVIVAL RATE IS MOST LIKELY RELATED TO:
        A. Careful repeated evaluation of respiratory sufficiency
        B. Electric stimulation of the nerves
        C. Antiviral drugs
        D. Freeing of trapped peripheral nerves

Blood gasses were carefully monitored and kept withing normal limits. On the 15th day, he spiked a temperature to 102 degrees F. Multiple blood cultures grew out proteus. Large doses of ampicillin were used. The patient became afebrile over the next 48 hours and the blood cultures became sterile. His strength improved slowly and physical therapy was started.

QUESTION:

17.   IF THE PATIENT SURVIVES THE ACUTE PHASE OF THE ILLNESS, HE STILL HAS LITTLE CHANCE OF COMPLETELY RECOVERING:
        A. True
        B. False

CASE STUDY #51

Two months after his illness began, he no longer required ventilatory assistance, the tracheostomy tube was removed and the site healed well. The patient was eating a regular diet by mouth. His strength still was markedly impaired with most movements only possible against gravity. He was given many months of intensive physical therapy. The steroids were tapered and stopped. His strength returned gradually so that first he walked with assistance and support, then with a walker, then with two canes and bilateral foot lifts. At the end of one year, his muscles were flabby with mild atrophy but his strength was normal except for bilateral foot drop. His deep tendon reflexes remained absent.

QUESTIONS:

18. AT PRESENT, THE ETIOLOGY OF THIS SYNDROME IS DEFINITELY KNOWN:
     A. True
     B. False

19. IMPORTANT ETIOLOGICAL THEORIES PROPOSED INCLUDE:
     A. Fat microemboli
     B. An immunological response to a virus
     C. An immunological response to foreign protein injection
     D. All of the above

20. RECENT PATHOLOGICAL STUDIES OF THE PERIPHERAL NERVOUS SYSTEM IN THIS SYNDROME REVEALED:
     A. No inflammation
     B. Inflammation
     C. No demyelination
     D. Demyelination

ANSWERS AND DISCUSSION:

1. CDEF   The most common cause of foot drop is a lesion of the common peroneal nerve, due to trauma, diabetes, or other etiologies of mononeuropathy. Fifth lumbar root lesions may be associated with foot drop. The familial degenerative process called peroneal muscular atrophy or the syndrome of Charcot-Marie-Tooth has foot drop and wasting of the muscles of the anterior calf compartment as an early manifestation. Distal myopathy was first described by Gowers. It is a relatively benign form of dystrophy beginning in the distal hand and the tibial muscles.

2. C   Sensory abnormalities are not found in myopathies or myasthenia gravis. The patient did not show any increase in strength with successive muscular contractions, as might be seen in the myasthenic syndrome associated with cancer. With spinal cord disease, evidence of damage to the long motor and sensory tracts, as well as sphincter involvement is seen often. Diseases of the anterior horn cell, as spinal muscular atrophy and poliomyelitis, are unassociated with sensory abnormalities. In addition, poliomyelitis produces asymmetrical paralysis, and is often associated with signs of meningeal irritation. With brainstem involvement one would expect cranial nerve and long tract abnormalities. Disease of the basal ganglia is associated with abnormalities of posture, movements, coordination, and muscle tone. The "thalamic syndrome" includes sensory diminution or loss on the opposite half of the body, pain in this area, and ataxia and choreoathetoid movements of the contralateral limbs. The findings in cerebral cortical disease would

CASE STUDY #51

vary greatly depending on the extent and location of the disease. Unilateral cerebral cortical disease may produce abnormalities such as visual field cuts, aphasia if the dominant hemisphere speech areas are affected; and cortical sensory appreciation loss if the parietal lobe is involved.

3. CD   Multiple peripheral nerve conduction velocity measurements were markedly slower than normal. The electromyography pattern initially was normal. After two weeks, it was compatible with denervation in multiple extremity muscles tested. With acute nerve lesions, this time lag before electromyographic demonstration of denervation is typical.

4. A

5. E

6. ABCE   Chronic manganese intoxication causes a basal ganglia syndrome similar to Parkinson's syndrome. Mercury in high concentration causes irregular tremors of the facial and extremities with personality changes from mild to severe dementia. (Hat makers in Victorian England used mercury. The phrase "mad as a hatter" derives from this.) Neuropathy has also been described with mercury poisoning.

7. B   Lead poisoning in infants and most children causes an encephalopathy. Neuropathy usually is not seen in infants, but may be seen in older children or adults.

8. H

9. D   It is not present invariably, particularly at the onset of the illness.

10. E   The typical case has these features.

11. B

12. E

13. D   (See comments.)

14. ABC   Authorities agree that prophylactic antibiotics are not indicated. Instead, the patient is carefully evaluated each day for possible infection, appropriate culture studies are performed, and then the proper antibiotic for the particular infection is instituted.

15. B

16. A   As noted earlier, the death rate has been reduced by the prompt institution of therapy for respiratory insufficiency and treatment of intercurrent bacterial infections.

17. B   (See comments)

18. B

CASE STUDY #51

19. BC   The two major theories are viral and immunological. Although viruses have been isolated from various tissues, including cerebrospinal fluid and specific viral antibodies identified in some cases, no direct action of a virus has been proven. Polyneuropathy does occur following serum or vaccine injection in a small number of patients. An immunological etiology is suggested by: The time lag between the infection that usually begins the illness and the neuropathy; the microscopic pathology; the increase of immune globulin (gamma globulin) of the cerebrospinal fluid in some cases, and similarities to experimental allergic neuritis. Recently, Drachman et al. reported a patient receiving immunosuppressive drugs who developed a polyneuropathy. This casts doubt on the Landry-Guillain-Barré syndrome being invariably an autoimmune disease.

20. BD

COMMENTS: The problem of polyneuropathy of undertermined cause, often following a minor upper respiratory infection, is of great clinical, pathological and etiological interest. This syndrome may have multiple etiologies. It was first described in 1859 by Landry. He stressed the feature of progressive symmetrical paralysis of the extremities. In 1916, Guillain, Barré, and Strohl described similar cases with albuminocytologic dissociation of the spinal fluid. Today the syndrome is called infectious polyneuropathy, idiopathic polyneuritis, or the Landry-Guillain-Barré syndrome. The typical features have been described in the questions and answers. These include lack of sphincter involvement, progressive paralysis and paresthesias of the distal extremities and the protein-cellular dissociation of the spinal fluid. Sensory loss is less than motor. The motor loss is usually symmetrical. The VII cranial nerve is most commonly involved, although multiple cranial nerves may be affected.

The first step in differential diagnosis is to localize the disease process to the nerves, ruling out myopathies such as the periodic paralyses and acute polymyositis, neuromuscular junction disorders such as botulism, myasthenia gravis, and diseases of the spinal cord or other portions of the central nervous system. The second step is to differentiate "infectious polyneuropathy" from other acute neuropathic disorders such as heavy metal poisoning, porphyria, diphtheria, post vaccination neuropathy and tick paralysis. The disease follows an acute or subacute course. It usually progresses over 1-3 weeks, and then stabilizes with complete or almost complete recovery the rule. Recovery occurs in six months to a year. The distal muscles are the last to return to normal. Some patients are left with residual neurological deficits, occasionally with significant functional handicaps. The pathology is characterized by inflammation and demyelination which affects spinal nerves, roots and ganglia. The mortality in many series has been between 10-20% but there were no deaths in a large series at the University of Michigan between 1941 and 1963. Death usually results from respiratory insufficiency, intercurrent infection, or vasomotor collapse. In some patients, shortly after corticosteroids are started, dramatic improvement occurs. In other patients there is some improvement possibly related to the steroids, or improvement is equivocal or inapparent. Many neurologists feel that a trial of steroids may be indicated in the more severe cases. The value of corticosteroids, however, is very controversial. The prime reason for the decrease in mortality rate from this illness is careful attention to the problems of infection and respiratory insufficiency.

REFERENCES

1. Asbury, A.K., et al., The Inflammatory Lesions in Idiopathic Polyneuritis, Medicine 48:173, 1969.

2. Drachman, D.A., et al., Immunosuppression and The Guillain-Barré Syndrome, Arch Neurol 23:385, 1970.

3. Haymaker, W.E., and J.W. Kernahan, Medicine 28:59, 1949.

CASE STUDY #51

4. Marshall, J., The Landry-Guillain-Barré Syndrome, Brain 86:55, 1963.

5. McFarland, H.R. and G.L. Heller, Guillain-Barré Disease Complex, Arch Neurol 14:196, 1966.

6. Merritt, H.H., A Textbook of Neurology, 5th Ed., Lea and Febiger, 1973.

7. Munsat, T.L. and J.E. Barnes, Relation of Multiple Cranial Nerve Dysfunction to the Guillain-Barré Syndrome, J Neurol Neurosurg Psych 28:2, 115, 1965.

8. Osler, L.E. and A.D. Sidell, Guillain-Barré Syndrome; The Need for Exact Diagnostic Criteria, N Eng J Med 262:964, 1960.

9. Thomas, P.K., et al., Recurrent and Chronic Relapsing Guillain-Barré Polyneuritis, Brain 92:589, 1969.

10. Wiederholt, W.C., and D.W. Mulder, Cerebrospinal Fluid Findings in the Landry-Guillain-Barré-Strohl Syndrome, Neurology, 15:184, 1965.

11. Leneman, R., The Guillain-Barré Syndrome, Arch Intern Med 118:139, 1966.

12. Pleasure, D.E., R.E. Lovelace, and R.C. Duvoisin, The Prognosis of Polyradiculoneuritis, Neurology 18:1143, 1968.

13. Lichtenfeld, P., Autonomic Dysfunction in The Guillain-Barré Syndrome, Am J Med 50:772, 1971.

14. Eisen, A., and P. Humphreys, The Guillain-Barré Syndrome, Arch Neurol 30:438, 1974.

15. Goodall, J.A.D., J.C. Kosmidis, and A.M. Geddes, Effect of Corticosteroids on Course of Guillain-Barré Syndrome, Lancet 1:524, 1974.

16. Grose, C., et al., Primary Epstein-Barr Virus Infections in Acute Neurologic Diseases, New Eng J Med 292:392, 1975.

17. Emmons, P., et al., Cardiac Monitoring and Demand Pacemaker in Guillain-Barré Syndrome, Arch Neurology 32:59, 1975.

CASE STUDY #52

A Man with Spells of Unawareness

HISTORY: A 36 year-old man was in good health until the age of 26, when he began experiencing attacks of loss of awareness. During these attacks he would stare ahead, smack his lips, and if writing at his desk, would continue to make writing motions with his pen, although he would not write or draw anything understandable during the spell.

QUESTION:

1. STEREOTYPED ACTIVITY OF THIS SORT IS KNOWN AS:
   A. Writer's cramp
   B. Micrographia
   C. Polygraphia
   D. An automatism
   E. Main en griffe (claw hand)

With some of the attacks his body would briefly stiffen. At no time were tonic posturing or clonic movements observed by others. He was never incontinent, nor did he bite his tongue. The frequency of his attacks was extremely variable, from seven to eight a week to one or two a month. He was unable to relate this

CASE STUDY #52

variation in frequency to any definite factors. He had been diagnosed at another
hospital, when his episodes began, as having "petit mal epilepsy." He was treated
initially with phenobarbital in various doses, then with diphenylhydantoin. His
seizures had never been well controlled.

QUESTIONS:

2. DO YOU THINK THAT HE HAS PETIT MAL EPILEPSY?
   A. Yes
   B. No

3. MATCH THE MANIFESTATION WITH THE PROBLEM:
   A. ____ Petit mal epilepsy   E. Stereotyped activity
   B. ____ The hyperventilation syndrome   F. Brief staring spell
   C. ____ Psychomotor seizures   G. Tonic-clonic movements
   D. ____ Generalized (grand mal)   H. Light headedness, tingling
           epilepsy   digital paresthesias

4. PSYCHOMOTOR SEIZURES ALWAYS BEGIN IN CHILDHOOD:
   A. True
   B. False

   TRUE OR FALSE:

5. Petit mal seizures have a longer duration than psychomotor seizures.

6. After a petit mal seizure the patient is fully alert.

7. VISCERAL SYMPTOMS (NAUSEA, HUNGER, VOMITING):
   A. Are common in psychomotor epilepsy
   B. Are common in petit mal epilepsy

   MATCH THE EPILEPSY TYPE AND THE APPROPRIATE ANSWER:
8. ____ Psychomotor epilepsy   A. Synonymous with temporal lobe
                                         epilepsy
9. ____ Petit mal epilepsy   B. Synonymous with absence attacks
                                     C. Forced thinking, hallucinations
                                        (olfactory, visual, auditory)
                                     D. Affective disturbances (anger,
                                        fear) during attack
                                     E. No structural lesions of central
                                        nervous system
                                     F. Structural lesions frequently
                                        found
                                     G. Aura

10. MATCH THE SEIZURE TYPE AND THE ELECTROENCEPHALOGRAM
    PATTERN:
    A. ____ Petit mal epilepsy   C. 3 cycle per second spike and
                                        wave
    B. ____ Psychomotor epilepsy   D. Temporal lobe spikes and sharp
                                        waves

For the last one and one-half years, he had felt a strange "sensation that begins
as a vibration in my stomach." This was sometimes followed by a seizure.

CASE STUDY #52

11. IMPORTANT HISTORY MIGHT INCLUDE:
    A. Family history of epilepsy
    B. History of difficult birth and delivery in the patient
    C. History of encephalitis
    D. Adult head injury antedating the onset of his symptoms
    E. All of the above
    F. None of the above

He had a distant maternal cousin with epilepsy of unknown type. He believed he was the product of a normal pregnancy and delivery; denied any illness suggesting encephalitis or any significant head injury.

EXAMINATION: A muscular but slender male who appeared in good health. He was oriented, alert and cooperative, but spoke with moderately slow speech. He had flattening of affect combined with intermittent inappropriate laughter. The remainder of the physical examination was completely normal.

QUESTIONS:

12. "SLOW SPEECH" CAN BE SEEN IN THE PATIENT:
    A. Taking large doses of phenobarbital
    B. Taking large doses of diphenylhydantoin
    C. With brain damage from a number of causes
    D. All of the above

13. IF THIS WAS AN ANTICONVULSANT DRUG EFFECT, HE MIGHT EXHIBIT ALSO ON EXAMINATION:
    A. Gait ataxia
    B. Incoordination of the limbs
    C. Nystagmus
    D. Weakness
    E. Actual slurring of speech

14. NYSTAGMUS SECONDARY TO DRUG EFFECT IS USUALLY:
    A. Present only when looking to the right
    B. Present when looking in all fields of gaze
    C. Rotary in character
    D. Accompanied by diplopia

He was hospitalized for further tests.

15. WHICH OF THE FOLLOWING TESTS ARE INDICATED?
    A. Lumbar puncture
    B. Skull X-rays
    C. Brain scan
    D. EEG
    E. Computer assisted tomography
    F. All of the above

LABORATORY DATA: CBC, fasting and 2 hour postprandial sugar, serum electrolytes, BUN, calcium and phosphorus: Normal. All of the tests mentioned in question 15 were normal, except for the electroencephalogram, which was abnormal. The CAT test was not yet available when this patient was seen.

Electroencephalogram interpretation: "Right temporal spikes and intermittent 3-5 cycle per second slow waves." The electroencephalogram specimen (Fig. 63) shows an example of the right temporal spikes. (T_3-C_z).

CASE STUDY #52

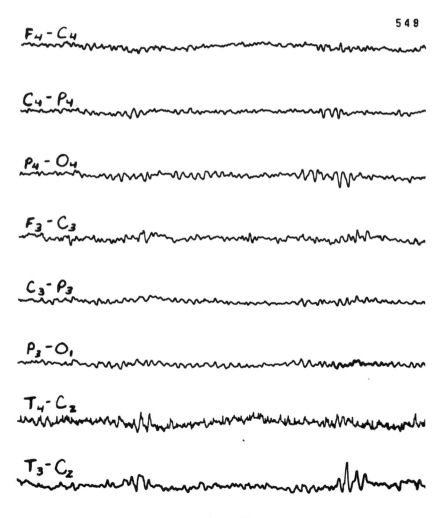

Figure 63

CASE STUDY #52

16. WOULD YOU NOW PERFORM:
   A. A right carotid angiogram
   B. A left carotid angiogram
   C. A pneumoencephalogram
   D. A brain biopsy
   E. A myelogram
   F. No further tests

17. IF THAT TEST WERE NORMAL, ONE MIGHT THEN CONSIDER:
   A. Brain biopsy
   B. Pneumoencephalogram
   C. Electromyogram
   D. None of the above

The pneumoencephalogram and bilateral carotid angiograms were normal. While in the hospital, his medications were changed. The phenobarbital was stopped and the diphenylhydantoin increased to more therapeutic levels.

QUESTION:

18. IN ADDITION TO DOSE APPROXIMATIONS BY PATIENT BODY WEIGHT, DIPHENYLHYDANTOIN LEVELS MAY BE MEASURED IN THE SERUM:
   A. True
   B. False

He became seizure free at that time, but subsequently, as an outpatient, he required the addition of primidone to control the seizures. He continues to do well with this combination of drugs, except when he neglects to take the medication as scheduled. His neurological examination continues to be unremarkable.

QUESTIONS:

19. MEDICATIONS TEND TO BE LESS EFFECTIVE WITH:
   A. Major motor epilepsy
   B. Petit mal epilepsy
   C. Psychomotor epilepsy

20. THE MOST COMMON AREA FOR PATHOLOGY IN TEMPORAL LOBE EPILEPSY IS:
   A. Lateral temporal lobe
   B. Medial temporal lobe
   C. Both of the above
   D. Neither of the above

21. ELECTROENCEPHALOGRAM WITH SCALP ELECTRODES:
   A. May be normal while deep temporal cortical electrodes reveal abnormalities
   B. May be normal with abnormal discharges from sphenoidal or nasopharyngeal electrodes
   C. Always reveals temporal lobe seizure discharges
   D. Sometimes may be normal during a seizure

22. TO INTELLIGENTLY TREAT SEIZURES, THE DOCTOR SHOULD KNOW EACH DRUG'S:
   A. Anticonvulsant action
   B. Effectiveness with different seizure types
   C. Metabolism
   D. Dosage
   E. Side reactions and toxicity

CASE STUDY #52

23. DETERMINATION OF EACH PATIENT'S SEIZURE TYPE:
    A. Is important in determining work-up
    B. Is unimportant
    C. Is important in deciding the type of drug to be used

24. MATCH THE DRUG WITH THE SEIZURE TYPE AGAINST WHICH IT MAY BE
    EFFECTIVE: (ONE DRUG MAY BE USED MORE THAN ONCE.)
    A. _____ Phenobarbital   1. Major motor seizures
    B. _____ Diphenylhydantoin (Dilantin)   2. Psychomotor seizures
    C. _____ Primidone (Mysoline)   3. Petit mal seizures
    D. _____ Ethosuximide (Zarontin)
    E. _____ Carbamazepine (Tegretol)

ANSWERS AND DISCUSSION:

1. D

2. B   See following answers for reasons.

3. A---F
   B---H
   C---E
   D---G

4. B   Psychomotor seizures may begin either in childhood or adulthood.
              That psychomotor seizures may begin in childhood has been em-
              phasized by Falconer. Petit mal epilepsy almost always begins
              in childhood.

5. False   Petit mal attacks usually last 3 to 10 seconds. Much less fre-
              quently they may last 20 to 30 seconds. Rarely, the attacks occur
              very close together for minutes or even hours in petit mal status.
              Psychomotor seizures may be very brief. Usually they last 1 to
              2 minutes, although the duration may vary from 30 seconds to 4 or
              5 minutes. The "usual" patient with psychomotor seizures has
              longer spells than the "usual" patient with petit mal epilepsy.

6. True

7. A   In addition, autonomic nervous system changes may be observed
              during the seizure. These include blood pressure changes, pupil
              dilatation or contraction, and respiratory arrest.

8. ACDFG

9. BE

10. A---C
    B---D   Therefore, the electroencephalogram is often further help in
              differentiating between these two seizure types.

11. E   All of the above answers could be related to his type of seizure.

12. D

13. ABCE

14. B

CASE STUDY #52

15. F   The tests are indicated to try and localize the seizure discharges to one temporal lobe, and to help evaluate for a possible temporal lobe structural lesion. The computer assisted tomogram is a new radiologic procedure of enormous value. The technique involves passing X-rays through the head in several planes; these X-rays are then recorded by special detector crystals, instead of on a conventional X-ray film. The results are then analyzed by a computer. An extraordinary range of normal anatomical structures and pathological foci may be visualized with this noninvasive method. Thus, intracranial masses of almost any nature are seen - neoplasms, abscesses, hematomas, infarcts and cysts.

16. A   A right carotid angiogram would be the preferred contrast procedure in view of the right temporal spike and slow wave focus on the EEG.

17. B

18. A   This may be used in helping to discover the patient who is not following a proper dosage schedule, taking less or more diphenylhydantoin than prescribed. It is helpful also in the unusual patient who metabolizes the drug more rapidly or at a slower rate in the liver than the average patient.

19. C   It is estimated that approximately 35% of patients with temporal lobe epilepsy will not be able to achieve complete freedom from their seizures.

20. B

21. ABD   Therefore, a normal electroencephalogram cannot be taken as absolute proof that the patient does not have psychomotor seizures, particularly in the interictal recording. Sphenoidal and nasopharyngeal electrode placement is done in the EEG laboratory.

22. ABCDE Only by knowledge of all of these factors can the doctor hope to have success in treating the patient.

23. AC

24. A. 1,2,3
    B. 1,2
    C. 1,2
    D. 3   Phenobarbital is more effective against major motor seizures
    E. 1,2   than in temporal lobe or petit mal epilepsy.

COMMENTS: Temporal lobe epilepsy (psychomotor seizures) is one of the focal types of epilepsy. It is a partial seizure with complex symptoms. Typically, the patient is unaware during the spell, but may continue to function and respond to a limited degree. The spells may be of varying length, but are usually between one and two minutes. If they are very transient, they may be confused with petit mal epilepsy. The differentiation should be possible when the patient's age, the frequency of seizures and the electroencephalogram are considered. The patient often has abnormal visceral sensations as part of his seizures. These are most frequently described as emanating from the abdomen or stomach. The patient may describe the subsequent spread of the sensation to the head, often with a feeling of choking. The phenomena of deja vu (feeling that the experience has occurred before) or of unreality are part of some patients' temporal lobe seizures. In addition to the seizure, patients with this form of epilepsy tend to exhibit emotional and behavioral abnormalities at other times.

CASE STUDY #52

Temporal lobe seizures are associated with a high frequency of neuropathological abnormalities of which mesial temporal sclerosis is the most common. There is debate about the pathogenesis of the neuronal loss and gliosis in mesial temporal sclerosis. Theories include anoxia occurring during infantile or childhood seizures and brain damage during molding of the head at birth. Other less common pathological findings include neoplasms, arteriovenous malformations, scars or structural anomalies. Depth electrode studies have shown that a clinical temporal lobe seizure almost always originates electrically in the hippocampus or the hippocampal gyrus, rarely in the amygdala rather than from the temporal lobe convexity cortex.

The doctor caring for a patient with temporal lobe epilepsy has two major tasks. The first is to evaluate the patient for a possible underlying lesion that needs treatment, such as a tumor. Tests for evaluating this have already been discussed. Although the EEG may be helpful in localization, mirror foci can exist and transmission across commissures can confuse localization. The second task is to control the seizures with medication, usually diphenylhydantoin or primidone. If this is not possible, and the problem can be localized to one temporal lobe, an anterior temporal lobectomy should be considered.

REFERENCES

1. Falconer, M.A., Significance of Surgery for Temporal Lobe Epilepsy in Childhood and Adolescence, J Neurosurg 33:233, 1970.

2. Green, J.R., and D.G. Schutz, Surgery of Epileptogenic Lesions of the Temporal Lobe, Arch Neurol 10:135, 1964.

3. Griggs, W.L., III, Modern Treatment 8:258-276, Harper and Row, 1971.

4. Schmidt, R.R., and B.J. Wilder, Epilepsy, F.A. Davis Co., 1968.

5. "Temporal Lobe Epilepsy", Brit Med J 3:320-321, 1971.

6. Walter, R.D., Clinical Aspects of Temporal Lobe Epilepsy: A Review, Calif Med 110:325, 1969.

7. Falconer, M.A., Genetic and Related Etiological Factors in Temporal Lobe Epilepsy; A Review, Epilepsia 12:13, 1971.

8. Margerison, J.H., et al., Epilepsy and the Temporal Lobes; A Clinical, Electroencephalographic and Neuropathological Study of the Brain in Epilepsy, With Particular Reference to the Temporal Lobes, Brain 89:499, 1966.

9. Falconer, M.A., Reversibility by Temporal Lobe Resection of the Behavioral Abnormalities of Temporal-Lobe Epilepsy, NEJM 289:451, 1973.

10. Geschwind, N., Editorial: Effects of Temporal Lobe Surgery on Behavior, NEJM 289:480, 1973.

11. Computer Assisted Tomography, Editorial, British Medical Journal June 22, 1974.

12. Kistler, J.P., et al., Computerized Axial Tomography: Clinicopathologic Correlation, Neurology 25:201, 1975.

CASE STUDY #53

A Little Girl with Episodes of Staring and Poor Schoolwork

HISTORY: A seven year-old girl was referred because of difficulty with her lessons at school. Her teacher described her as: "very quiet and tends to be withdrawn and doesn't try."

QUESTION:

1. CONDITIONS THAT COULD PRODUCE THIS BEHAVIOR INCLUDE:
    A. Autism
    B. Mental retardation
    C. Deafness
    D. All of the above

The mother described intermittent episodes lasting about 2 seconds in which her daughter's eyes rolled up and she appeared to be unaware of her surroundings.

QUESTION:

2. THESE EPISODES SUGGEST AN ALTERATION OF CONSCIOUSNESS:
    A. True
    B. False

These first had been noticed at least one year earlier. The frequency was variable. Some days she would have several; on others apparently more than ten. Several episodes might occur within minutes. At other times none would be noticed for several days.

QUESTION:

3. THIS CHILD'S SPELLS MOST LIKELY ARE DUE TO:
    A. Narcolepsy
    B. Transient cerebral ischemia secondary to atherosclerosis
    C. Carotid sinus hypersensitivity
    D. Reactive hypoglycemia
    E. All of the above
    F. None of the above

The mother felt that these usually occurred while her daughter was under stress.

The patient was the product of a normal twin pregnancy, but her sibling died at birth. She appeared in good health in the first year of life with normal milestones: walking at fourteen months, talking intelligible words and phrases at the same time. The family felt that her coordination was normal and that she was developing similarly to her older siblings except for her spells and "quietness."

FAMILY HISTORY: Maternal cousin had one grand mal seizure at age six years, while at a moving picture. Now aged 12 years, she takes an unknown medication three times a day. No other history is available.

PHYSICAL EXAMINATION: A quiet girl who is cooperative, often stating "I can't do that" before attempting to follow the examiner's requests. There was bilateral tonsillar hypertrophy without exudate or hyperemia. Bilateral small lymph nodes were palpated anteriorly and posteriorly in the neck. These were firm, movable, and nontender.

CASE STUDY #53

NEUROLOGICAL EXAMINATION: She is right handed. The exam was completely normal, including copying pictures in a modified Bender-Gestalt test. When hyperventilating for approximately twenty-five seconds, she suddenly stopped over-breathing, her eyes rolled up slightly, conjugately, followed by a "blank look." She then shook her head one time and became responsive.

QUESTIONS:

4. THIS TEST PROVES THAT SHE HAS THE HYPERVENTILATION SYN-
   DROME:
   A. True
   B. False

5. WITH THE HISTORY AND THIS EXAMINATION, HER ENTIRE PROBLEM
   COULD BE CLASSIFIED BEST AS:
   A. Major motor epilepsy
   B. Psychomotor epilepsy
   C. Petit mal (absence) epilepsy
   D. Focal motor epilepsy
   E. The hyperventilation syndrome

6. WITH THE INFORMATION TO DATE, ONE SHOULD PROCEED
   IMMEDIATELY TO:
   A. Carotid angiography
   B. Pneumoencephalography
   C. Institutionalization in a mental hospital
   D. None of the above
   E. All of the above

7. THE TEST MOST LIKELY TO BE HELPFUL IS:
   A. Lumbar puncture
   B. Radio-isotope brain scan
   C. Electroencephalogram
   D. Echoencephalogram

LABORATORY DATA: Fasting blood sugar, BUN, complete blood count, ESR, calcium, skull X-rays: All normal.

EEG INTERPRETATION: 8 cycle per second moderate amplitude alpha pre-dominated from the posterior head regions. Bilaterally synchronous 3 cycle per second generalized spike and wave paroxysmal bursts are seen without clinical seizures (Fig. 64). With hyperventilation, higher voltage slow waves occur and there are further seizure discharges. Several are associated with clinical seizures.

IMPRESSION: This little girl was felt to have petit mal epilepsy, and ethosuximide (Zarontin) was started.

QUESTION:

8. DRUGS CONVENTIONALLY USED IN TREATING PETIT MAL EPILEPSY:
   A. Usually help little with other epilepsy types
   B. Are helpful with other epilepsy types
   C. Must be given by injection
   D. Require careful supervision by the physician in charge of the patient

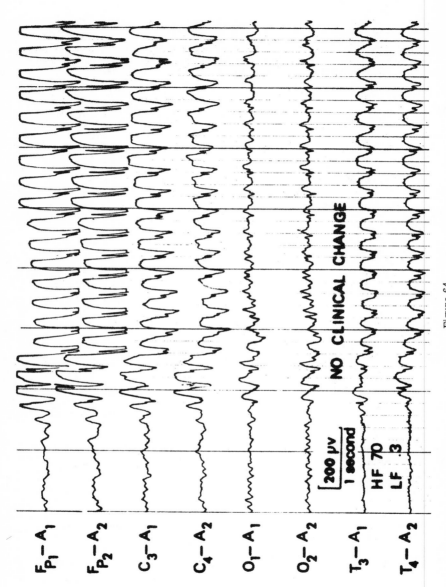

Figure 64

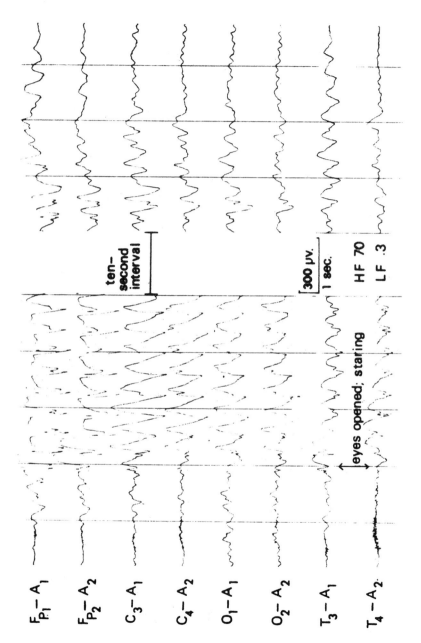

Figure 65

CASE STUDY #53

QUESTIONS:

9. CLASSES OF DRUGS USED IN PETIT MAL INCLUDE:
    A. Succinimides
    B. Oxazolidinediones (diones)
    C. Hydantoins
    D. Phenothiazines
    E. Carbonic anhdrase inhibitors
    F. Amphetamines

10. SIDE EFFECTS ARE MORE COMMON WITH THE SUCCINIMIDES THAN
    WITH THE OXAZOLIDINEDIONES (DIONES):
    A. True
    B. False

11. MATCH THE DRUG USED IN ABSENCE ATTACKS WITH ITS SIDE
    EFFECTS:
    A. ___ Trimethadione (Tridione)   E. Yellow skin
    B. ___ Ethosuximide (Zarontin)   F. Gastrointestinal upset, headache,
    C. ___ Amphetamines   skin rash
    D. ___ Quinacrine (Atabrine)   G. Insomnia, irritability, anorexia
                                         H. Skin rash, light hypersensitivity
                                             (visual), bone marrow depression

12. A SIGNIFICANT PERCENTAGE OF PATIENTS WITH PETIT MAL
    EPILEPSY MAY:
    A. Have fewer or no absence attacks at all as they enter the late teens
    B. Develop major motor (grand mal) epilepsy attacks
    C. Have underlying brain tumors
    D. Have mild mental retardation
    E. All of the above
    F. None of the above

13. IT IS COMMON FOR ADULTS TO HAVE ALTERATIONS OF
    CONSCIOUSNESS DUE TO PETIT MAL ATTACKS BEGINNING IN ADULT
    LIFE:
    A. True
    B. False

14. PETIT MAL EPILEPSY DISCHARGES ARISE IN THE CEREBRAL CORTEX:
    A. True
    B. False

ANSWERS AND DISCUSSION:

1. D   Autism is a psychosis thought to begin in infancy. It is
             characterized by the child's inability to relate to people and
             situations. The child's behavior is withdrawn and non-
             communicative.

             The diagnosis of retardation or deafness may be overlooked
             until the child is evaluated further because of school difficulties.

CASE STUDY #53

2. A   This raises new diagnostic implications. First, it is important to determine that she has actual alterations of consciousness. Then the form of this alteration must be analyzed carefully for proper diagnosis and correct treatment. No previous physician who had seen this girl obtained this vital information.

3. F   Narcolepsy is a syndrome of apparently uncontrollable periods of sleep. Transient cerebral ischemia presents usually with focal neurological symptoms and signs. It would be highly unlikely in this age group, except in rare instances such as children with progeria. Carotid sinus hypersensitivity causes reflex slowing of the heart, and the blood pressure falls when one or both carotid sinuses are massaged. It particularly occurs in the elderly. They may describe their symptoms occurring with sudden head turning, particularly when wearing a tight collar. Reactive hypoglycemia usually causes symptoms such as weakness, hunger, tachycardia, and sweating, following several hours after a large carbohydrate meal. Loss of consciousness is unusual.

4. B

5. C   Some patients with psychomotor epilepsy have episodes that are very brief, without automatisms. In general psychomotor seizures begin at a later age than petit mal, may be associated with an aura, and last longer than petit mal seizures. She has none of the signs of major motor (grand mal) seizures, such as tonic posturing or clonic movements, incontinence, tongue biting, post-ictal confusion or somnolence. Focal motor epilepsy is not suggested by the history or examination. The symptoms of the hyperventilation syndrome include light headedness; tingling of the digits and, occasionally, around the mouth; anxiety and less frequently actual syncope.

6. D   All of the evidence thus far suggests that she has petit mal epilepsy. Nothing suggests a structural lesion of the nervous system. Therefore, the potential risk of contrast procedures is not justified.

7. C   Primary interest is in any seizure discharges and their pattern in the electroencephalogram.

8. AD   This stresses again the importance of proper diagnosis so that correct therapy will be given.

9. ABEF   The diones and succinimides are the major drugs used to treat absence attacks. Carbonic anhydrase inhibitors and amphetamines are used when necessary as adjuncts.

10. B   The succinimides are effective in controlling seizures in the majority of patients with petit mal epilepsy. The succinimides have a much lower incidence of side effects than the diones. Most authorities consider them to be the drugs of choice at the present time in absence attacks. Ethosuximide (Zarontin) is the most used drug of this class.

CASE STUDY #53

11. A---H
     B---F
     C---G
     D---E

12. ABD   Most series agree that petit mal seizures usually stop when the
                  patient enters his late teens or early twenties. However, a
                  significant percentage of children with absence attacks will have
                  major notor seizures as they become older. Centrencephalic
                  (sub-cortical) petit mal epilepsy is not associated with cerebral
                  neoplasms. Recent psychometric studies have shown mild re-
                  tardation in 20% of a large group with petit mal epilepsy.

13. B

14. B   The abnormal discharges begin in the thalamic structures. Then
                they spread bilaterally simultaneously to the cerebral cortex.

COMMENTS: This girl represents a typical example of petit mal epilepsy. The
spell is clinically characterized by absence attacks during which the child stares
for a few seconds. The child also may have minor movements. These most commonly involve the eyes, the eyelids, or the arms. The child usually does not fall.
If the child is talking, speech arrest usually occurs. The petit mal seizure may
be more complex in some cases. Myoclonic and akinetic seizures in the past have
been related to absence attacks. It is now understood that, although some of these
seizure types are closely related to absence attacks, most are associated with
severe and progressive degenerative diseases of the brain. In the susceptible
patient, hyperventilation (causing low carbon dioxide), photic stimulation, and low
blood sugar frequently precipitate absence attacks. The typical electroencephalogram has three cycle per second spike and wave discharges beginning and ending
abruptly. The discharges are diffuse and not focal.

Seizure frequency varies among patients. However, 10-20 seizures a day is not
uncommon. Rarely, usually in the adult with a previous history of petit mal, petit
mal status occurs. Clinically, the patient appears confused. The electroencephalogram again has three cycle per second spike and wave discharges.

The abnormal discharges are thought to originate in deep midline structures, particularly the thalamus. The seizure is then projected diffusely to the cerebral
cortex. Pathologically, no specific lesions have been found associated with absence attacks. This is in marked contrast to the focal epilepsies, such as psychomotor epilepsy, in which focal lesions are frequently found, including neoplasms.
There is a strong genetic predisposition in petit mal epilepsy.

Treatment has been outlined in the answers. Because of the frequency of grand
mal seizures later developing in patients who began with petit mal seizures, there
is some controversy regarding treatment. Some authorities feel that the patient
with petit mal epilepsy who has had no grand mal seizures should be treated "prophylactically" against grand mal, usually with phenobarbital.

CASE STUDY #53

REFERENCES

1. Carter, S., and A. Gold, Convulsions in Children, NEJM 278:315-317 (Feb.) 1968.

2. Charlton, M.H., Borderlands of Petit Mal, Am J Psych 122:669-672, (Dec.) 1965.

3. Charlton, M.H., and M.D. Yahr, Long Term Follow-up of Patients with Petit Mal, Arch Neurol 16:595-598, 1967.

4. Costeff, H., Convulsions of Childhood. Their Natural History and Indications for Treatment, NEJM 273:140-143, 1965.

5. Currier, R.D., K.A. Kooi, and L.J. Saidman, Prognosis of "Pure" Petit Mal; Follow-up Study, Neurology 13:959-967, 1963.

6. Forster, F.M., The Epilepsies and Convulsive Disorders; in Baker, A.B., Clinical Neurology, Vol. 2, Harper and Row, 1971.

7. Jasper, H.H., A.A. Ward, Jr., and A. Pope, Basic Mechanisms of the Epilepsies, Little, Brown and Co., Boston, 1969.

8. Livingston, S., Drug Therapy for Epilepsy, Charles C Thomas, Springfield, 1966.

9. Livingston, S., The Epilepsies. Diagnosis and Treatment. Disease of the Month (July) 1967.

10. Livingston, S., et al., Petit Mal Epilepsy, JAMA 194:227-232, 1965.

11. Merritt, H.H., A Textbook of Neurology, V Ed., Lea and Febiger, Philadelphia, 1973.

12. Metrakos, J.D., and K. Metrakos, Genetics of Convulsive Disorders, I. Introduction, Problems, Methods, and Baselines, Neurology 10:228-240, 1960.

13. Metrakos, J.D., and K. Metrakos, Genetics of Convulsive Disorders, II. Genetic and Electroencephalographic Studies in Centrencephalic Epilepsy, Neurology 11:474-483, 1961.

14. Schmidt, R.P., and B.J. Wilder, Epilepsy, F.A. Davis Co., Philadelphia, 1968.

15. Holowach, J., D.L. Thurston, and J. O'Leary, Prognosis in Childhood Epilepsy, NEJM 286:169, 1972.

16. Rabe, E.F., Editorial: Anticonvulsant Therapy: To Stop or Not to Stop, NEJM 286:213, 1972.

CASE STUDY #54

Unconsciousness in the Sun

HISTORY: A 22 year-old single welder's health was good when he began a fishing vacation preceded by considerable sleep deprivation. In the early afternoon of a hot summer day, he developed a headache beginning in the back of his head. He lay down, looked up at the sun and that is the last he remembered for several hours. Witnesses reported that his body and extremities stiffened and then shook for several seconds. He lay still briefly, then had a much more prolonged tonic-clonic episode, in which he bit his tongue and was incontinent of urine.

QUESTIONS:

1. THE HISTORY IS THAT OF A:
   A. Faint (syncope)
   B. Narcolepsy
   C. Generalized (grand mal) seizure
   D. Psychogenic disturbance
   E. Transient cerebral ischemia
   F. Petit mal epilepsy
   G. Psychomotor epilepsy
   H. Focal motor epilepsy without generalization
   I. All of the above
   J. None of the above

2. FACTORS THAT MAY INFLUENCE SEIZURE THRESHOLD INCLUDE:
   A. Sleep deprivation
   B. Photic stimuli
   C. State of hydration
   D. The use of psychotropic medications
   E. Withdrawal from heavy alcohol ingestion
   F. All of the above
   G. None of the above

3. HISTORY OF POSSIBLE IMPORTANCE AND RELEVANCE INCLUDES:
   A. Family history of epilepsy
   B. Recent other neurological symptoms
   C. A focal component to the seizures
   D. Exposure to toxins
   E. Significant head trauma
   F. All of the above
   G. None of the above

4. COMPLETE HISTORY OF AREAS IN WHICH THE PATIENT HAS RESIDED OR VISITED IS NECESSARY:
   A. True
   B. False

He had no other known neurological symptoms or health problems. The seizures were generalized without focality. There was no known exposure to toxins and he did not drink alcohol to excess. He had lived in California all his life including several visits to the San Joaquin Valley. His father had died two years previously, age 44, of a malignant brain tumor. The father's twin sister had epilepsy, onset at age 13. Her seizures were major motor in type and very difficult to control.

CASE STUDY #54

QUESTION:

5. EPILEPSY MAY BE CLASSIFIED AS EITHER "IDIOPATHIC" OR
   "SYMPTOMATIC":
   A. True
   B. False

PHYSICAL EXAMINATION: A muscular, mildly obese man with a sunburn, in no
distress. He seemed to have slightly below average intelligence. His neck was
supple. He had negative Kernig's and Brudzinski's tests.

QUESTION:

6. WHY ARE THESE TESTS IMPCRTANT HERE?

The skull was normal to palpation; there were no bruits over the eyes, head, and
neck; and the carotid arteries were normal to palpation. There were no cardiac
murmurs.

QUESTION:

7. VALVULAR DISEASE OF THE HEART MAY PRESENT WITH
   CONVULSIONS:
   A. True
   B. False

The lungs were clear and the remaining physical examination was normal, except
for a mild laceration of the tip of the tongue.

NEUROLOGICAL EXAMINATION: Completely normal.

LABORATORY DATA: CBC: Normal. Urinalysis, VDRL, electrolytes, LDH,
prothrombin time, heterophile test, Watson-Schwartz test for porphobilinogen,
skull X-rays: all within normal limits. SGOT: 38 units. Total bilirubin: 1.6
three days after admission; five days after admission: 1.0. Alkaline
phosphatase: borderline three days after admission, normal two days later.

QUESTIONS:

8. THE HETEROPHILE TEST WAS OBTAINED:
   A. Because heterophiles often have convulsions
   B. Because infectious mononeucleosis occasionally causes encephalitis
   C. To rule out parasites
   D. All of the above
   E. None of the above

9. THE URINE WAS EXAMINED FOR THE PRESENCE OF PORPHO-
   BILINOGEN BECAUSE:
   A. Acute intermittent porphyria may present with convulsions
   B. The patient had abnormal liver chemistries
   C. If he had porphyria, a barbiturate anticonvulsant would be
      contraindicated
   D. All of the above
   E. None of the above

CASE STUDY #54

Two hour post-prandial glucose: 170 mg% of glucose; urine positive at one and two hours for glucose.

QUESTION:

10.   SEIZURES ARE OFTEN SEEN IN PRE-DIABETIC PATIENTS WITH REACTIVE HYPOGLYCEMIA:
      A.   True
      B.   False

EEG: Right fronto-temporal slowing; single and poly spikes from the right frontal and temporal electrodes.

Brain scan was negative.

QUESTION:

11.   ISOTOPE SCANS OF THE BRAIN MAY BE A VALUABLE DIAGNOSTIC PROCEDURE IN THE PATIENT WITH EPILEPSY:
      A.   Who has a subdural hematoma
      B.   Who has a CNS neoplasm
      C.   Who has a cerebral infarction
      D.   All of the above
      E.   None of the above

Chest X-ray was normal.   Fasting blood sugar normal.   Spinal fluid: No WBC; one RBC; sugar 70 mg% (concomitant blood sugar 130 mg%); protein 36 mg%.

QUESTION:

12.   THE RATIO BETWEEN SPINAL FLUID AND BLOOD SUGAR OBTAINED AT APPROXIMATELY THE SAME TIME IS:
      A.   Of no diagnostic use
      B.   Of potential help in determining meningeal infection
      C.   Of potential help in determining meningeal carcinomatosis
      D.   Normally that the CSF value approximates 2/3 the blood value
      E.   All of the above
      F.   None of the above

HOSPITAL COURSE: He had symptoms of an upper respiratory infection.   For the first four hospital days he spiked a fever between 100 and 101 degrees Fahrenheit.   Repeated general and neurological examinations were unremarkable otherwise.   He was started with diphenylhydantoin 300 milligrams a day.   He tolerated this well.

QUESTIONS:

13.   SIDE EFFECTS OF DIPHENYLHYDANTOIN:
      A.   Include skin rash in approximately 5% of patients in the first two weeks of therapy
      B.   Include gastric upsets in some patients
      C.   Early in its administration may feature anxiety and insomnia
      D.   All of the above
      E.   None of the above

CASE STUDY #54

14. SERUM DIPHENYLHYDANTOIN LEVELS:
A. Help to determine the patient who is omitting his medication
B. Help to discover the patient taking more medication than prescribed
C. Are useful in finding the rare patient who hypo- or hypermetabolizes the drug
D. Correlate well with symptoms of toxicity
E. All of the above
F. None of the above

On the morning of the seventh day after his first convulsion he began having frequent and repetitive convulsions without regaining consciousness between the seizures. On several occasions these began with movements of the left upper extremity and then became generalized.

QUESTIONS:

15. SEIZURES WITH A FOCAL ONSET:
A. Suggest structural disease of the central nervous system
B. Are frequent in idiopathic epilepsy
C. Suggest pseudo-seizures in hysterics
D. May become generalized through subcortical systems
E. All of the above
F. None of the above

16. WHAT IS CONSIDERED PRESENTLY TO BE THE ANTICONVULSANT DRUG OF CHOICE IN STATUS EPILEPTICUS?:
A. Phenobarbital
B. Diphenylhydantoin (Dilantin)
C. Diazepam (Valium)
D. Primidone (Mysoline)
E. Ethosuximide (Zarontin)

This drug was given intravenously with cessation of the seizures.

QUESTIONS:

17. THIS ANTICONVULSANT, WHEN USED IN THE TREATMENT OF STATUS EPILEPTICUS:
A. Is given orally
B. Is usually given intravenously
C. Has a usual dose of approximately 10 mgs
D. May have side effects of orthostatic hypotension, rarely cardiac arrest associated

18. DANGERS OF STATUS EPILEPTICUS INCLUDE:
A. Hyperpyrexia--deepening coma--death
B. Therapy may lead to cardiac or respiratory arrest
C. Permanent neuronal damage
D. All of the above
E. None of the above

19. SEIZURES ORIGINATE IN:
A. Gray matter
B. White matter

CASE STUDY #54

20. STRUCTURAL LESIONS OF THE NERVOUS SYSTEM ASSOCIATED WITH
    SEIZURES INCLUDE:
    A. Arteriovenous malformations
    B. Primary cerebral neoplasms
    C. Metastatic cerebral neoplasms
    D. Cerebral abscess
    E. All of the above
    F. B, C, D, but not A

SUBSEQUENT EXAMINATION: Petechiae over the posterior pharynx and uvula,
bitten tongue, and extensor plantar response on the left, flexor on the right.

LABORATORY DATA: 14,000 WBC's, 88% segmented polymorphonuclear
leukocytes. All subsequent CBC's: normal. CSF crystal clear, with normal
sugar, no cells, protein 19 mg%. CSF, bacterial and fungal cultures: no growth.
Tissue culture of spinal fluid: no virus isolated. Serum electrolytes, calcium,
phosphorous, repeat blood sugar, serology, blood urea nitrogen, heterophile
test, ESR, blood cultures: all normal. Acute and convalescent viral
serological studies: no rise in titer. All liver chemistries were normal, except
for one SGOT determination of 38 units (normal less than 20 units). Right carotid angiogram: normal. Brain scan: normal. An EEG taken 24 hours after the
last seizure was interpreted as showing a right temporal slow wave focus with
generalized slowing and bilateral fronto-temporal sharp activity.

HOSPITAL COURSE: For three days he ran a low grade fever, never over 100.2
degrees. He was oriented and alert but irritable. He had no further convulsions.
Repeated neurological examinations were normal. From the fourth hospital day
until discharge he was afebrile, and he was no longer irritable. His subsequent
convalescence was unremarkable. He has continued to take phenobarbital and
diphenylhydantoin without side effects. He has had no further seizures.

QUESTIONS:

21. SEIZURES ASSOCIATED WITH FEVER (BUT WITHOUT CNS INFECTION
    OR OTHER CNS PATHOLOGY):
    A. May occur at any age
    B. Rarely occur after 5 years of age
    C. Occur more frequently in children with strong epileptic family history
    D. All of the above
    E. None of the above

22. CONVULSIONS OCCUR IN WHICH OF THE VIRAL INFECTIONS BELOW?:
    A. Poliomyelitis
    B. Herpes simplex
    C. Japanese encephalitis
    D. Rabies
    E. All of the above
    F. None of the above

23. PATIENTS WITH ENCEPHALITIS:
    A. May have convulsions with the acute illness
    B. May convulse as a late complication
    C. May develop a glial scar in the cerebral cortex
    D. May be left with other signs and symptoms of nervous system damage
    E. All of the above
    F. None of the above

CASE STUDY #54

ANSWERS AND DISCUSSION:

1. C   Brief clonic movements, usually of the upper extremities, may occur in syncope. Prolonged tonic and clonic movements are not compatible. The patient with syncope rarely is incontinent. Narcolepsy is a syndrome characterized by repeated episodes of an uncontrollable need to sleep, brief loss of muscle tone, and inability to move when awakening. The tonic posture and then clonic movements are the hallmark of a generalized seizure. Tongue biting and incontinence often result. Although hysterical pseudo-seizures may be very difficult to differentiate from a generalized seizure, in most patients the movements are inconsistent, and pain may arouse them from supposed unconsciousness. Tongue biting and incontinence are rare. The brief staring spells of petit mal attacks are not suggested by the history. Psychomotor epileptics have clouding of consciousness, rarely fall, may smack their lips or chew, have repetitive, seemingly purposeful, movements, and rarely bite their tongues or are incontinent. A focal motor attack without generalization will produce clonic movements of an extremity or part of it without the loss of consciousness or other signs in the history.

2. F

3. F   Recent other neurological symptoms and a focal component to the seizure both suggest a possible underlying structural lesion of the nervous system.

4. A   This is true particularly in this age of rapid travel. Had he come recently from Southeast Asia, malaria with cerebral symptoms would have to be ruled out. Residence in Mexico would suggest the possibility of cysticercosis. As noted in the next paragraph, he had visited the San Joaquin Valley which is a particular reservoir of coccidioidomycosis which may present with cerebral symptoms.

5. A   This is the major thrust of evaluation of the patient with a seizure, whether it is due to an abnormal cerebral discharge without a structural basis that can be demonstrated by present methods of evaluation, or whether the seizures are secondary to structural disease of the nervous system.

6.   Both of these tests for meningeal irritation are important here in evaluating the patient for the presence of meningeal infection, subarachnoid hemorrhage, and, although less likely at his age, the possibility of neoplastic infiltration of the meninges.

7. A

8. B

9. D

10. B   Seizures may occur with hypoglycemia secondary to insulinoma, but are rare in reactive "functional" hypoglycemia, where the symptoms are usually sweating, irritability and nervousness, weakness, hunger and tachycardia.

CASE STUDY #54

11. D — This easily performed and well tolerated test may be of great help in demonstrating any of these structural lesions of the central nervous system.

12. BCD — Although the cerebrospinal fluid sugar follows the blood sugar with a time lag of approximately two hours, for practical reasons the blood sugar is usually drawn just before lumbar puncture when it is felt that the cerebrospinal fluid sugar may be an important determination. If the spinal fluid sugar determination is important, and the patient's status is such that he will suffer no ill effects from delay in doing the lumbar puncture, the most accurate determination of both blood sugar and spinal fluid would be performed in the fasting state. As an example, a spinal fluid sugar of 50 mg% which is "normal" may be actually abnormally low if the patient's blood sugar at the same time is 250 mg%. This illustrates the potential extreme importance of doing both determinations.

13. D — For these reasons the patient should be warned of the possible side effects. The medicine may be better tolerated if taken with meals or if taken at bedtime with a glass of milk. Further common side effects of diphenylhydantoin include gingival hyperplasia and hirsutism. Less common are liver disease, megaloblastic anemia, exfoliative dermatitis, and granulocytopenia. Recent evidence suggests that bone marrow depression may be dose related. Rarely the drug has been linked with aplastic anemia, a lupus erythematosus syndrome, generalized lymphadenopathy, and a lymphoma syndrome that may or may not reverse with cessation of the drug. Peripheral neuropathy may develop. It has been suggested that long term use leads to coarsening of the facial features. Possible teratogenic effects are under investigation. Diphenylhydantoin interacts with certain other drugs, such as dicoumarol, isoniazid, phenothiazines and aminosalicylic acid. This may depress normal hepatic metabolism and lead to toxic reactions. Nystagmus and ataxia are the most common signs of overdosage, beginning to appear at serum levels of 20 micrograms/milliliter or higher of diphenylhydantoin. Diphenylhydantoin tends to crystallize after intramuscular injection and is poorly and unevenly absorbed.

14. E — Serum diphenylhydantoin and phenobarbital levels now may be determined with accuracy by gas-liquid chromatography. The most practical application of this test occurs in the patient who swears he is taking the prescribed diphenylhydantoin correctly, but whose seizures are not being controlled and who has a low blood level of the drug. This is compatible with undermedication due to not taking the medicine in prescribed amounts in all except the rare instances of the patient who metabolized the drug unusually rapidly in the liver. The converse is the patient who presents with slurred speech, ataxia, and falling, suggesting over-medication, and who claims to be taking the proper dose, but whose Dilantin level is elevated into the toxic range.

15. AD

16. C — Phenobarbital prior to the use of diazepam was one of the drugs most frequently used for status epilepticus, along with paraldehyde and even massive doses of diphenylhydantoin by some workers. As Valium is not invariably effective against patients in status epilepticus, other drugs may have to be used on occasion. These include phenobarbital and paraldehyde. On rare occasions general anesthesia is used.

CASE STUDY #54

17. BCD

18. D

19. A

20. E

21. BC   In the adult, fever and seizures suggest intracranial pathology, par-
            ticularly infections such as viral encephalitis, meningitis, cerebral
            abscess and venous sinus thrombosis. In children under five years,
            often with a family history of epilepsy, seizures may occur associated
            with fever without any evidence of intracranial pathology.

22. BCD

23. E

COMMENTS: The physician with a patient who has a probable seizure disorder
should be aware of the features of the common seizure types, be able to elicit
relevant historical information, and perform an adequate neurological examination.
He then must use this information for accurate seizure classification, formulation
of differential diagnosis and treatment plan. Seizure classification may be difficult
and there are many different classifications in use. The differential diagnosis is
first between seizures and other paroxysmal disorders such as syncope and cerebral ischemia. If the patient is thought to have seizures, it must be determined
whether the seizure type is generalized or partial and focal, and whether they are
idiopathic or secondary to focal or diffuse intracranial disease or to extracranial
factors.

Idiopathic generalized epilepsy is related to genetic factors that influence the
brain's seizure threshold. Intracranial lesions that may be associated with seizures include trauma, infection, degeneration, vascular lesions and neoplasm.
Extracranial causes include anoxia, endocrine disorders, and endogenous or exogenous toxins. This patient clearly had seizures. The major problems were:

    1. Determining if there was an underlying structural lesion of the central
nervous system or an extracranial etiology causing his seizures.

    2. Controlling his seizures.

Several factors that may precipitate seizures in a susceptible individual should be
considered here, e.g., sleep deprivation, a heavier alcohol intake than admitted
to the examining physicians, and photic stimulation caused by intermittent eye
blinking while lying in the sun. The low grade fever continuing for several days,
the upper respiratory infection and the abnormal liver chemistries suggested the
possibility of another process occurring, in particular, a viral infection. The
patient appeared to be doing well, with no symptoms, no fever, and return to normal of all of his laboratory tests excepting the electroencephalogram, when he
went into status epilepticus. The focal onset of some of his seizures, left Babinski response, and the right frontotemporal slow wave focus of the EEG further
suggested the possibility that he was suffering from an underlying structural lesion
of the central nervous system, such as encephalitis secondary to a viral agent, a
cerebral abscess, a cerebral neoplasm, or arteriovenous malformation. No definite etiology was found, but a viral encephalitis remained most likely. Cells are
usually found in the spinal fluid in viral encephalitis, particularly with meningeal
involvement, but the absence of cells does not rule out encephalitis. For a 7 year
follow-up period he has been seizure free with normal neurological examinations.
Repeat EEG's have all been normal. Intravenous diazepam (Valium) helped stop
his status epilepticus. Long-term seizure control was attained with diphenylhydantoin and phenobarbital.

CASE STUDY #54

In summary, the patient exemplifies the necessity for careful and repeated neurological, general physical, laboratory and special procedural examinations, in a
search for specific anatomical or biochemical lesions, and to solve the problems
of acute and chronic seizure control.

REFERENCES

1. Griggs, W. L. III, Modern Treatment 8:258-276, Harper and Row, New York,
1971.

2. Merritt, H. H., A Textbook of Neurology, 5th Ed., Lea and Febiger, Philadelphia, 1973.

3. Millichap, J. G. (ed.), Modern Treatment 6:1177, 1275, Harper and Row,
New York, 1969.

4. Nicol, C. F., J. C. Tutton, and B. H. Smith, Parenteral Diazepam in Status
Epilepticus, Neurology 19:332, 1969.

5. Prensky, A. L., et al., Intravenous Diazepam in the Treatment of Prolonged
Seizure Activity, New Eng J Med 276:779, 1967.

6. Schmidt, R. P., and B. J. Wilder, Epilepsy, F. A. Davis Co., Philadelphia,
1968.

7. Kutt, H., and F. McDowell, Management of Epilepsy with Diphenylhydantoin
Sodium, JAMA 203:969, 1968.

8. Buchanan, R. A., et al., Diphenylhydantoin (Dilantin) Following Once-Daily
Administration, Neurol 22:126-130, February 1972.

9. Johnson, L. C., et al., Diagnostic Factors in Adult Males Following Initial
Seizures, Arch Neurol 27:193, 1972.

10. Solow, E. B., and J. B. Green, Simultaneous Determination of Multiple Anticonvulsant Drug Levels by Gas-Liquid Chromatography, Neurol 22:540-550,
May 1972.

11. Gunderson, C. M., and P. B. Dunne, Sleep Withdrawal Seizures, Neurol
23:678, 1973.

12. Sherwin, A. L., et al., Anticonvulsant Drugs in Human Epileptogenic Brain.
Correlation of Phenobarbital and Diphenylhydantoin Levels with Plasma,
Arch Neurol 29:73, 1973.

13. Wilensky, A. J., Inadequate Serum Levels After Intramuscular Administration
of Diphenylhydantoin, Neurology 23:318, 1973.

CASE STUDY #55

A Woman with Tingling Fingers

HISTORY: This 43 year-old housewife and professional house cleaner was in good
health until three years ago when she first experienced pain in her right hand while
bowling. She did not recall the exact location of the pain or its quality. Since that
time, she felt intermittent sensations of "pins and needles in the thumb, index,
and middle fingers."

QUESTION:

1. THE PERIPHERAL NERVE THAT SUPPLIES SENSATION TO THESE DIGITS
IS:
A. The ulnar nerve
B. The median nerve
C. The peroneal nerve
D. The musculo-cutaneous nerve
E. The radial nerve

CASE STUDY #55

The pins and needles sensations initially occurred after she arose in the morning, but for several weeks the sensations were so intense that they awakened her. She noted several weeks of vague discomfort in the wrist. When she tried to use her fingers in the morning, they were stiff and she was unable to close her hand. It took her approximately one hour to work out the stiffness so that her hand and fingers were normally flexible.

QUESTION:

2. IF THE DIGITAL PAIN WAS ACCOMPANIED BY BLANCHING OF THE FINGERS:
   A. This would be important to know
   B. It is not important to know
   C. This would suggest Raynaud's phenomenon
   D. All of the above
   E. None of the above

She characteristically sleeps on her stomach with the right extremity hanging over the side of the bed in dependent position.

QUESTION:

3. THIS POSITION COULD:
   A. Compress the neuro-vascular bundle entering the right arm
   B. Stretch the cervical nerve roots
   C. Cause edema of hand and digits
   D. Cause a "Saturday night palsy"
   E. All of the above
   F. None of the above

The only other times that she noted the problem was when driving her automobile with the right hand cocked-up on top of the steering wheel, and when her work on the job required repetitive hyperextension of the wrist.

She denied any significant past illness, and specifically denied diabetes, thyroid disease, any form of arthritis or trauma. The family history was not contributory. She took no medications other than aspirin.

QUESTIONS:

4. WHAT MEDICATION(S) CAN CAUSE TINGLING DIGITS?
   A. Acetazolamide (Diamox)
   B. Ergot alkaloids
   C. Methysergide (Sansert)
   D. Calcium gluconate
   E. Vincristine
   F. All of the above
   G. None of the above

CASE STUDY #55

5.   IN THE ABOVE PROBLEMS, DIGITAL SYMPTOMS:
      A. Usually involve all the digits
      B. Usually involve one or two digits

EXAMINATION: A muscular, tall woman in no distress. BP - 130/84, both
arms equal. Pulses were equal, with normal thoracic outlet tests and negative
cervical root compression tests, and with full range of motion of the cervical
spine.

QUESTIONS:

6.   IF HER PROBLEM WERE DUE TO CERVICAL ROOT DISEASE:
      A. In most cases pain is produced by neck hyperextension
      B. The pain would not go to the fingers
      C. There usually is decreased range of motion of the neck
      D. The most common cause is a cervical disc protrusion
      E. All of the above
      F. None of the above

7.   PAIN FROM INVOLVEMENT OF WHICH ROOT USUALLY RADIATES
      INTO THE THUMB ?:
      A. C4
      B. C5
      C. C6
      D. C7
      E. C8
      F. T1

8.   THIS ROOT IS INVOLVED BY DISC PROTRUSION AT WHICH
      INTERSPACE?:
      A. C2-3
      B. C3-4
      C. C4-5
      D. C5-6
      E. C6-7
      F. C7-8

9.   IF THAT ROOT WERE INVOLVED, ONE MIGHT FIND WEAKNESS IN
      WHICH MUSCLE(S)?:
      A. In the biceps
      B. In the brachioradialis
      C. In the triceps
      D. In the small hand muscles
      E. All of the above
      F. None of the above

10.   IF THESE SAME MUSCLES WERE INVOLVED IN PERIPHEREAL NERVE
      LESIONS:
      A. A radial nerve lesion could do this
      B. An ulnar nerve lesion could do this
      C. Only a combined musculo-cutaneous nerve and radial nerve lesion
          could cause this
      D. A musculo-cutaneous lesion alone could cause this

PHYSICAL EXAMINATION: Inspection and palpation of both wrists appeared to
be normal. There was no definite atrophy of the hand muscles on either side.

CASE STUDY #55

NEUROLOGICAL EXAMINATION: Strength - normal except for: slight weakness in opposition and flexion of the right thumb. Sensation: mild decreased perception of pin and temperature, more than touch, of the first three digits, most marked in the plantar pad of the thumb. Percussion with a soft rubber hammer over the median nerve in the wrist on the right produced tingling and pain in the first three digits. There was no response to percussion over the left median nerve. She experienced increasing discomfort and numbness and tingling paresthesiae with flexion of the right wrist for 60 seconds. A blood pressure cuff was inflated at a level between her systolic and diastolic blood pressure and held at that level for two minutes. This produced pain and tingling in the first three digits of the right hand, but was without effect on the left.

QUESTIONS:

COMPARE AND CONTRAST NERVE ROOT DISEASE WITH PERIPHERAL NERVE DISEASE BY MATCHING (ANSWER MAY BE ONE, BOTH, OR NEITHER):

11. ___ Pain or paresthesias intensified often by cough or sneeze   A. Root disease

12. ___ Pain or paresthesias distally produced by percussion over a nerve   B. Peripheral nerve disease

13. ___ May have dermatome sensory loss   C. Neither

14. ___ Atrophy of muscle

15. ___ Weakness of muscles   D. Both

16. ___ Reflex loss or diminution

17. IF THIS PATIENT HAD ATROPHY SECONDARY TO INVOLVEMENT OF THE MEDIAN NERVE:
A. All the small muscles of the hand would be affected
B. It would be in the lateral part of the thenar eminence
C. It would be seen to involve all the small hand muscles except the lateral thenar group
D. All of the above
E. None of the above

18. ATROPHY OF ALL OF THE SMALL MUSCLES OF THE HAND:
A. Occurs in polyneuropathy
B. Occurs in motor neuron disease (amyotrophic lateral sclerosis)
C. Can be seen in combined eighth cervical and first thoracic root lesions
D. All of the above
E. None of the above

19. WHAT BLOOD TESTS WOULD YOU LIKE TO OBTAIN?

20. WHAT ELECTRICAL TESTS WOULD YOU LIKE TO OBTAIN?

LABORATORY DATA: Nerve conduction velocities were measured for both the right and left median nerve. For the right median nerve, the terminal latency was delayed at 6.3 milliseconds. For the left median nerve it was 3.3 milliseconds. There was no nerve action potential recordable at the wrist with stimulation of the right third finger. In contrast, stimulation of the right fifth finger resulted in a normal 10 microvolt nerve action potential at the wrist. (An electrical stimulus is applied distally to a digital nerve. Recording electrodes are placed on the skin over the appropriate median or ulnar nerve, and the action potential is measured.) EMG was compatible with partial denervation of muscles supplied by the median nerve.

CASE STUDY #55

QUESTIONS:

21.   THESE FINDINGS WOULD BE COMPATIBLE WITH:
        A. Right ulnar nerve palsy
        B. Right median nerve compression at the elbow
        C. Right median nerve compression at the wrist
        D. Left median nerve compression at the wrist
        E. All of the above
        F. None of the above

22.   THIS COMMON PROBLEM IS KNOWN AS THE:
        A. Carpal tunnel syndrome
        B. Thoracic outlet syndrome
        C. Scalenus anticus syndrome
        D. Shoulder-hand syndrome

COURSE: It was elected to treat this patient first with a removable splint that
held her wrist in the "neutral" position, neither flexed nor extended. It was
particularly urged that she wear this while sleeping. She continued her heavy
work, and found only slight relief from her symptoms. Therefore, she was
injected with 40 milligrams of methylprednisolone after sterile preparation.

QUESTIONS:

23.   YOU WOULD WANT TO MAKE THIS INJECTION:
        A. Into the right carpal tunnel
        B. Into the right olecranon bursa
        C. Into the thenar eminence
        D. Into the finger tips

Despite continuing with her work and wearing the neutral position splint only at
night, she experienced complete relief of her symptoms.

24.   A HIGH PERCENTAGE OF PATIENTS TREATED THIS WAY EXPERIENCE
        INITIAL COMPLETE RELIEF OF SYMPTOMS:
        A. True
        B. False

25.   IF MULTIPLE INJECTIONS ARE NOT HELPFUL:
        A. Nothing further can be done for the patient's problem
        B. The transcarpal ligament may be severed surgically
        C. The nerve may be surgically translocated anteriorly
        D. All of the above
        E. None of the above

26.   IN THE CARPAL TUNNEL SYNDROME:
        A. Clinical tests may be within normal limits (percussion of the nerve in
            the wrist, hyper-extension or flexion of the hand)
        B. Clinical tests are always abnormal
        C. Even with normal clinical examination, the electromyogram may be
            abnormal
        D. Even with abnormal clinical examination, the electromyogram may be
            normal
        E. All of the above
        F. None of the above

CASE STUDY #55

ANSWERS AND DISCUSSION:

1. B

2. AC   Cyanosis of the digits suggests Raynaud's phenomenon, and implies peripheral vascular spasm or occlusion.

3. ACD   "Saturday night palsy" is weakness of muscles supplied by the radial nerve secondary to mechanical compression of the nerve and its blood supply as it winds around the humerus. It occurs most often in people who fall asleep after excess drug or excess alcohol ingestion with one arm draped over the back of the chair. (See case 15.)

4. ABCE   The ergot alkaloids and methysergide may be associated on occasion with serious vascular spasm and occlusion. Vincristine is an anti-metabolite used in the chemotherapy of cancer. It can cause paresthesias and neuropathy.

5. A

6. ACD

7. C

8. D   In the cervical region the nerve roots emerge from the spinal canal superior to the vertebral body of the same number. Below the cervical region, because of the presence of an 8th cervical nerve root with only seven cervical vertebra, the nerve roots emerge via their foramina below their numbered vertebral body.

9. AB

10. C   This contrasts a C6 root lesion which could cause weakness in the biceps and brachio-radialis muscles with functional weakness of supination and flexion of the forearm. This can be distinguished easily from weakness of the brachio-radialis due to radial nerve involvement. That would cause weakness also of extension of the wrist and of the digits of the hand, and if the involvement was sufficiently proximal, weakness of the triceps. An isolated lesion of the musculo-cutaneous nerve would cause weakness of the biceps muscle.

11. A

12. B

13. A

14. D

15. D

16. D

17. B

18. D

CASE STUDY #55

19.   Sedimentation rate. Rheumatoid test, thyroid tests such as a
                     T_3 and T_4, and a two hour postprandial sugar.

20.   Electromyography with motor and sensory nerve conduction
                     tests.

21. C

22. A

23. A

24. A   Unfortunately, this initial relief may be of short duration.

25. B   This maneuver releases pressure on the median nerve in most
                     cases. It is accompanied by relief of symptoms in a high
                     percentage of patients.

26. ACD   This makes it mandatory for the examining physician to
                     carefully evaluate all of the evidence before making or
                     discarding the diagnosis.

REFERENCES

1.   Robbins, H., Anatomical Study of the Median Nerve in the Carpal Tunnel:
     Etiologies of the Carpal Tunnel Syndrome, J Bone Joint Surg 45:953-966,
     1963.

2.   Phillips, R.S., Carpal Tunnel Syndrome as a Manifestation of Systemic
     Disease, J Bone Joint Surg 48:588, 1966.

3.   Phalen, G.S., Reflections on Twenty-one Years Experience with the
     Carpal Tunnel Syndrome, JAMA 212:1365-1367, 1970.

4.   Phalen, G.S., The Carpal Tunnel Syndrome: Seventeen Years Experience
     in Diagnosis and Treatment of Six Hundred Fifty-four Hands, J Bone Joint
     Surg 48-A:211-228, 1966.

5.   Roos, D.B., and J.C. Owens, Thoracic Outlet Syndrome, Arch Surg 93:71,
     1966.

6.   Thomas, J.E., et al., Electrodiagnostic Aspects of the Carpal Tunnel
     Syndrome, Arch Neurol 16:635-641, 1967.

7.   Hamlin, E., Jr., and R.A.W. Lehman, Carpal Tunnel Syndrome, NEJM
     276:849-850, 1967.

8.   Thompson, W.A.L., and H.P. Kopell, Peripheral Entrapment
     Neuropathies of the Upper Extremity, NEJM 260:1261-1265, 1959.

9.   Cervical Rib or Carpal Tunnel? Lancet 1:588, 1971.

CASE STUDY #56

A Woman with Fever, Stupor, and Seizures

HISTORY: A 54 year-old woman complained of a diffuse headache on the way home from an evening of square dancing. Her friends said that her speech "didn't make sense." The next day her speech was normal, but she had a fever of 102 and was brought to the hospital. She had been previously well except for chronic otitis media.

In the emergency area she had a seizure, consisting of twitching of the right arm and leg and turning of the head and eyes to the right, lasting several minutes; temperature was 102. General physical examination was negative, except for a perforation of the right tympanic membrane. She was sleepy, but easily aroused. She replied "I don't know" to all questions. Deep tendon reflexes were increased in the right arm and leg; there was a right Babinski sign, right hemiparesis and right hemianopsia. She had neither nuchal rigidity nor a Kernig sign.

QUESTIONS:

1. THIS PATIENT'S LESION IS IN THE:
   A. Mesencephalon
   B. Left cerebral hemisphere
   C. Pons
   D. Cerebellum

Skull films and an echoencephalogram were normal. Lumbar puncture was performed.

2. IF UPON ENTRY OF THE LUMBAR PUNCTURE NEEDLE INTO THE SUBARACHNOID SPACE, THE CEREBROSPINAL FLUID EMERGED VERY RAPIDLY FROM THE NEEDLE TIP, THIS WOULD SIGNIFY INCREASED INTRACRANIAL PRESSURE, AND THE LUMBAR PUNCTURE SHOULD BE IMMEDIATELY DISCONTINUED.
   A. True
   B. False

The fluid was clear. Opening pressure was 90 mm H_2O. There were 6 RBC and 452 WBC/cu. mm. 30% of the white cells were polymorphonuclear, 70% mononuclear. Sugar was 65 mgm%, total protein 66 mgm%. Gram stain negative. Blood count and blood sugar were normal.

QUESTIONS:

3. AT THIS POINT, IMPORTANT DIAGNOSTIC POSSIBILITIES INCLUDE:
   A. Tuberculous meningitis
   B. Acute pyogenic meningitis
   C. Bacterial cerebritis
   D. Brain abscess
   E. Viral meningoencephalitis

4. IF THE SPINAL FLUID SUGAR HAD BEEN 20 MGM%, WHICH OF THE ABOVE LIST OF DIAGNOSTIC POSSIBILITIES WOULD HAVE BEEN EXCLUDED?

5. THE BEST WAY TO MANAGE THE SEIZURE PROBLEM NOW WOULD BE WITH:
   A. Intramuscular Dilantin
   B. Intramuscular phenobarbital
   C. Either of the above

CASE STUDY #56

6. OTHER USEFUL TESTS AT THIS POINT WOULD BE:
   A. Electroencephalogram
   B. Brain scan
   C. Computerized Axial Tomography
   D. Ophthalmodynanometry
   E. Electromyogram

Electroencephalogram showed a focus of 3-5cps slow activity over the left temporal lobe with lesser degrees of slowing over the entire left hemisphere. Brain scan showed a large zone of increased uptake in the left temporal lobe. Left carotid arteriogram was normal.

COURSE: Multiple cultures were taken, and the patient was started on high doses of penicillin and chloromycetin. Blood and spinal fluid cultures were negative. Over the next week, she remained obtunded with a right hemiparesis. A repeat carotid angiogram was normal. Lumbar puncture now showed 53 WBC/cu. mm., all mononuclear, protein 24 mgm%, sugar normal, india ink preparation negative; chest film showed bilateral pneumonia; bitemporal delta slowing was seen on the electroencephalogram. A repeat brain scan again showed a focus of increased uptake in the left temporal lobe. Right focal and major motor seizures continued intermittently in spite of anticonvulsant therapy; she remained mute and obtunded. Both plantar responses were extensor. Antibiotics were discontinued after two weeks of treatment. A repeat spinal tap now was entirely normal. She gradually became comatose and would react to painful stimuli with decerebrate posturing.

QUESTIONS:

7. WHAT DO YOU THINK IS THE PROBABLE DIAGNOSIS?

8. WHAT DIAGNOSTIC STEPS WOULD YOU TAKE TO PROVE IT?

The patient was found dead in bed six weeks after admission. Antibody titer to herpes simplex had risen from 1:4 several days after admission to 1:64 two weeks later; antibody titers to a variety of other viruses did not rise. The general autopsy showed pulmonary emboli and aspiration pneumonia. Grossly the brain showed striking destruction and softening in the left temporal lobe. (See Fig. 66)

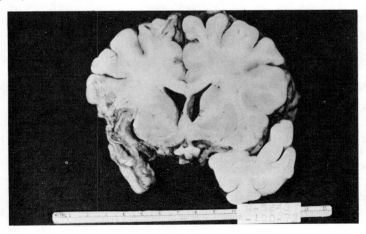

Figure 66

CASE STUDY #56

Microscopically there was necrosis of the left temporal lobe cortex with some extension into the white matter, perivascular round cell cuffing and gliosis. No inclusion bodies were seen. The meninges showed only rare focal accumulations of round cells.

QUESTIONS:

9. THE DRUG WHICH HAS BEEN USED MOST OFTEN IN THE TREATMENT OF THIS DISEASE HAS BEEN:
   A. L-Dopa
   B. Antilymphocyte globulin
   C. Idoxuridine
   D. Tetrabenazine
   E. Gentamicin
   F. Interferon

10. TOXICITY AND SIDE EFFECTS OF THIS DRUG INCLUDE:
    A. Thrombocytopenia
    B. Leukopenia
    C. Alopecia
    D. Secondary infection
    E. Stomatitis
    F. All of the above

ANSWERS AND DISCUSSION:

1. B   The focal seizure and hemianopsia localize the lesion to the contra-lateral cerebral hemisphere. Occasionally one sees hemiparesis or hemianopsia as "false localizing signs" ipsilateral to a cerebral lesion, due to shifting of the brain and compression of the contra-lateral cerebral peduncle or posterior cerebral artery against the tentorial edge.

2. B   The rate of spinal fluid flow from the needle cannot be used as a gauge of intracranial pressure. A slow flow may be caused by the needle tip lying against a nerve root, or a more rapid flow may be seen in a tense patient who is tightening his abdominal muscles and increasing intraabdominal pressure.

3. CDE In untreated acute purulent meningitis there is a low sugar and poly-morphonuclear preponderance in the spinal fluid. If the bacterial meningitis has been partially treated with antibiotics, however, the spinal fluid sugar may be normal. Tuberculous meningitis typically shows a lymphocytic white cell preponderance and decreased sugar. Although brain abscess is an important diagnostic consideration in a patient with chronic ear infection, fever, and hemiparesis, the short, one day history of neurological symptoms prior to admission is against this diagnosis.

4.   A low spinal fluid sugar would not absolutely exclude any of the given diagnoses. The spinal fluid sugar is usually normal in brain abscess unless bacteria have invaded the meninges. In rare instances of viral meningitis, the spinal fluid sugar may be low. This has been reported with various viruses, including mumps, herpes simplex and herpes zoster. The rarity of this finding, however, emphasizes that when the spinal fluid sugar is low then the diagnosis of viral men-ingitis can only be made after vigorous exclusion of all of the other more probable (and treatable) alternatives.

5. B   Dilantin is poorly absorbed from intramuscular sites. Even if given intravenously, very large doses of about 1000 mgm are necessary to achieve adequate anticonvulsant blood levels rapidly.

CASE STUDY #56

6. ABC

9. C

10. F

DISCUSSION: Herpes simplex encephalitis is the most common type of sporadic encephalitis in this country. Fever, psychosis, and focal neurological symptoms and signs are a frequent clinical triad. Seizures, coma and papilledema may be present. Brainstem or myelitic clinical presentations have been reported.[3,11] The spinal fluid usually shows a few to several hundred white cells/cu. mm. with a round cell preponderance, moderate increase in protein, and with very rare exceptions, a normal sugar. The EEG may show diffuse or asymmetrical and focal slowing or periodic complexes against a diffuse slow wave background. Brain scan and angiography may show a focal mass lesion, and the possibility of tumor or abscess may not be ruled out until after craniotomy.

Pathological findings include hemorrhagic necrosis of grey and white matter, mononuclear perivascular cuffing and intranuclear inclusions within neurons and glial cells. Although all areas of the brain may be affected, the orbital region of the frontal lobe and the inferior and mesial portions of the temporal lobe are particularly susceptible to this disease for reasons that are not understood.

Specific diagnosis is confirmed by the pathological findings at brain biopsy, immunofluorescent identification of viral antigen, and isolation of the virus from the brain. Serum antibody rises to H. simplex virus support the diagnosis, but are not completely reliable, as increases in antibody titer to herpes simplex have been reported with other infections perhaps due to nonspecific activation of latent or intercurrent herpesvirus.

Recent reports[14] of immunofluorescent demonstration of viral antigens in cells in the spinal fluid are encouraging and this technique may permit rapid and specific diagnosis without brain biopsy.

The overall mortality in herpes simplex encephalitis is about 50%. The prognosis is worse for the comatose patient. Permanent neurological abnormalities in survivors are common.

Idoxuridine and cytosine arabinoside have been the most commonly used drugs in the treatment of herpetic encephalitis. There are many reports in the literature involving small numbers of patients with either optimistic or pessimistic conclusions about the value of these drugs. A recent controlled study concluded that idoxuridine was both highly toxic and clinically ineffective. Adrenal corticosteroids have been reported to be of benefit possibly via the mechanism of decreasing cerebral edema.

REFERENCES

1. Case Records of the Massachusetts General Hospital, New Eng J Med 271:1313, 1964.

2. Kent, T., and D. Nicholson, Herpes Simplex Encephalitis, Am J Dis Children 108:644, 1964.

3. Encephalitis Due to Herpes Simplex Virus, Editorial, New Eng J Med Aug. 12, 1965.

CASE STUDY #56

4. Encephalitis Caused by Herpes Simplex Virus, Editorial, New Eng J Med 277:1315, 1967.

5. Meyer, J.S., et al., Herpesvirus Hominis Encephalitis, Arch Neurol 23:438, 1970.

6. Van Welsum, R., et al., The Protein Composition of the Cerebrospinal Fluid in Acute Necrotizing Encephalitis, Neurology 20:996, 1970.

7. Hanshaw, J., Idoxuridine in Herpesvirus Encephalitis, New Eng J Med 282:47, 1970.

8. Gurwith, M., et al., Approach to Diagnosis and Treatment of Herpes Simplex Encephalitis, Calif Med 115:63, 1971.

9. Fishman, M., et al., Failure of Idoxuridine Treatment in Herpes Simplex Encephalitis, Am J Dis Child 122:250, 1971.

10. Rappel, M., et al., Diagnosis and Treatment of Herpes Encephalitis, J Neurol Sci 12:443, 1971.

11. Dayan, A., et al., Brain Stem Encephalitis Caused by Herpesvirus Hominis, Brit Med J Nov. 18, 1972.

12. Johnson, K., et al., Herpes Simplex Encephalitis, Arch Neurol 27:103, 1972.

13. Klastersky, J., et al., Ascending Myelitis in Association with Herpes Simplex Virus, New Eng J Med 287:181, 1972.

14. Dayan, A., Rapid Diagnosis of Encephalitis by Immunofluorescent Examination of Cerebrospinal Fluid Cells, Lancet Jan. 27, 1973.

15. Farris, W., et al., Cytarabine Treatment of Herpes Simplex Encephalitis, Arch Neurol 27:99, 1972.

16. Weinstein, L., et al., The Chemotherapy of Viral Infections, New Eng J Med 289:725, 1973.

17. Nolan, D., et al., Idoxuridine in Herpes Simplex Virus Encephalitis, Ann Int Med 78:243, 1973.

18. Sarubbi, F., Herpesvirus Hominis Encephalitis, Arch Neurol 29:268, 1973.

19. Rennick, P., et al., Neuropsychologic and Neurologic Follow-up After Herpesvirus Hominis Encephalitis, Neurology 23:42, 1973.

20. Serrano, E., et al., Plasma Diphenylhydantoin Values After Oral and Intramuscular Administration of Diphenylhydantoin, Neurology 23:311, 1973.

21. Wilensky, A., Inadequate Serum Levels After Intramuscular Administration of Dilantin, Neurology 23:318, 1973.

22. Wallis, W., et al., Intravenous Diphenylhydantoin in Treatment of Acute Repetitive Seizures, Neurology 18:513, 1968.

23. Wolf, S.M., Decreased Cerebrospinal Glucose Level in Herpes Zoster Meningitis, Arch Neurol 30:109, 1973.

CASE STUDY #56

24. Rosenthal, M.S., Viral Infections of the Central Nervous System, Med Clin N Am 58:593, 1974.

25. Boston Interhospital Virus Study Group, Failure of High Dose 5-Iodo-2-Deoxy-uridine in the Therapy of Herpes Simplex Virus Encephalitis, New Eng J Med 292:599, 1975.

26. Elian, M., Herpes Simplex Encephalitis, Arch Neurology 32:39, 1975.

27. Harford, C., Isolation of Herpes Simplex Virus from the Cerebrospinal Fluid in Viral Meningitis, Neurology 25:198, 1975.

CASE STUDY #57

A Physician with a Dilated Pupil

HISTORY: While dining by candlelight, a young physician's wife noted that her husband's left pupil was widely dilated. They had been married for five years and neither had been previously aware of a difference in the size of his pupils. The following day he was examined by a neurologist.

QUESTION:

1. A UNILATERAL DILATED PUPIL MAY BE CAUSED BY:
   A. A lesion in the mesencephalon
   B. Interruption of the third nerve beneath the brain stem
   C. A lesion in the superior cervical ganglion
   D. Eyedrops
   E. Any of the above

The patient's only other complaint was intermittent, right-sided, throbbing head-aches. These were not associated with nausea, vomiting, visual disturbances or any other neurological symptoms. He had been free of headache for several months before the anisocoria was noted. He had never experienced diplopia, weak-ness of the extremities or any change in vision. He did not use eyedrops.

EXAMINATION: He was fully alert. His neck was supple. Neurologic examina-tion was negative, except for the size and behavior of the pupils. The right pupil measured 2 mm. in diameter, the left 5 mm. Both were round and regular. The right pupil reacted briskly to light, both directly and consensually; the left did not react, either directly or consensually. Extraocular movements were normal.

QUESTIONS:

2. THIS PATTERN OF PUPILLARY BEHAVIOR INDICATES INTERRUPTION OF THE:
   A. Afferent arc of the light reflex on the right
   B. Afferent arc of the light reflex on the left
   C. Efferent arc of the light reflex on the right
   D. Efferent arc of the light reflex on the left

CASE STUDY #57

3. BASED ON THE INFORMATION AVAILABLE SO FAR, THE MOST PROBABLE
   DIAGNOSIS IS:
   A. Aneurysm of the posterior communicating artery
   B. Third nerve palsy due to diabetes mellitus
   C. Ophthalmoplegic migraine
   D. A brain tumor causing transtentorial herniation of the temporal lobe with
      pressure on the third nerve
   E. Weber's syndrome
   F. Benedikt's syndrome
   G. Idiopathic third nerve palsy
   H. None of the above

EXAMINATION CONTINUED: The right pupil reacted briskly in convergence, but
the left did not change size. When convergence was sustained, the left pupil constricted slowly and steadily until it grew smaller than the right. When the convergence effort was relaxed, it took 45 seconds for the left pupil to return to its
original size.

QUESTIONS:

4. AT THIS POINT A DEFINITIVE PHARMACOLOGIC TEST WAS DONE. THE
   SUBSTANCE USED WAS:
   A. Cocaine   D. Atropine
   B. Tensilon (Edrophonium)   E. Epinephrine
   C. Mecholyl (Methacholine)

5. THIS WAS ADMINISTERED:
   A. IM   D. Topically
   B. IV   E. Any of the above
   C. Subcutaneously

6. THE EXPECTED (AND OBSERVED) REACTION WAS:
   A. The left pupil dilated   D. The right pupil constricted
   B. The right pupil dilated   E. Both pupils dilated
   C. The left pupil constricted   F. Both pupils constricted

   MATCH THE NUMBERED DIAGNOSIS WITH THE APPROPRIATE LETTERED
   DESCRIPTIVE FEATURES OF THE PUPIL.

7._ Argyll-Robertson pupil
8._ Tonic pupil (Adie's syndrome)
9._ Horner's syndrome
10._ Third nerve palsy due to aneurysm of circle of Willis

        A. Large   G. Reacts slowly in convergence
        B. Small   H. Usually unilateral
        C. Regular   I . Usually bilateral
        D. Irregular   J. Constricts after instillation of
        E. Reacts normally to light   mecholyl
        F. Reacts normally in convergence K. Associated with ophthalmoplegia

11. THE PROBABLE SITE OF THE LESION IN THIS PATIENT IS:
    A. Thalamus   C. Ciliary ganglion
    B. Pretectum   D. None of the above

CASE STUDY #57

ANSWERS AND DISCUSSION:

1. ABD   A lesion in the superior cervical ganglion causes Horner's syndrome, with homolateral ptosis and miosis.

2. D

3. H   An aneurysm of the circle of Willis or ophthalmoplegic migraine will almost never produce isolated pupillary dilation. Invariably, other components of third nerve paralysis are evident. Headache is prominent in both these conditions.

Transtentorial herniation of the temporal lobe is ruled out by the patient's alertness, the absence of headache, and the negative neurological examination. Weber's syndrome consists of a third nerve palsy and contralateral hemiparesis, due to a lesion of the third nerve as it courses through and emerges from the mesencephalic cerebral peduncle which contains the corticospinal tract. Benedikt's syndrome is also due to a mesencephalic lesion involving the third nerve and the red nucleus, resulting in ophthalmoplegia and contralateral tremor or choreoathetoid movements of the extremities.

In addition to a fixed, dilated pupil, and "idiopathic" third nerve palsy is associated with ptosis of the upper eyelid and/or weakness of some or all of the four extraocular muscles supplied by the third nerve. A "diabetic" third nerve palsy presents also with weakness of extraocular muscles supplied by that nerve. The size and reactivity of the pupil is usually normal.

4. C

5. D   A 2.5% solution of mecholyl is used. This has no effect on a normal pupil.

6. C

7. BDFI

8. ACGHJ

9. BCEFH

10. ACHK

11. C

DISCUSSION: Physicians are generally aware that a fixed dilated pupil may have sinister diagnostic implications. Hence, the patient with a tonic pupil may sometimes be subjected to needless neurologic or even neurosurgical investigations. It should be emphasized that these patients look and feel well. The normal alertness, absence of headache, extraocular muscle weakness or visual impairment, and the slow, but full, response to accommodation all suggest the correct diagnosis. Occasionally, for reasons unknown, the knee or ankle jerks may be diminished or absent. This is part of Adie's syndrome, a benign condition. Appropriate testing of the abnormal pupil, with emphasis on the mecholyl test, should quickly dispel all apprehension. The patient may then be reassured and dismissed. A syndrome of transient benign unilateral pupillary dilation in younger adults has recently been described. This differs from the Adie pupil in that there may be recurrent episodic pupillary dilation lasting several hours to days; there is no hypersensitivity to methacholine, nor any alteration in the deep tendon reflexes.

CASE STUDY #57

REFERENCES

1. Adie, W.J., Tonic Pupils and Absent Tendon Reflexes: A Benign Disorder Sui Generis: Its complete and Incomplete Forms, Brain 55:98-113, 1932.

2. Adler, F.H. and H.G. Scheie, The Site of the Disturbance in Tonic Pupils, Trans Am Ophthalmol Soc 38:183-192, 1940.

3. Goldstein, J., and D.G. Cogan, Diabetic Ophthalmoplegia with Special Reference to the Pupil, Arch Ophthalmol 64:592-600, 1960.

4. Friedman, A.P., D.H. Harter and H.H. Merritt, Ophthalmoplegic Migraine, Arch Neurol 7:320-327, 1962.

5. Green, W., et al., Neuro-Ophthalmologic Evaluation of Oculomotor Nerve Paralysis, Arch Ophthalmol 72:154, 1964.

6. Walsh, F.B., and W.F. Hoyt, Clinical Neuro-ophthalmology, 3rd Ed., Williams and Wilkins Co., 1969.

7. Thompson, H.S., et al., The Fixed Dilated Pupil, Arch Ophthal 86:21, 1971.

8. Edelson, R.N., and D.E. Levy, Transient Benign Unilateral Pupillary Dilation in Young Adults, Arch Neurol 31:12, 1974.

CASE STUDY #58

Headaches and Hemiparesis in a Man with Cancer

HISTORY: A 78 year-old man was admitted to the hospital because of headaches and forgetfulness. Cancer of the prostate had been diagnosed 12 years earlier, and he was treated with orchiectomy and stilbestrol. Three weeks prior to admission, he began to complain of bifrontal, severe steady headaches, not relieved by aspirin. A week later, his family noted that he was confused and forgetful.

Examination revealed a thin, alert, elderly man with prominent gynecomastia. He spoke slowly and did not know the month or year. There was a right hemiparesis, and the deep tendon reflexes were increased in the right extremities. There were no pathological reflexes. The cranial nerves and the remainder of the neurological examination were normal.

QUESTIONS:

1. THE LESION IS PROBABLY IN THE:
   A. Peripheral nerves
   B. Brachial and lumbosacral plexus
   C. Spinal cord
   D. Brain stem
   E. Cerebral hemispheres

2. WITH CEREBRAL DISEASE, A HEMIPARESIS LOCALIZES THE LESION TO THE CONTRALATERAL HEMISPHERE:
   A. Always
   B. Usually, but not necessarily
   C. About half of the time

CASE STUDY #58

3. IN CEREBRAL DISEASE, A HEMIANOPSIA LATERALIZES THE LESION TO
   THE CONTRALATERAL HEMISPHERE:
   A. Always
   B. Usually
   C. About half of the time

4. WITH A CEREBRAL LESION, A FIXED AND DILATED PUPIL IS A BETTER
   LATERALIZING SIGN THAN EITHER HEMIANOPSIA OR HEMIPARESIS.
   A. True
   B. False

5. IN THIS PATIENT, WHAT DO YOU THINK IS THE MOST PROBABLE DIAG-
   NOSIS?

6. THE FOLLOWING TESTS ARE INDICATED TO DETERMINE THE ETIOLOGY
   OF THIS PATIENT'S CONFUSION AND HEMIPARESIS:
   A. Isotope cisternogram
   B. Electromyogram
   C. Pneumoencephalogram
   D. Slit lamp examination of the eyes
   E. Serum magnesium
   F. None of the above

LABORATORY DATA: X-rays of the skull and chest, and a skeletal survey for
bony metastases, were all normal. An echoencephalogram was normal. The
electroencephalogram showed small amounts of 5-7cps slowing in the left parietal
area. A brain scan revealed a large focus of increased activity in the left parietal
area. Blood count, serum sodium, calcium, alkaline and acid phosphatase, and
bilirubin were all normal.

COURSE: During the next two weeks, the hemiparesis became progressively more
severe. He became more confused and obtunded.

QUESTIONS:

7. WHAT DO YOU THINK IS THE MOST PROBABLE DIAGNOSIS NOW THAT
   YOU HAVE SEEN THE LABORATORY FINDINGS?

8. THE MOST APPROPRIATE COURSE OF ACTION NOW WOULD BE:
   A. Morphine every 4 hours to relieve pain and anxiety
   B. A course of dexamethasone
   C. A course of glycerol
   D. Cerebral angiography
   E. Pneumoencephalography
   F. A course of "whole-head" radiation
   G. A course of anticancer chemotherapy

A left carotid arteriogram was performed. (See Figures 67 and 68)

CASE STUDY #58

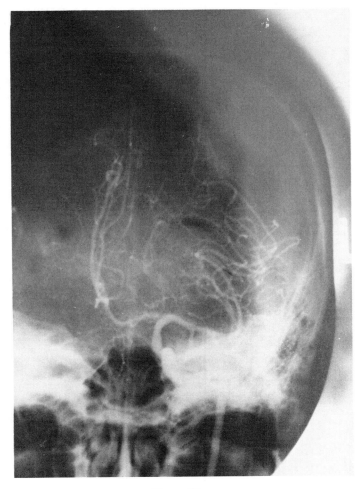

Figure 67

CASE STUDY #58

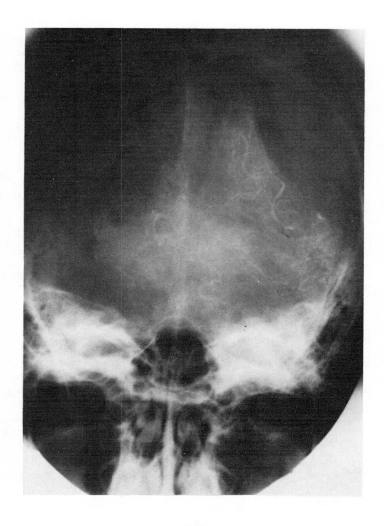

Figure 68

CASE STUDY #58

9. THIS IS THE CLASSIC ANGIOGRAPHIC PATTERN OF A:
   A. Metastatic tumor   C. Cerebral infarct
   B. Subdural hematoma   D. Meningioma

At craniotomy, 200 cc of fluid and clotted blood was removed from the subdural space. The hematoma appeared about 1-2 months old. Postoperatively he was much more alert with gradual improvement of mental and motor functions.

ANSWERS AND DISCUSSION:

1. E   The weakness on one side of the body associated with hyperactive deep tendon reflexes points to a lesion of the central nervous system involving the corticospinal tract. The prominent mental symptoms indicate intracranial disease. Although lesions in the posterior fossa can impair intellectual function - as for example in hydrocephalus due to obstruction of the 4th ventricle or aqueduct - this patient has no symptoms of cranial nerve or cerebellar dysfunction. The lesion thus is most likely in the left cerebral hemisphere.

2. B

3. B

4. A   Hemiparesis or hemianopsia ipsilateral to a cerebral mass lesion are known as false localizing signs. The explanation is that the mass pushes the upper brainstem in the opposite direction, pressing the contralateral cerebral peduncle or posterior cerebral artery against the tentorial edge. If the function of the opposite pyramidal tract in the cerebral peduncle is impaired, hemiparesis ipsilateral to the original lesion will result. If the contralateral posterior cerebral artery is compressed, ischemia of the occipital lobe may cause a hemianopsia ipsilateral to the original lesion. A fixed and dilated pupil may result from herniation of the temporal lobe through the tentorial notch with compression of the third cranial nerve. This is usually on the same side as the mass lesion and is called a Hutchinson pupil.

6. F   An isotope cisternogram is one of the tests used in the diagnosis of "normal pressure" hydrocephalus and would not be indicated when the primary clinical suspicion is of a mass lesion. A PEG is neither an "initial" test, nor is it the preferred contrast study when a lateralized cerebral lesion is suspected.

8. D   The major decision to be made is whether further diagnostic procedures are to be done. Although the clinicians caring for the patient thought that he may have had a metastasis from the prostatic cancer, they were concerned about ruling out alternative possibilities.

9. B   Note the dark area between the skull and the vessels of the cerebrum.

COMMENT: This case illustrates the risk in assuming that cerebral dysfunction in a patient with cancer must be due to metastases. Other treatable infectious and metabolic complications of cancer which cause cerebral symptoms, such as inappropriate secretion of antidiuretic hormone and hypercalcemia, have been discussed with earlier cases. The decision to do contrast studies in a patient with cancer and a cerebral lesion depends on the particular circumstances of an individual patient. The patient in this case had a relatively good prognosis and no evidence of widespread metastases. At the other end of the spectrum might be a patient with cancer of the lung which very commonly metastasizes to the brain, with evidence of systemic spread of the cancer. This patient might then not have contrast studies to evaluate a focal cerebral lesion because of the poor prognosis for life, as well as the very high probability of cerebral metastasis.

CASE STUDY #58

Another very important lesson taught by this case is that although subdural hematomas are most often seen following serious head trauma, often the history of trauma is poor, and there are certain groups of people who may develop a subdural hematoma with trivial or no history of head trauma. These include infants, the elderly, patients with blood dyscrasias, on anticoagulants or hemodialysis. The elderly patient in this case had no history of head trauma.

REFERENCES

1. McKissock, W., et al., Subdural Hematoma, Lancet 1:1365, 1960.

2. Dejesus, P., and C. Poser, Subdural Hematomas, A Clinicopathologic Study of 100 Cases, Postgraduate Medicine 44:172, 1968.

3. Talalla, A., and M. Morin, Acute Traumatic Subdural Hematoma: A Review of One Hundred Consecutive Cases, J Trauma 11:771, 1971.

4. Clinical Pathological Conference, New Eng J Med 286:650, 1972.

5. Bechar, M., et al., Subdural Hematoma During Long Term Hemodialysis, Arch Neurol 26:513, 1972.

6. Thomas, L., and E. Gurdjian, Intracranial Hematomas of Traumatic Origin, in Neurological Surgery, Youmans, J. Ed., W.B. Saunders Co., 1973.

7. Bender, M., et al., Nonsurgical Treatment of Subdural Hematomas, Arch Neurol 31:73, 1974.

CASE STUDY #59

A Stuporous Young Man with a Twitching Hand

HISTORY: A 27 year-old man had been told several years previously that he had diabetes mellitus. He did not receive any treatment, but was well until three weeks before admission, when he noted increasing thirst and urination. A week later his left hand began to shake uncontrollably. The shaking spread up the arm to the shoulder. The episode lasted about three minutes. His left arm subsequently felt numb.

QUESTION:

1. THIS EPISODE WAS A:
   A. Focal seizure
   B. Transient ischemic attack
   C. Either
   D. Neither

On the day of admission, he had a similar episode which progressed to a grand mal seizure. He had no headache or other neurological symptoms. Past medical history was otherwise negative.

Examination several hours after the seizure revealed a stuporous obese young man. Vital signs were normal. The deep tendon reflexes were symmetrically hypoactive. Response to pinprick in the left arm was decreased. No other abnormalities were noted.

LABORATORY DATA: Blood sugar was 666 mgm%; Urine glucose was 4 plus; Blood and urine acetone negative; Blood sodium, chloride, potassium, CO_2 content normal. Hemoglobin, calcium, skull films, echoencephalogram, brain scan were all normal. Spinal fluid was normal, except for increased sugar content. Electroencephalogram showed minimal amounts of 5-7cps slowing in the right temporal region.

CASE STUDY #59

QUESTIONS:

2. THE BEST DIAGNOSIS ON THE BASIS OF THE AVAILABLE INFORMATION IS:
   A. Lactic acidosis
   B. Diabetic ketoacidosis
   C. Brain tumor
   D. Nonketotic hyperglycemia
   E. Arteriovenous malformation
   F. Brain abscess

3. THE MOST IMPORTANT DRUG TO GIVE NOW WOULD BE:
   A. Dilantin
   B. Amytal
   C. Mannitol
   D. Decadron
   E. Insulin
   F. Penicillin

COURSE: He was treated with fluids and insulin. No further seizures occurred and he became normally alert and coherent. The blood sugar became normal. Polyuria and polydipsia disappeared. The numbness and decreased pin sensation in the left arm disappeared after several days.

QUESTION:

4. THE NEXT STEP IN MANAGEMENT SHOULD BE:
   A. Carotid angiography
   B. Continuous anticonvulsant treatment with Dilantin or phenobarbital
   C. Discharge from the hospital on an antidiabetic diet and drug regimen
   D. Pneumoencephalography

When seen in clinic several months later, he was asymptomatic and neurologically normal. A repeat electroencephalogram was normal.

QUESTIONS:

5. FOCAL SEIZURES ARE ALMOST ALWAYS SIGNS OF A STRUCTURAL CERE-BRAL LESION. SOME METABOLIC CONDITIONS, AS HYPEROSMOLAR NON-KETOTIC COMA MAY, HOWEVER, PRESENT WITH FOCAL SEIZURES OR EVEN WITH HEMIPARESIS WHICH DISAPPEARS AS THE METABOLIC AB-NORMALITY IS CORRECTED. THESE INCLUDE:
   A. Hyponatremia
   B. Hepatic encephalopathy
   C. Hypoglycemia
   D. All of these

6. DRUGS WHICH HAVE BEEN ASSOCIATED WITH THE PRECIPITATION OF HYPEROSMOLAR NONKETOTIC COMA HAVE INCLUDED:
   A. Thiazides
   B. Steroids
   C. Dilantin
   D. All of these

7. COMA IN A DIABETIC PATIENT MAY BE DUE TO:
   A. Hypoglycemia
   B. CNS infection
   C. Ketoacidosis
   D. Cerebral hemorrhage or thrombosis
   E. Any of these

ANSWERS AND DISCUSSION:

1. A   The spread of twitching from the hand up the arm is a typical description of a focal Jacksonian seizure. Shaking of an extremity is a useful differential diagnostic point in distinguishing a focal seizure from a transient ischemic attack.

2. D

3. E

CASE STUDY #59

4. C   Although recognizing the possibility that the patient might harbor a focal lesion such as an arteriovenous malformation or brain tumor, the clinicians caring for this patient decided, in view of the frequent association of focal seizures with nonketotic hyperglycemia, not to subject the patient to the risks of major contrast studies unless further seizures or evidence of a progressive neurological deficit occurred. Also, since the seizures were attributed to the metabolic problem, chronic anticonvulsant medications were not given.

5. D

6. D

7. E

DISCUSSION: In a recent review of the literature, Singh found that 25% of 158 cases of nonketotic hyperglycemia had seizures, the majority of which were focal motor. These were often followed by transient neurological focal deficits such as aphasia, hemianopia, hemiparesis or hemisensory loss. The reason for the high frequency of seizures is unclear. Seizures and focal neurological signs are very rare in ketoacidotic hyperglycemia, despite similar hyperosmolality and hyperglycemia. Perhaps ketosis protects against seizures, as in the treatment of some forms of epilepsy with a ketogenic diet. Some have theorized that acidosis may also have an anticonvulsive effect by increasing the concentration of gamma amino butyric acid (GABA), an inhibitory neurotransmitter, in the brain. Some of the autopsied cases of hyperglycemic nonketotic coma have shown small cerebral infarcts located in areas that would explain the focal seizures, and opinions vary in the literature as to whether the metabolic abnormality can itself account for the focal seizures and signs or whether it causes an otherwise "silent" structure lesion to become symptomatic.

REFERENCES

1. Maccario, M., et al., Focal Seizures as a Manifestation of Hyperglycemia Without Ketoacidosis, Neurology 15:195, 1965.

2. Vastola, E., et al., Activation of Epileptogenic Foci by Hyperosmolality, Neurology 17:520, 1967.

3. Maccario, M., Neurological Dysfunction Associated with Nonketotic Hyperglycemia, Arch Neurol 19:525, 1968.

4. Cohen, P., et al., Hyperosmolar Coma: A Medical Emergency, Med Ann DC 37:258, 1968.

5. Shavelle, H., Cerebral Syndromes of Diabetes Mellitus, Calif Med 110:283, 1969.

6. Daniels, J., et al., Anacidotic Hyperglycemia and Focal Seizures, Arch Int Med 124:701, 1969.

7. Espinas, O., and C. Poser, Blood Hyperosmolality and Neurologic Deficit, Arch Neurol 20:182, 1969.

8. Gerich, J., et al., Clinical and Metabolic Characteristics of Hyperosmolar Nonketotic Coma, Diabetes 20:228, 1971.

9. Singh, B., et al., Nonketotic Hyperglycemia and Epilepsia Partialis Continua, Arch Neurol 29:187, 1973.

10. Arieff, A., and H. Carroll, Cerebral Edema and Depression of Sensorium in Nonketotic Hyperosmolar Coma, Diabetes 23:525, 1974.